PRAISE FOR
ANCIENT WISDOM, MODERN KITCHEN

"We have a lot to learn from how other cultures approach health and medicine. *Ancient Wisdom, Modern Kitchen* not only offers mouth-watering Asian recipes and lore about food, it also provides a new way to look at what makes up a healthy diet—a refreshing antidote to the way many of us in America eat today."

—Paul W. Miller, MD, adjunct professor,
Exercise and Nutritional Science Department, San Diego State University

"I have been waiting for this book for 20 years. Finally, respected authorities in the field, Dr. Yuan Wang and Warren Sheir, LAc, have written a book on food therapy with writer Mika Ono that will appeal to both practitioners of traditional Chinese medicine and anyone who is interested in harnessing an Eastern approach to the power of food for better health."

—Jack Miller, LAc, MA (Education),
president of Pacific College of Oriental Medicine

"Part cookbook, part introduction to Chinese medicine, *Ancient Wisdom, Modern Kitchen* embraces a holistic approach to food that is second nature in China and essential to medical practice there. I will be sharing this exceptional work with both my patients and colleagues."

—Guohui Liu, MS, MB/BS, LAc, faculty member at
Oregon College of Oriental Medicine and National College of Naturopathic Medicine,
and author of Warm Pathogen Diseases

ANCIENT WISDOM
MODERN KITCHEN

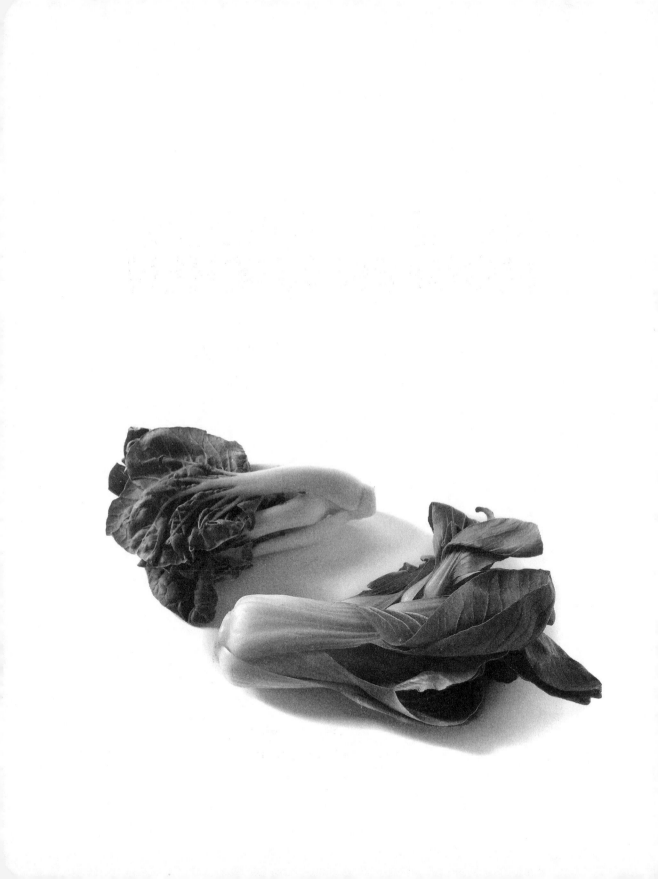

ANCIENT WISDOM,
MODERN KITCHEN

*Recipes from the East for Health,
Healing, and Long Life*

Yuan Wang, Warren Sheir, and Mika Ono

A Member of the Perseus Books Group

Designed by Pauline Brown
Set in 10 point Berkeley Book by the Perseus Books Group

Cataloging-in-Publication data for this book is available from the Library of Congress.

First Da Capo Press edition 2010
ISBN: 978-0-7382-1325-5

Published by Da Capo Press
A Member of the Perseus Books Group
www.dacapopress.com

Note: The information in this book is true and complete to the best of our knowledge. This book is intended only as an informative guide for those wishing to know more about health issues. In no way is this book in-tended to replace, countermand, or conflict with the advice given to you by your own physician. The ultimate decision concerning care should be made between you and your doctor. We strongly recommend you follow his or her advice. Information in this book is general and is offered with no guarantees on the part of the authors or Da Capo Press. The authors and publisher disclaim all liability in connection with the use of this book. The names and identifying details of people associated with events described in this book have been changed. Any similarity to actual persons is coincidental.

Da Capo Press books are available at special discounts for bulk purchases in the U.S. by corporations, insti-tutions, and other organizations. For more information, please contact the Special Markets Department at the Perseus Books Group, 2300 Chestnut Street, Suite 200, Philadelphia, PA, 19103, or call (800) 810-4145, ext. 5000, or e-mail special.markets@perseusbooks.com. For information and updates on the authors, visit http://www.ancientwisdommodernkitchen.com.

10 9 8 7 6 5 4 3 2 1

CONTENTS

CONTENTS

CONTENTS

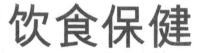

PREFACE
THREE PATHS TO THE
HEALING POWER OF FOOD

Although we have dramatically different backgrounds, the three authors of this book have all come to embrace the potential of food to promote health and healing. Here are our stories.

YUAN'S STORY

I LEARNED TO COOK from my mother, who came from a large and ancient family in southern China. She was in charge of cooking for the family, and, as the oldest daughter, I would help by peeling the garlic, cleaning the vegetables, and keeping her company while she worked. We enjoyed preparing meals together for the whole family—often dozens of people.

My mother was also a Chinese medical doctor. When I was a teenager I developed skin problems that Western medicine couldn't diagnose. I suffered until I started taking a traditional herbal preparation that completely cleared up the condition. When it was time to pursue my education, my mother told me, "Chinese medicine makes a lot of good sense. You will be able to help people." It was easy to take her advice, because I was fascinated by traditional Chinese medicine and had seen for myself what kind of relief it could bring.

I studied at Chengdu College of Traditional Chinese Medicine for a bachelor's degree, then at the Tianjin Institute of Traditional Chinese Medicine for a master's. Mao's Cultural Revolution meant that all high school students were required to spend time in the countryside. For me, this part worked out well, and I spent four years learning about local plants and herbal medicine, which supplemented my textbook and clinical work.

I went on to become a lecturer, researcher, and physician-in-charge for the Departments of Medicine, Kidney Diseases, Digestive Diseases, and the Research Institute of Blood Diseases at the Chengdu Traditional Chinese Medicine Hospital. I also participated on research teams investigating stroke, cancer, diabetes, and menstrual disorders. I helped design course curricula and textbooks for the Chengdu College of Traditional Chinese Medicine, was on the editorial board of Great China Encyclopedia Column of Medicine, and published a number of academic articles.

In 1995, I moved to the United States, although I still go back to China to visit my mother (who is still cooking fabulous meals). After teaching at the International Institute of Chinese Medicine in Santa Fe for five years, I moved to San Diego, California, where I now teach at the Pacific College of Oriental Medicine and see patients in my private practice, The Source, in Poway.

Many of my patients suffer from one of the "high three": high blood pressure, high glucose levels, or high cholesterol. These conditions, so widespread in the West, are all related to diet, and eating right can pave the way to better health. One of the questions I hear most frequently in my practice is, "What should I eat?" We have written this book to help answer that question.

WARREN'S STORY

I AM THE CULINARY REBEL IN MY FAMILY (okay, my family calls me a "picky eater," especially given my long-standing intolerance of dairy). As soon as I left for college, I realized the world of food was at my fingertips—I could eat whatever I wanted! When I was a kid, I used to sneak jelly doughnuts from the bakery, a dozen at a time, when my mother wasn't looking. But in college I found something much better—macrobiotics, an approach toward food developed by Japanese educator George Ohsawa (1893–1966).

I became fascinated by the connection between heath and diet. To me, it made complete sense that what you put in your body would affect how you felt. I took workshops from macrobiotic leaders Michio Kushi, Herman Aihara, and Noburo Muramoto, who spoke on the benefits of a traditional Japanese diet of whole grains, seaweed, and vegetables, as well as the medicinal effects of various foods. My commitment to whole foods and fresh produce was enhanced by my involvement in the very early days of Eden Foods (back when it was just two rooms upstairs from a bicycle shop) and my work in a number of high-end restaurants, including that of renowned chef Rick Bayless, whose artistry and respect for fresh ingredients has remained an inspiration.

During those many years as a "starving" student at the Cleveland Institute of Music/Case Western Reserve University, then as a "starving" musician, I ate extraordinarily well! I found that contrary to common opinion (and the insinuations of ads for packaged foods) it is not expensive or time consuming to eat fresh, healthy food. Over the years, I have come to apply macrobiotics much less strictly, but still embrace its principles of a largely plant-based and whole-grain diet. I don't think it's any accident that the Japanese have one of the longest life spans in the world, and I worry about the effects on health of the unprecedented consumption of refined and processed foods in the West.

As a student and then faculty member at the Pacific College of Oriental Medicine in San Diego, I gained a Chinese perspective on food and healing, including the theoretical constructs behind Chinese medicine (also influential in other parts of Asia) and a broader knowledge of medicinal herbs and their applications.

I still eat better than almost anyone I know. The recipes in this book are some of my favorites, drawing on the Chinese tradition of healing herbs, a Japanese aesthetic of simplicity, and an American sense of convenience, practicality, and fun. Bon appétit!

MIKA'S STORY

IT TOOK SOME THIRTY-FIVE YEARS for the world to catch up with my father. In 1970, he moved the family from a gray suburb to a semirural area outside of Toronto, Canada (Laskey Village, between King City and Nobleton, for those who know that part of the world), where he set up a garden—not just any garden but a front fence to back fence ¾-acre plot with different varieties of tomatoes, beans, pumpkin, squash, lettuce, chard, potatoes, corn, strawberries, dill, mint, basil, mizuna, burdock, and whatever caught his fancy in the seed catalog.

Every spring, when he wasn't teaching or working in his vision research lab at York University or on sabbatical in Japan, he would rototill, plant, compost, and weed, and the garden would return the favor by producing its bounty—a little different every year depending on what my father had been inspired to plant, the weather, and who had the upper hand for the moment in the long-running battle between ingenious squirrels and ingenious gardeners. We kept Rhode Island Red hens, which would loudly proclaim their accomplishment to the world every time they laid another fresh, brown egg, and a pony would sometimes help "mow" the lawn. My mother was very much part of this scene as well, cooking, freezing, and pickling the harvest, and embracing the virtues of organic whole foods at a time when the idea was considered controversial.

Of course, as a kid with fresh produce and whole foods flowing into the family kitchen, I took them completely for granted and the big city seemed more appealing. There was little in the general culture to convince me otherwise.

But the tide has now turned, and, in this age that has become ever more dominated by processed foods and supermarkets, a connection to the earth and to fresh produce has become a rarity. Some young people are taking up natural food production as a cause and a number of popular books are exploring just how far we have drifted from our food sources, the negative effects of this divide on our body and our planet, and what we should do to remedy this condition.

Here, the Asian tradition has something to say. Because balance in our body and with the seasons has been a central tenet of Asian thought for millennia, I believe this is a fruitful direction to look for transplants to grow a more wholesome, healthful, and fulfilling Western lifestyle. Yoga, meditation, and acupuncture have already become commonplace in the West. The kitchen is the next frontier.

医食同源

INTRODUCTION:
DELICIOUS RECIPES, HEALTHY LIFE

EASTERN TRADITIONS are now part of the Western lifestyle. We go to yoga classes after work to relax, use feng shui to create a welcoming space in our living room, and consult an acupuncturist to relieve our lingering shoulder pain. Yet parts of the Eastern tradition are still to be discovered in the West. One of these is the potential of Chinese herbs and other natural foods to promote health and longevity through everyday cooking.

The recipes in this book are simple and easy to prepare. They comprise healthy East Asian dishes such as egg-drop herbal soup—still largely unknown in the West, but begging to cross the cultural divide—as well as recipes that might seem familiar, but that have an unexpected twist, such as oatmeal with walnuts and goji berries or chicken soup with ginseng. Drawing on family recipes, years of study of traditional Chinese medicine at institutions in China and in the United States, and experience in treating patients in a traditional Chinese medical clinic, we want to put

healthy recipes at your fingertips to enhance your life, promote a sense of well-being, and increase your longevity.

ADD EAST AND WEST, STIR VIGOROUSLY

FOR THOUSANDS OF YEARS, the Chinese have been seeking the secret to health and healing. Unlike in the West, traditional Chinese medicine makes no clear distinction between food and medicine. As the Chinese say, food and medicine are from same source (*yi shi tong yuan*). Respect for the healing properties of food is woven into the fabric of everyday cuisine. Although some herbs are particularly potent and used only for severe illnesses, many herbs and other beneficial ingredients are as common in Chinese cuisine as ketchup and mustard are in America.

The West has its own home remedies. We prepare chicken soup when we have a stuffy nose, reach for a drink of ginger ale to sooth an upset stomach, warm up milk to lull us back to sleep in the middle of the night, and tell our children to eat their vegetables "because they are good for you." We marvel when the latest scientific study comes out supporting these remedies, and, in the meantime, savor these foods and beverages through sickness and health.

Recently, the idea of selecting foods for their specific healthful properties has become even more popular in the West, as "superfoods" or "functional foods"—which offer benefits beyond basic nutrition—have caught on. Already gracing the aisles of natural food stores are goji berries, soy products, and green tea—all part of the East Asian healing and culinary traditions.

Traditional Chinese medicine celebrates the relationship between food and health. Instead of a few simple home remedies, the tradition offers a highly developed system of using the intrinsic properties of different herbs and foods to maximize each individual's well-being in a changing environment, enhancing the body's own natural powers for health, healing, and rejuvenation. In this tradition, too, science is lending support to ancient notions of the healing properties of many traditional Chinese ingredients—cinnamon, curcumin, and ginger, to name only a few.

In China, a respect for the power of food seems to be everywhere. Whole restaurants—perhaps analogous to American juice bars or establishments offering California cuisine—specialize in preparing dishes for their healing properties. In one such restaurant in Sichuan Province, for example, big jars of herbs line the entranceway, while families of young and old alike gather around tables, ordering favorite dishes to heal their ills and

enhance their well-being. In Japan, this tradition of cooking with healing foods and herbs is called *yakuzen*.

For specific ailments and more serious conditions, the system of traditional medicine is widespread and well accepted in many parts of Asia. Thousands of practitioners each year, mostly in China, Taiwan, Korea, and Japan, but now also in the United States, Canada, Europe, and other parts of the world, train in the use of herbs and acupuncture—the two major instruments in Chinese medicine's toolbox—in large schools of traditional medicine, research institutes, and teaching hospitals. Currently, some fifty schools of traditional Chinese medicine have been accredited or are in the process of accreditation in the United States and Canada.

In China, clinics specializing in traditional medicine coexist side-by-side with Western-style clinics, sometimes even in different wings of the same hospital. Patients feel free to take advantage of both traditions; for example, someone with cancer might undergo chemotherapy but also use traditional herbs to help manage side effects, such as nausea, and to increase the body's immunity to fight off disease.

Similarly, this book embraces a holistic approach in which a perspective from the East works hand-in-hand with Western medicine. Both traditions have much to learn from each other. Whereas Western medicine tends to treat the body like a machine, Eastern medicine approaches it more as a garden, to be tended rather than engineered. Eastern medicine shines in disease prevention; Western medicine's strengths lie in acute care. We believe that the best Chinese medicine is practiced with an awareness of what is going on in Western medicine. Similarly, the best Western medicine draws on a more Eastern respect for the importance of prevention, the body's own healing powers, and the complexity of individuals acting in their environment.

None of the recipes in this book are intended as a substitute for consulting with a physician. Instead, this book offers a window into a different tradition of health and healing to support your efforts to remain vital and well.

BALANCE—THE MISSING INGREDIENT

WHAT UNDERLIES THE EAST ASIAN approach to herbal cooking?

Balance and interrelatedness rule. In this tradition, herbal healing and cooking seek to bring balance to our meals, and thus to our body and mind.

And in the West? Unfortunately, balance is often the first casualty in the single-minded pursuit of another goal, usually weight loss. Who hasn't tried the grapefruit diet, the cabbage soup diet, the carb-free diet, the fat-free diet, or another such diet that includes restrictions from entire food groups? Yes, you will probably lose weight (at least temporarily) if you eat nothing but grapefruit. But will you be healthier? Extend your life span? Increase your sense of well-being? Or in the end, will you simply shudder at the thought of facing another darned citrus?

Vitamins and other supplements are another popular form of "insurance" in the West for those concerned with health, and, depending on circumstances, these may have something to offer. However, it's easy to get lulled into a false sense of security. Taking a handful of supplements every morning doesn't mean you are getting what you need in the form your body needs it. You still face the challenge of eating well.

The East Asian tradition offers another way— one based on whole foods and herbs, in rich variety. All foods, flavors, colors, and temperatures have their time and place on the table. No single ingredient is vilified, nor consumed to excess. The key is that the pieces work together as part of a whole.

In addition, foods can bring the individual in harmony with natural cycles and other parts of the environment, as the act of eating is in itself a regular and profound interaction with one's surroundings. Certain seasonal dishes can bring a person in line with the time of year. Particular foods are thought to counteract an individual's own personal tendency toward, say, lethargy or restlessness. Different dishes are recommended for different phases of a woman's monthly cycle. And our best choices change as we age. The East Asian view of the body as an ever-changing ecosystem goes hand-in-hand with a dynamic approach to food and health.

DEEP ROOTS, FLOWERING BRANCHES

TRADITIONAL CHINESE MEDICINE IS based on a coherent system of thought refined by critical thinking and clinical observation throughout the millennia, from contributions by Taoist hermits seeking the ultimate goal of immortality to modern-day scientists illuminating the effects of herbal substances. Traditional Chinese medicine originated in China, as the name would suggest, then spread through East Asia to countries that include Korean, Japan, and Vietnam, where it not only influenced the approach to food and medicine in these regions, but was also enriched by local ingredients, preferences, and culture.

In the earliest times, in Asia (like most of the world) people believed that disease was caused by evil spirits or angry ancestors. However, like Hippocrates of ancient Greece, who rejected the idea that supernatural forces caused illness, early Chinese scholars began to consider the revolutionary idea that health and sickness could be explained by natural laws and observable phenomena.

By the time of the Eastern Han Dynasty (25–220 CE) and the Three Kingdoms Period (220–280 CE), scholars were contributing important classics to the field of traditional Chinese medicine. These works include the *Divine Farmer's Materia Medica* (*Shen Nong Ben Cao*), which describes more than 365 medical substances, one for each day of the year, as well as the *Treatise on Cold Diseases* (*Shang Han Lun*), the first major prescription manual, and *The Essentials from the Golden Cabinet* (*Jin Gui Yao Lue*), both written by Zhang Zhong Jing. *The Yellow Emperor's Classic of Internal Medicine* (*Huang Di Nei Jing*) laid out the philosophical foundations of traditional Chinese medicine. In later centuries, other key contributors, such as Sun Si Miao and Li Shi Zhen, followed.

The philosophy of Chinese medicine spread to neighboring Korea and Japan in the sixth and seventh centuries, as government envoys exchanged medicine as well as diplomacy. By 702 CE, the Japanese government was so taken with the Chinese approach, it issued an imperial order to copy the Tang Dynasty's medical educational system. Later, the Japanese standardized and

simplified Chinese herbal therapies into a system known as *kampo* (occasionally *kanpo*; literally "Han (Chinese) people prescription"), which is currently integrated into the Japanese national health-care system. Chinese medical thought also had great influence on the area now known as Vietnam, and traditional medicine in that region (dubbed "Dong Y" in the seventeenth century to distinguish it from Western medicine) coevolved with and contributed to Chinese practice.

China's exchange with surrounding regions was a two-way street. Many herbs in the Chinese herbal medicine cabinet can be traced to an origin outside the country, and the famed Silk Road brought fruits, vegetables, spices, and herbs to China—and to Chinese medicine—that are now an integral part of this tradition.

Today, throughout East Asia, herbal medicine accounts for more than one billion clinical visits a year, according to Tufts University School of Medicine's Evidence-Based Approach to Complementary and Alternative Medicine group, overshadowing other traditional approaches such as acupuncture and massage. Out of some ten thousand herbs officially described and classified, a few hundred have become first-line therapies, usually prescribed in specific combinations thought to create unique therapeutic effects.

Food therapy is often used to support herbal treatments, and to continue the treatment after the course of herbal therapy is done. Foods and dishes targeting a specific problem are often eaten regularly for a few days or a few weeks to support the body's healing process, then included in the diet occasionally to prevent future recurrences.

While herbal medical practice has been more or less standardized within some regions, therapeutic foods are another matter. Partly because East Asia—and China itself—covers such a vast area, healing dishes are influenced by local variation, family tradition, the availability of ingredients, and the whims of the cook. Nevertheless, this general approach expresses the principles of traditional East Asian medicine and a consistent underlying approach toward food.

CHINESE MEDICINE IN A NUTSHELL

THE BIG PICTURE of what East Asian herbal medicine has to offer us today is easy to grasp—a rich tradition of healing and clinical observation, a variety of herbs and foods, a philosophy of balance, an emphasis on context, and a respect for individual differences. While Eastern and Western systems both look for natural phenomena to explain illness, Western medicine today relies heavily on microscopic observations and biochemistry, whereas East Asian medicine depends on an approach based on context and examination of the patient as a whole.

Westerners who are curious about the particulars of an East Asian approach should get ready for a mind-opening experience. Some central concepts of Chinese medicine make sense according to our worldview, but others challenge us to see the world from a completely fresh perspective. In many ways, entering the world of traditional Chinese medicine is like learning a foreign language. When you learn a language, say, French, you also learn a whole new way of thinking. You may encounter phrases that are difficult to translate literally, such as *"Zut alors!"* or *"Vive la difference."* The same is true for the language of traditional Chinese medicine.

To learn to "speak" traditional Chinese medicine, it helps to know a few central concepts.

These include: yin and yang, vital substances, the five elements, and the six evils. Sound intriguing?

Yin and Yang: Dynamic Harmony

You'll probably recognize the symbol of yin and yang, now commonplace in the West. The differing areas of the circle underline the importance of seeing parts in relation to the whole, and express the dynamic ebb and flow between complementary opposites. Keep in mind that yin and yang do not express a simple duality—instead, both yin and yang are rooted in each other and contain a piece of each other; there is no up without down, no man without woman, no back without front. A reference to yin and yang is found in the *I Ching* (*Book of Changes*) as early as 700 BCE.

Yin and yang reflect the natural world, as in the interplay between high tide and low tide or day and night. Yin—whose character originally meant the shady side of the slope—is associated with cold, interior, moisture, density, stillness, downward movement, and substance. Yang—whose character originally meant the sunny side of a slope—relates to heat, exterior, dryness, movement, upward motion, and function.

In Chinese medicine, yin and yang offer one of the most important touchstones for understanding health and disease. Health and well-being flourish when yin and yang are in balance. But if there's too much yin in the body, a person will come down with an illness that involves weakness, slowness, coldness, or lethargy. If there's too much yang, an individual is susceptible to illnesses expressed with quick, forceful movement, heat, or hyperactivity. Chinese medicine advises that an excess of yin should be countered with more yang, and vice versa. Also, a deficiency of yin should be addressed by supplementing yin; a deficiency of yang should be addressed by supplementing yang.

In this tradition, one way to restore balance to the body is through diet. So, if you feel weak, yang dishes (such as Longevity Mushrooms with *He Shou Wu*) may be therapeutic; if you are tense or hyperactive, yin dishes (such as Breathe-Easy Fritillaria Pear) may help. The proper balance of yin and yang promotes and restores health, helping your body ward off disease.

Vital Substances: Wellsprings of Health

According to traditional Chinese medicine, several "vital substances"—qi, Blood, *jing*, and body fluid—are also wellsprings of health.

Qi (pronounced "chee") is another ancient and central concept in Chinese philosophy. While difficult to translate, qi can be understood as the life force or energy flowing through all things, the basic substance of the universe. Its ideograph can mean "vapor," "steam," or "uncooked rice"—tying this idea back to food, a major source of qi. Qi circulates in channels called meridians on the body's surface, as well as in pathways inside the body. According to the Chinese worldview, illnesses take hold when the flow of qi is disturbed, unbalanced, or blocked. To restore health, Chinese medical practitioners seek to free and realign the flow of qi, with acupuncture or with herbs and food.

Blood, which is propelled by qi, is also vital, circulating through the body to nourish organs, skin, muscles, tendons, and bones, as well as to support memory and mental activities. In the Chinese tradition, much importance is placed on replenishing Blood lost due to injury, menses, or childbirth. This is accomplished with appropriate food and herbs. Proper flow of Blood is also important.

Jing, or essence, refers to a refined and precious substance that forms the organic basis for all life. *Jing* influences our constitution, reproduction, growth, and development—and our longevity. *Jing* comes in (at least) two forms, prenatal *jing* and postnatal *jing*. Traditional Chinese medical practitioners advise you to conserve your prenatal *jing* as much as possible, as everyone is endowed with a fixed amount. You can use yours judiciously by approaching life's activities—including diet, work, and sexual activity—with balance and moderation to prolong your mental and physical health. Postnatal *jing* can be enhanced by eating the proper diet.

Last (and, in fact, probably least on the hierarchy of importance according to Chinese medicine) is a substance roughly translated as body fluid, which includes saliva, gastric fluid, joint cavity fluid, tears, sweat, urine, and so on. Derived from food and drink, body fluid serves to warm and nourish the muscles, moisten the skin, lubricate the joints, moisten the orifices, and surround the brain. One type of disharmony of the fluids is expressed by dryness of the skin and eyes.

Chinese medical practitioners will look to certain foods and herbs to help enhance and direct these vital substances, according to the needs of each individual. Dishes such as Classic Chinese Ginseng-Chicken Soup or Fish Dish for Vigor can help strengthen qi. Dishes such as Five-Spice Powder Chicken or Wasabi Fish Cooked in Sake will move the qi, countering qi stagnation. Other foods and herbs are considered especially effective for nourishing or moving the Blood, for example those in Triple-Mushroom Mélange and Steadying Spinach Egg Drop Soup, respectively. If body fluids are depleted, preparations such as Five-Fruit Dessert Potage, Simple Peach Kanten, or watermelon juice can help.

The Five Organs: The Dance of Life

To help understand the body, traditional Chinese medical practitioners draw on a view of dynamic, interrelated systems that reflect other relationships found in nature. In the natural world, Chinese philosophers identified five elements (also known as "five phases")—wood, fire, earth, metal, and water—which support or restrain each other in continuous patterns.

As in the game of Rock-Paper-Scissors, each element has its strengths and weaknesses in relation to other elements. Water can put out Fire; Fire melts Metal; Metal (as in a saw) can cut Wood;

Wood (as in a shovel) can overcome Earth; and Earth (as in a dam) can divert Water. Or, expressed in a different sequence, Water nurtures Wood (as in trees); Wood can be used to make Fire; Fire generates Earth (ashes); Earth brings forth Metal; and Metal, when heated, produces Water (steam). Many other aspects of the world are explained with similar dynamics, including the five tastes (sour, bitter, sweet, spicy, and salty), the five colors (blue-green, red, yellow, white, and black), and the five emotions (anger, joy, worry, grief, and fear).

In the body, five "organs"—the Liver, Heart, Spleen, Lung, and Kidney—also coexist and provide support or restraint for each other's functions. Even though similar words are used in Western medicine, keep in mind that in Chinese medicine these terms refer less to the physical organs themselves, and more to the nature they embody and their influence on the system as a whole. Here are some of the contributions of each organ:

CHART: THE IMPORTANCE OF FIVE

ELEMENT	WOOD	FIRE	EARTH	METAL	WATER
SEASON	SPRING	SUMMER	LATE SUMMER	AUTUMN	WINTER
CLIMATE	WIND	HEAT	DAMPNESS	DRYNESS	COLD
TASTE	SOUR	BITTER	SWEET	SPICY	SALTY
COLOR	GREEN/BLUE	RED	YELLOW	WHITE	BLACK
EMOTION	ANGER	JOY	WORRY	GRIEF	FEAR
YIN ORGAN	LIVER	HEART	SPLEEN	LUNG	KIDNEY
YANG ORGAN	GALL BLADDER	SMALL INTESTINE	STOMACH	LARGE INTESTINE	BLADDER
SENSORY PART	EYES	TONGUE	MOUTH	NOSE	EARS
TISSUE	TENDONS	BLOOD VESSELS	FLESH	SKIN	BONES

- **THE LIVER** ensures the smooth flow of qi throughout the body, controls and nourishes the tendons and ligaments, and stores and regulates the Blood. Symptoms such as muscle spasms, dry eyes, and blurry vision are associated with problems with the Liver.
- **THE HEART** governs the Blood and blood vessels, as well as the consciousness and spirit. Symptoms such as insomnia and dream-disturbed sleep as well as palpitations and poor circulation are associated with problems with the Heart.
- **THE SPLEEN** oversees digestion, controls the muscles and limbs, and houses the intellect. Symptoms such as lack of appetite, obesity, weakness, and fatigue are associated with dysfunction of the Spleen.
- **THE LUNGS** govern qi, control respiration, direct the passage of water, and relate to the hair, skin, and pores. Symptoms such as cough, nasal congestion, a hoarse voice, sweating irregularities, and skin rashes are associated with problems with the Lungs.
- **THE KIDNEYS** store essence, govern human reproduction, growth, and development, control water metabolism, and produce bone marrow. Symptoms such as brittle bones, poor hearing, urinary problems, and premature aging are associated with malfunctions of the Kidneys.

When these systems work well individually and are in balance with one another, health and vitality flourish.

In Chinese medicine, the five elements and their relationships can help guide food choices for your health and well-being. The tastes, colors, and properties of foods and herbs can support their counterparts in the body. For example, in the Wood sphere, leafy green vegetables can support the influence of the Liver, and its domain of the eyes, tendons, and ligaments. In the Metal sphere, foods such as pears can support and soothe the functions of the Lungs. In the Fire domain, meat and other foods can strengthen the Heart and enhance its influence in the body. In the Earth domain, foods such as buckwheat can support the Spleen and its functions regulating energy. And in the Water sphere, foods such as seaweed can influence the Kidneys and their connections to the bladder, bones, and ears, and to longevity.

The Six Evils: Trouble at Your Door

No, the six evils aren't your relatives from New Jersey (at least not in this book). In Chinese medicine, the six evils, also sometimes translated as the "six pernicious influences" or the "six pathogenic factors," are environmental forces that can spring from inside or outside the body to play a part in disease. If your body is weakened by imbalance, you become susceptible to the harmful effects of one of these influences.

The six evils are:

- **WIND.** Analogous to wind in nature, the concept of Wind in Chinese medicine embodies movement and change. Diseases caused by Wind often have migratory symptoms, sudden onset, and rapid progression, or other features associated with movement such as spasms, tremors, twitching, or dizziness. These diseases tend to affect the upper and outer parts of the body. Wind, prominent in the spring but appearing in any season, is the one evil that rarely appears by itself. Instead, it promotes the invasion of the body by one of the other influences.

● COLD. Like cold in nature, Cold in Chinese medicine is associated with contraction, obstruction, slower movement, and underactivity. An individual influenced by Cold will feel cold and will typically seek warmth with sweaters or blankets. To the observer, this person's body may appear pale and feel cold to the touch. Cold, which often appears in the winter but is not limited to this season, is associated with symptoms such as chills, headache, and body aches. Cold can lead to pain, which tends to be sharp or cramping.

● HEAT. Most closely associated with summer, Heat (also known as Fire) can take hold and produce symptoms such as high fever, a red face, red eyes, thirst, dark urine, inflammation, and reddish eruptions of the skin. Heat is often associated with problems of the upper body, such as headaches. Like Wind, Heat causes movement, but Heat's movement has a sudden and abrupt quality, associated with states like delirium and irritability.

● DAMPNESS. Like damp weather and sometimes associated with it, in Chinese medicine Damp is heavy, wet, and turbid. Diseases caused by Damp tend to linger and be difficult to cure. Like Cold, Dampness can cause pain, but Damp pain is heavy and protracted, rather than sharp and cramping. Damp is associated with sticky secretions and tends to attack lower portions of the body. Damp disorders can

include water retention (edema), especially in the legs or abdomen, as well as indigestion and diarrhea.

● DRYNESS. Sometimes appearing with Heat or Cold, dryness is associated with dehydration and scant body fluids. Its symptoms can include dry nostrils, lips, and skin. Dryness can affect the Lung, for example as a dry cough, asthma, or chest pain.

● SUMMER HEAT. Summer Heat occurs only in summer with exposure to extreme heat. Its symptoms may include sudden high fever, heavy sweating, exhaustion, dry mouth, and thirst.

How can you ward off these evils? Food and herbs provide some help.

Promote Healing, Avoid Harm

In contrast to Western medicine, which tends to view food through the lens of protein, fat, carbohydrate, and vitamin content, traditional Chinese medicine looks at food according to properties that include temperature, taste, and function. These qualities can help guide the selection of the best foods and herbs to eat depending on your condition, your constitution, and your environment, as well as which are best to avoid.

Temperature is front and center. This includes both the physical temperature of the food (piping hot or ice cold) and the thermal effects on the body (increasing metabolism until you break a sweat or cooling until you feel the tingle of chills). On the warmer end of the spectrum are foods and herbs such as ginger, chili peppers, cinnamon, turmeric, nutmeg, green onions, and walnuts. On the cooler end of the spectrum are foods and herbs such as peppermint, citrus, tofu, milk, lettuce, celery, cucumber, and tomato. (While across East Asia there is general agreement on the temperature classification of most ingredients, there also can be regional differences. For example, peach is sometimes classified as cool and sometimes as warm.) Cooking methods can influence the nature of the end product. Blanching, steaming, pickling, and boiling have a cooling influence, whereas grilling, frying, roasting, smoking, searing, simmering, and cooking with alcohol make a dish more warm.

Hot and warm foods dispel Cold, warm the interior, and fortify yang. Cold and cool foods clear Heat, relieve toxicity, and enrich yin. Neutral foods moderate the effects of either. To restore balance, someone experiencing an attack of Cold would want to choose warm and warming dishes, such as a steaming bowl of chicken ginger soup, and avoid foods that generate more Cold, such as chilled lettuce, ice water, and frozen desserts. Likewise, someone experiencing too much Heat would want to restore balance by choosing cooling foods, such as a cucumber salad, and by avoiding those that are warming.

An individual's constitution can also guide food choices in this regard. Some people tend to run warm, rarely needing a sweater and generally feeling energetic and active. These individuals benefit by gravitating toward cooler foods to balance these characteristics (and avoiding overconsumption of warmer foods so as not to exacerbate any imbalance). People with a cool constitution, who tend to feel cold and have a propensity toward fatigue, benefit from selecting more warming foods and avoiding meals with too many foods that are cooling.

According to traditional Chinese medicine, another important feature of a food or herb is taste, which can include sour, bitter, sweet, spicy, salty, bland, and/or fragrant. Each taste is linked to a general type of therapeutic effect:

- **SOUR**, which is associated with the Liver, tends to constrict and consolidate. Sour foods and herbs are used to counteract symptoms such as diarrhea and excessive sweating. Too many sour foods should be avoided, however, in cases when there is already too much contraction, such as when there is cold weather or a person is suffering from arthritis. The astringent taste acts similarly to the sour taste.
- **BITTER**, which is associated with the Heart, tend to improve appetite, move qi downward, and dry Dampness. Bitter foods are used to treat fever, constipation, and some types of cough, as well as addressing conditions such as arthritis. Too many bitter foods, however, are thought to cause diarrhea and to damage fluids.
- **SWEET**, which is associated with the Spleen, strengthens, improves, moistens, and harmonizes many systems of the body. Some sweet foods are used to address conditions involving weakness, dry cough, and thirst. Too many sweet foods, however, can cause conditions such as fatigue, recurrent bronchitis, and obesity.
- **SPICY/PUNGENT**, which is associated with the Lung, tends to disperse and circulate qi and invigorate Blood. Some spicy foods and herbs are used to treat a type of common

cold. Too many spicy foods, however, can cause skin problems, restlessness, and sleep disorders.

- **SALTY**, which is associated with the Kidneys, tends to soften firm masses. Some salty foods are used to address cysts, inflammatory masses, or connective tissue accumulation. Too many salty foods, however, damage fluids, muscles, and the vascular system.
- **BLAND** can play a role in regulating fluids. Bland foods may be used to help counteract swelling and puffiness.
- **FRAGRANT** can revive the Spleen and transform Dampness, so fragrant foods are used to help with digestive problems. Too many fragrant foods, however, can have a drying effect.

Foods and herbs are also known for additional functions, for example, acting on certain parts of the body (Upper, Lower, Interior, Outer Surface), and promoting certain types of movement (Ascending, Descending, Floating, and Sinking).

Meals for All Seasons

In East Asia, much attention is placed on eating according to the season, to help bring the body into harmony with the environment. Of course, all seasons call for a balanced diet. In China, a balanced diet is thought to consist of *fan*—the more fundamental, main, or primary food, necessary to any meal such as rice, wheat, or other grain—and *cai*—meats, fruits, and vegetables that make the meal more tasty and balanced. In general, though,

the East Asian approach suggests that people can optimize health with meals that support yang in the spring, clear Heat and generate body fluids in the summer, nourish yin in the autumn, and warm the body in the winter. In the spring and summer, yang rises to the surface of the body and needs to be replenished. In the fall and winter, cold, dry weather provides extra challenges for the body to stay warm and moist.

In the spring, a season of birth and new growth, people want to support the natural tendencies of their bodies by strengthening the Liver and its regulation of qi, as well as fortifying against external attacks of Wind, common in the spring, which can lead to irritability, insomnia, headaches, and dizziness. Good spring foods include onions, leeks, Chinese yam, wheat, cilantro, mushrooms, sprouts, and spinach and other leafy green vegetables.

In the summer, a season in which qi and Blood tend to be vigorous throughout the body and external Heat can be a problem leading to diarrhea and sunstroke, food can support the Heart and help cool and moisten the body. Foods with sour and salty flavors can help to ease irritability and insomnia from excess sweating. Fruits and vegetables help provide sufficient fluids and promote digestion. Other summer foods that help keep the body cool and balanced include watermelon, tomatoes, mung beans, cucumber, lotus root, coix, bean sprouts, and ocean fish.

In the late summer or in hot and rainy areas, Dampness can also be a problem that leads to gastrointestinal disorders, skin problems, and joint pain, and you can help your body stay healthy by eating more bland foods that help regulate fluid balance, such as coix, soy milk, and pine nut porridge. Some soups, such as mung bean seaweed soup, are thought to be especially good at counteracting Summer Heat.

In the fall, the body turns inward to prepare for winter and Dryness often dominates in the environment, which can prompt a dry cough, dry eyes, and dry skin. You can support your body by supplementing the Lung and promoting the production of body fluids with foods such as lily bulb, white wood ear, pear, pumpkin, nuts and seeds, honey, and soy milk. Sour foods, such as apple and lemon, can also be helpful in preventing the loss of body fluids.

In the winter, the body slows down and Cold appears in the environment, which can result in fatigue and sexual dysfunction. You can help build strength and counteract Cold by adding foods in moderation that support the Kidney and warm the body. Good winter foods include lamb, beef, Chinese yam, sesame, chestnuts, mushrooms, leeks, and nuts.

A Tale of Two Medicines

Let's take a look at how Chinese and Western medicine would provide different perspectives on a single patient.

Tammy, who lives in Malibu, California, and loves the outdoors, decides one fall day that she will drive out to the desert for some camping and mountain biking. For a while, she enjoys the wide-open spaces and the broad horizon, but she notices that the hot, dry Santa Ana winds are picking up from the East. The next morning, Tammy comes down with a fever and chills, then soon after, a dry cough. A few days later, she feels better and goes back to work, but the dry cough lingers for weeks.

A Western medical perspective would tell us that Tammy came down with the pesky common cold, caused by a virus. Since antibiotics won't kill viruses, Tammy might be encouraged to reach for some over-the-counter cough syrup as well as some aspirin or Tylenol to control her fever. Typically, a doctor would recommend drinking lots of fluids and getting some rest. As for the lingering cough, the doctor would assure Tammy that it was just a matter of time before she managed to shake it.

A Chinese medical perspective would give us a different story. Because of internal imbalance, Tammy was susceptible to an attack of external Warm-Dryness, which she encountered in the desert. Her fever and chills reflect her body's reaction to these external evils, and the cough resulted from the Warm Dry pathogen depleting the yin fluids of her Lung. A Chinese medical practitioner would initially prescribe a cool, moistening herbal beverage made from mulberry leaf, apricot kernel, and other herbs. After the fever and chills subside, the practitioner would recommend replenishing the yin fluids of the Lung with foods such as pear and herbs such as fritillaria.

And Tammy might be interested in taking advantage of both points of view, using aspirin for the fever and chills, then addressing the lingering cough by adding ripe pears to her diet.

If you are interested in learning more about the many intricacies of Chinese medicine and philosophy, you may want to look to the bibliography in the back of this book for additional sources, as here we only skim the surface of this deep art. In the United States and Canada today, graduate schools in Chinese medicine typically require four rigorous years of study. Luckily, producing excellent and healthy results in the kitchen isn't nearly so hard! And we've provided tips at the bottom of each recipe about each dish's special qualities according to Chinese medicine, so you don't have to study for that degree unless you really want to.

What About Science?

The modern scientific method is a wonderful thing and has led to new insights into some elements of traditional Chinese medicine.

Chinese wormwood (*Artemisia annua* or *qing hao*), for example, has been used by Chinese medical practitioners for more than a thousand years as a treatment for fever and certain skin conditions. In 1971, scientists found that extracts from the leaves had antimalarial activity in primate models. In 1972, Chinese scientist Tu Youyou isolated the active ingredient, artemisinin, and described its chemical structure. Artemisinin was fashioned into a therapy known as ACT (artemisinin-based combination therapy), which the World Health Organization currently recommends as the antimalarial treatment of choice in areas where multi–drug resistant strains of an organism *Plasmodium falciparum* that causes malaria, are common. Artemisinin is also under investigation as an anticancer agent.

Although not all results will be as positive, the panoply of herbs used in Chinese medicine contain a rich source of potential discoveries for the future. Remember, many drugs in our medicine cabinet today originally came from natural sources—aspirin originated from the bark of a willow tree, penicillin was discovered by accident from a mold growing in a petri dish, and the expectorant guaifenesin (a key ingredient in cough syrup) was derived from the guaiac tree.

The scientific method has provided evidence that other herbs used in traditional Chinese medicine offer promise. The U.S. National Institutes of Health's National Center for Complementary and Alternative Medicine (NCCAM) assesses and comments on a number of these, including:

- **ASIAN GINSENG**, which "may lower blood glucose" and provide "possible beneficial effects on immune function"
- **ASTRAGALUS**, for which preliminary studies suggest "may benefit heart function and help the immune system fight infections"
- **GARLIC**, which "may slow the development of atherosclerosis (hardening of the arteries)"
- **GINGER**, which "can safely relieve pregnancy-related nausea and vomiting"
- **GINKGO LEAF**, which has yielded "some promising results" in the treatment of Alzheimer's disease, tinnitus, and other conditions
- **GREEN TEA**, which has produced laboratory studies suggesting it "may help protect against or slow the growth of certain cancers"
- **LICORICE ROOT**, which "might reduce complications from hepatitis C in some patients"
- **PEPPERMINT OIL**, which "may improve symptoms of irritable bowel syndrome"
- **SOY**, which with daily intake "may slightly lower levels of LDL ("bad") cholesterol" and which some studies suggest "may reduce hot flashes in women after menopause"
- **TURMERIC**, which preliminary findings from animal and laboratory studies suggest contains a chemical—called curcumin that "may have anti-inflammatory and anti-cancer properties."

As NCCAM points out, in most cases more research is needed to establish a scientific consensus. At the same time, funding for such studies is tight and variables in the diet are notoriously difficult to control. Many studies have offered suggestive rather than conclusive evidence, for example, showing effectiveness of a compound in the test tube or in animal models without extensive and expensive human trials. But even human trials have their limitations.

With interrelated factors of genetics, behavior, and society, it is difficult to tease apart the contribution of one dietary element on a complex condition such as heart disease, diabetes, or cancer. The phytochemicals plants have to offer vary according to season, variety, and growing conditions. An heirloom plant grown in rich soil and picked in the late summer won't be the same as a plant variety bred for mass production harvested from poor soil in the spring. That's not to mention what happens to the produce after harvest—a strawberry eaten fresh simply is not the same as one consumed after being shipped across the country, then sitting a few days in a supermarket aisle.

In addition, in traditional Chinese medicine, herbs are rarely recommended in isolation. Instead, they are prescribed as part of herbal formulas, sometimes with as many as a dozen or more herbs. This type of polypharmacy, although sometimes studied in China, has rarely been tackled by investigators in the West. To complicate matters further, a central tenet in Chinese medicine is to tailor herbal formulas according to each individual's age, constitution, and symptoms. Only a few studies have tried to evaluate Chinese herbalism as practiced with this kind of rich variety.

It's worth noting, though, that a provocative November 2007 study in the American Chemical Society's *Journal of Chemical Information and Modeling* has lent support to the idea that East Asian herbalism has a chemical basis. Analyzing a database of chemical compounds, the study found that herbs in categories of traditional Chinese medicine (say, to strengthen qi, drain Dampness, or eliminate Wind Heat) do in fact demonstrate distinct patterns of association based on their chemistry. The authors also suggest how each of the categories might be translated into the language of Western medicine—herbs that strengthen qi, for example, are comparable with modern endocrine agents and immunostimulants. A number of ongoing projects, including a fifteen-year Chinese effort dubbed the Herbalome Project, aim to build bridges between biochemistry and traditional East Asian herbalism.

But it's easy to get lost among the myriad details. Keep in mind the most powerful and consistent message that the body of Western scientific evidence has to offer about diet—you increase your chances for a long life by eating a diet rich in a variety of fruits, vegetables, and whole grains, limiting your consumption of saturated fats, and avoiding junk food (and don't forget to exercise). We embrace this message wholeheartedly and find it marvelously compatible with East Asian kitchen therapy and the recipes in this book.

Keeping this big picture in mind, we encourage you to try the tasty dishes we offer, using your common sense, best instincts, and personal observations about your own health and well being as your guide.

HOW TO USE THIS BOOK

IN THIS BOOK, we present recipes from China, Japan, and Korea that use healthful ingredients from the East Asian tradition. We have tried to bring a delicious sampling of dishes to your table, selecting recipes that represent the East Asian approach, while recognizing that not all traditions easily cross the cultural divide (we are happy to offer recipes that call for tofu, lotus root, or ginseng, for example, but have avoided those with jellyfish or chicken feet). While we often provide a "slow cook" approach, we also offer tips to help make cooking easy and variations that can save time—just because the ancients didn't have a food processor or rice cooker doesn't mean you can't use one.

We encourage you to experiment with the recipes to adapt them to your tastes and circumstances. Some people prefer red miso to white, shiitake mushrooms to enokis, fresh thyme to dried, or less soy sauce to more. Find out what works for you. The substitution and conversion charts in the back of this book can help in this regard.

Similarly, we encourage you to use the recipes in a way that makes sense with your lifestyle. In general, traditional Chinese medicine discourages abrupt changes, so ideally new dishes supporting your specific health concerns and goals will be gradually integrated into your everyday diet (which is already basically healthy, right?). Occasionally, more sudden and comprehensive dietary changes are called for, but these cases are largely outside the scope of this book and are best accomplished under the guidance of a qualified health professional.

To help you make the most out of this book and to help bridge the gap between Western and Eastern medicine, after each recipe we have provided a list of heath conditions and concerns that the dish could address, using both Western terms and the language of traditional Chinese medicine. In the back section of this book, we have also provided a list of recipes grouped by health concerns. When using these tools, it is important to remember that Western diagnoses do not match Chinese medical diagnoses on a one-to-one basis. What is thought of as a single condition in the West can correspond to multiple patterns in traditional Chinese medicine. For example, the Western concept of insomnia can correspond in traditional Chinese medicine to sleep difficulties due to Heart Blood deficiency, Heart and Kidney yin deficiency, Heart or Liver fire, and so on, each calling for a different treatment. Those who want to take full advantage of the traditional Chinese medical approach should seek an individual diagnosis based on their own unique signs, symptoms, and constitution.

While our recipes are written to support health, not all ingredients are appropriate for all people. Pregnant and nursing women will want to avoid *dang gui* (angelica sinensis root) for example, and patients on blood thinners will want to consume wood ear in moderation. The perspective of traditional Chinese medicine also advises caution in certain circumstances; if you are afflicted with a condition involving Cold, for example, consuming large quantities of cold food and herbs will be counterproductive. As common sense would dictate, if you suffer from food allergies or intolerances, continue to avoid the offending ingredient. (Happily, one common source of food allergies and intolerances, dairy, is rarely used in East Asian cooking, and you can steer clear of wheat with relative ease, if necessary.) It's always a good idea to touch base with your physician about any questions regarding your own situation.

We recommend following the dosage guidelines in the recipes for herbs—for almost anything there is a point at which too much becomes harmful. (One of us vividly remembers a news story about a man in Great Britain who fell ill after eating nothing but carrots.) The herbs used in cooking—ginger, garlic, sesame seeds, green onions, and the other ingredients in this book (yes, including carrots)—are usually benign when used with even a dash of common sense. (Can the same be said of Twinkies and diet soda?) Of course, follow all the standard food preparation guidelines on refrigeration and washing. We're also advocates of buying organically grown produce and organically raised meat whenever possible to avoid the hazards of pesticides and other chemicals (and you'll help preserve the planet, too).

To help you shopping for and cooking with Chinese herbs and other Asian ingredients that might not be familiar to you, the "One Hundred Healthful Asian Ingredients" section provides details about foods and herbs that appear throughout this book. Also look to the color photographs to help you identify unfamiliar ingredients. Before we delve into some offerings for your table, here are a few additional practical notes on cooking with and shopping for East Asian herbs.

The How of Herbs

When the recipes in this book call for Chinese herbs, they often refer to dried herbs, which are typically rinsed and then soaked before cooking (although if you're making a soup, you can skip the soaking). In many dishes, the herbs are cooked with other ingredients and then removed before serving, as you would use a bay leaf. If several herbs are used this way in a dish, you can put them together in an empty tea bag or tie them in a piece of cheesecloth for easy removal before serving. This method can be used for herbal beverages as well, although it is often easier to simply strain out the herbs, as you would tea leaves.

Similar to herbs used in Western cooking, the cooking times for Chinese herbs vary—some herbs need to be cooked a long time, others are added toward the end of cooking to preserve their delicate character (think garlic versus basil).

In China, many people use earthenware herb cookers to prepare herbal mixtures. This piece of cookware has a spout to let out some steam while the liquid boils. Although an herb cooker is nice if you have it, you can simulate the process by covering a pot and leaving the lid open a crack, as we recommend in many of the recipes in this book. It is traditional to avoid using metal cookware with many of the herbs, but in a modern kitchen this is often difficult. If you need to use metal cookware, we recommend stainless-steel or enameled pots.

Over the past decade, concentrated herbal granules have become popular as a substitution for the dried form of herbs in therapeutic formulas. Granules are prepared with modern equipment that distills the herbs into a convenient and concentrated preparation that dissolves in warm water. However, granules need to be prescribed by a licensed Chinese herbalist; in this book we call for the herbs in a more natural state.

Don't confuse granules with herb powders, though—powders are simply dried herbs put through a grinder. In many cases, we recommend whole or sliced dried herbs over powders for cooking, as powders have a tendency to clump. However, powders can be useful when an herb is used as a thickener or flour, or when an inconveniently long cooking time would be required for larger pieces.

The same basic herb can come in many shapes—not only powdered, but also cubed, sliced, and in pieces of varying sizes. We have done our best to make measuring the herbs easy, by including the volume (such as tablespoons or number of pieces), as well as their weight. However, a kitchen scale will come in handy, especially for some of the more irregularly shaped herbs, such as wood ear. We have included grams as well as ounces for the herbs, as they are often sold in grams.

For other ingredients, such as vegetables, in this book we include approximate amounts to guide you. But when you're poised above a steaming pot, keep in mind that measurements are a modern addition to most East Asian cooking, so don't let unnecessary precision impede your creativity. Ancient recipes advise "a little bit of this" and "a little bit of that." Water isn't usually measured, but added until it is an inch or two over the solid ingredients. Don't the dishes come out a little different each time this way? Yes, but that makes it more interesting!

Shopping Tips

To help you while shopping, within each recipe we have included the Chinese name in pinyin (and sometimes the Japanese name) for herbs. Other names—often including alternative English names,

the Chinese character, and its Latin, Japanese, and Korean designations, are found in the "One Hundred Healthful Asian Ingredients" section. These may come in handy. Goji berries, for example, are also known as wolfberries and lycium fruit, and can be found in some Asian food stores and herb shops under their Chinese name, *gou qi zi*, or 枸杞子. Don't be shy about bringing along this book so you can show the shopkeeper or herbalist what you are looking for.

Hundreds of herbs are used in traditional Chinese medicine (and thousands discussed in the literature). In this book we focus on those easiest to find in the West, so shopping for them shouldn't require round-trip airfare to China, Japan, or Korea.

Pan-Asian food stores are a good bet to find many herbs and East Asian ingredients. Also, don't forget the smaller Asian food stores, which often have the advantage of having approachable help who can assist you in locating the ingredients. Almost anywhere there's a Chinatown, there's a well-stocked herb shop (worth stopping into even if you aren't shopping for herbs, for the sight of the rows of wooden drawers and the tantalizing smells of herbs wafting through the air). If you live in a major metropolitan center such as New York, San Francisco, or Chicago, locating an herb shop is probably as easy as looking up "Herbs" in the Yellow Pages or online.

Another local source for herbs is your neighborhood acupuncturist. Many acupuncturists are also trained in Chinese herbal medicine, as both healing arts are based on a common tradition. Even if your acupuncturist is not an expert in this field, he or she will most likely be able to direct you to a good source of herbs and East Asian foods. In fact, many acupuncturists are certified herbalists and run their own mini-herb shops.

In this electronic age, ordering online may be your choice—especially if you live far away from a center with a large Asian population. However, our experience is that there are more import-export companies that ship in bulk to traditional Chinese medicine practitioners, than outlets that sell small amounts to the individual consumer. So, pay attention to quantities when you order, or you may find you have inadvertently purchased a three-year supply! Look to the appendix for a list of online sources.

And for those with a green thumb, some herbs will grow in your garden or in a pot on your patio. Goji berries, for one, have become so popular that there's a nursery in Utah that specializes in distributing these seeds and plants. Another nursery in Athens, Ohio, specializes in Chinese medicinal plants in general—live plants as well as fresh and dried herbs—offering more than 130 species. Growing your own also gives you an appreciation for what goes into the herbs you buy at the market, where each herb has been harvested and preserved according to a method unique to each plant. In China, specialists train for years to identify the herbs, the best specimens, the optimal time of year to harvest them, as well as the best methods for preserving them.

Top Ten Herbs for Your Kitchen

You may want to keep the most delicious, nutritious, and commonly used Chinese herbs on hand—and you may be surprised to find you already have many of these in your refrigerator or cupboard. Here are some of our favorites, which happily appear frequently throughout the pages of this book:

- Garlic
- Ginger
- Green onion
- Mushrooms
- Seaweed
- Goji berries
- Ginseng
- Chinese red dates
- Coix (Job's tears)
- Cinnamon

Look to the next section for more information on these—and many other—healthy ingredients.

百味治百病

ONE HUNDRED
HEALTHFUL ASIAN INGREDIENTS

From almonds to winter melon, this section will help guide you through the ingredients that have noteworthy therapeutic properties according to traditional Chinese medicine and culture, as well as a few items that are ubiquitous in East Asian cooking. Some of these ingredients you know. Others will be more of an adventure. We've included alternative names when we think they will be helpful. These include the Chinese, Japanese, and/or Korean names for specialized ingredients you might be asking for in Asian grocery stores or herb shops (and the Chinese characters you can show shopkeepers) as well as alternative English names and the pharmaceutical Latin designations (or, if not available, then the botanical Latin) for ordering online and distinguishing among herbs.

Agar-Agar
See "seaweed."

Almonds
OTHER NAMES: *Prunus dulcis,* sweet almonds, *bian tao* 扁桃 or *xing ren zi* 杏仁子 in Chinese

Almonds are native to the Middle East and today are cultivated extensively in California, the Mediterranean, Australia, and South Africa. Rich in nutrients, they provide protein, fiber, B vitamins, vitamin E, calcium, iron, magnesium, phosphorus, and zinc, among other vitamins and minerals. Some scientific studies have suggested almonds can help lower LDL ("bad") cholesterol and increase HDL ("good") cholesterol. In Ayurvedic medicine, a system of traditional medicine practiced in India, almonds are used to promote a healthy brain and nervous system, as well as to increase longevity. In China, almonds are also considered a food with therapeutic properties, which can be used to counter a cough, especially with wheezing and dry throat (dryness with Lung deficiency), constipation (dryness in the Large Intestine), and lack of energy or appetite (Spleen deficiency). In the Chinese system, almonds are classified as sweet in taste and neutral in temperature. Try not to confuse almonds, the seeds from the fruit of the almond tree, with apricot kernels, sometimes called "bitter almonds" (see below).

Angelica Sinensis Root
See "dang gui."

Apricot Kernels

OTHER NAMES: *Armeniacae Semen,* bitter almonds, apricot almonds, apricot seed, *xing ren* 杏仁 in Chinese, *kyōnin* in Japanese, *haengin* in Korean

Apricot kernels are found within the apricot seed, and in the West are sometimes used in recipes for apricot jam, marzipan, and amaretto cookies and liqueur. You'll probably recognize the flavor when you cook with this ingredient. In the Chinese tradition, apricot kernels are considered a bitter, slightly warm medicinal herb (as well as a food), and are often used for coughs (especially dry coughs) and bronchitis, as well as to moisten the Intestines. Caution: This herb should be used only in small quantities, as like many other fruit seeds it can be toxic in large doses (more than forty raw seeds for adults, or as few as ten for children). In small, cooked amounts, however, apricot kernels are safe and a popular flavoring in cuisines around the world.

Asparagus

OTHER NAMES: *Asparagus officinalis, lu sun* 芦笋 in Chinese

The young shoots of the asparagus plant, a hardy perennial that is a member of the lily family, have been used as a food and a medicine for centuries, notably in ancient Egypt, Greece, and Rome, although probably a later introduction to East Asia. Asparagus, which is often harvested in the early spring, is high in vitamin K, folate, vitamin C, vitamin A, and fiber, among other nutrients. According to traditional Chinese medicine, asparagus, which is considered sweet, bitter, and cool, clears Heat and moistens the Lungs, addressing conditions such as chronic cough, high cholesterol, irritability, and depression.

Astragalus Root

OTHER NAMES: *Astragali Radix,* milk-vetch root, *huang qi* 黄芪 ("yellow leader") in Chinese, *ōgi* in Japanese, *hwanggwi* in Korean

Astragalus root comes from a plant native to northern China and the elevated regions of the Chinese provinces Yunnan and Sichuan, where it grows in dry, sunny locations. The root is usually harvested in the autumn when the plant is four to seven years old, and then dried. The roots are sliced before completely dry, producing a product that somewhat resembles tongue depressors. There are many types of astragalus (a member of the pea family)—more than two thousand, by some counts—but the Chinese version is distinctive. In addition to its use in cooking, astragalus root can be boiled in water and served as a tea; you might be able to find it packaged in the same section as herbal teas in a natural food store.

Astragalus root has been tested extensively for its healing properties. Some studies support the view that the herb stimulates the immune system, as well as lowering blood pressure and blood sugar levels. Shen Nong, the mythical founder of Chinese herbal medicine, gave astragalus the rank of "superior herb" in his classic *Divine Farmer's Materia Medica* (circa 100 CE). In fact, *huang qi* translates as "yellow leader," referring to the yellow color of the root and its status as one of the most important tonic herbs in traditional Chinese medicine. Astragalus root, which is considered sweet and slightly warm, is seen as acting on the Lung and Spleen channels to strengthen the immune system and improve digestion. The plant is often used in herbal formulas in combination with ingredients such as white atractylodes rhizome (a.k.a. *Atractylodes macrocephala* or *bai zhu* 白术) and Asian ginseng.

Azuki Beans

OTHER NAMES: *Phaseoli angularis Semen* or *Phaseoli calcarati Semen*, adzuki bean, rice bean, *chi xiao dou* 赤小豆 or *hong dou* ("red bean") in Chinese, *azuki* in Japanese, *pat* in Korean

Azuki beans are small, nutritious, russet-colored beans popular across East Asia, especially Japan where they are the second-most-common legume after the soybean. *Azuki* translates from the Japanese as "small bean," whereas soybean (*daizu*) translates as "large bean." Harvested from an annual vine, the beans are used in sweet red bean paste, dessert soups, and other dishes. Azuki bean sprouts are another popular option. Traditional Chinese medicine practitioners believe that azuki beans, which have a sweet and sour flavor and neutral temperature, enter the Heart and Small Intestine channels to drain Dampness and relieve toxicity; the beans are also considered useful in the management of diabetes.

Bamboo Shoots

OTHER NAMES: *Phyllostachys nigra* of *P. pubescens* of the grass family *Bambusoideae*, *zhu sun* 竹笋 in Chinese, *takenoko* in Japanese, *juksun* in Korean

Bamboo shoots are a popular vegetable in East Asia, eaten as a salad, in stir-fry dishes, or as part of a warm beverage. Available both fresh (from Asian markets) and canned (from almost any supermarket), bamboo shoots provide protein, fat, calcium, phosphorus, potassium, thiamine, riboflavin, and niacin. Fresh shoots are easiest to find in the spring; buy them only if they look firm and recently picked, and prepare them for cooking by cutting away the outer leaves (husk) and boiling them uncovered for 20 to 40 minutes to rid them of their bitter taste. From the perspective of traditional Chinese medicine, sweet, cooling bamboo shoots enter the Lungs, Stomach, and Large Intestine, clearing Heat and transforming phlegm and addressing such conditions as constipation, thirst, dry mouth, and certain types of cough.

Barley Malt

OTHER NAMES: *Maltosum*, maltose, barley malt sugar, *yi tang* 饴糖 in Chinese, *itō* in Japanese, *idang* in Korean

Barley malt is an ancient natural sweetener produced by the Chinese for at least two thousand years. The dark, thick, sweet liquid, which is sold in jars, is produced by a process that involves converting cereal starch to sugar ("malting"). Barley malt can be used to sweeten teas and other beverages and is one ingredient in Peking duck. Those thinking of using barley malt as a sugar substitute should note that the syrup has a distinctive flavor. In traditional Chinese medicine, barley malt, which is considered sweet and slightly warm, is thought to strengthen the Spleen and Stomach, helping to relieve digestive cramps, and moisten the Lungs, relieving coughs.

Bitter Melon

OTHER NAMES: *Momordica charantia*, bitter gourd, balsam pear, *ku gua* 苦瓜 in Chinese, *goya* in Japanese, *yeoja* in Korean

Bitter melon, a vegetable that often looks like a bumpy cucumber, appears in East Asian, Southeast Asian, and Indian cuisine. True to its name, this vegetable is bitter and it is often combined with ingredients (such as bean sauce, meat, onions, potatoes, or certain spices) that balance this flavor. It is also prepared in ways to curb its bitterness, such as using it while still green, before it begins to yellow and ripen; salting, then washing it; or salting it, exposing it to the sun, then squeezing and rinsing it several times. You'll find bitter melon in most Asian grocery stores. It is also available as a supplement. Bitter melon is high in vitamin C, and also offers folate, potassium, zinc, and other nutrients. Scientific studies have suggested that bitter melon contains a compound that moderates blood sugar, helping to control type 2 diabetes. The plant has also been associated with antiviral, anticancer, and antimalarial properties. In traditional Chinese medicine, the bitter, cold vegetable goes to the Stomach, Heart, and Liver channels, where it clears Heat, addressing thirst from a warm disease or Summer Heat, and treating visual problems with redness or pain in the eyes. The plant's seeds are used topically to treat sores that are slow to heal and swelling from sprains and fractures. Bitter melon is also used in Ayurvedic medicine. Caution: Avoid eating bitter melon if you are trying to conceive.

Black Wood Ear

OTHER NAMES: *Auricularia auricula*, black fungus, tree ear, *hei mu er* 黑木耳 in Chinese, *kikurage* in Japanese, *mogi beoseot* in Korean

Black wood ear is a mushroomlike fungus whose neutral taste adds little flavor to a dish, but whose texture offers a pleasant crunch. Native to Asia and some humid Pacific Ocean islands, this ear-shaped vegetable grows on the trunks of decaying trees. Wood ear is sold dried in Asian grocery stores and is relatively inexpensive compared with other specialized varieties of fungus. Store the dried pieces in a tightly covered heavy plastic

or glass container. When soaked in warm water, wood ear will expand to two to five times its original size, so a few pieces go a long way. Wood ear is frequently used in soups (such as hot and sour soup), stir-fried dishes, or salads, where it is cooked only briefly to maintain a crispy texture.

Wood ear contains fiber, and small amounts of the B vitamins thiamine, niacin, and riboflavin. Some scientific studies have suggested potential benefits of wood ear and other types of mushrooms in the diet, identifying a chemical that tends to inhibit blood clotting, which may help ward off vascular diseases such as strokes and heart attacks. In traditional Chinese medicine, the black wood ear, seen as sweet in taste and neutral in temperature, goes to the Lung and Stomach channels, nourishing the yin, moistening the Lungs, stopping bleeding, and generating fluids. Caution: People with hemorrhagic diseases or pregnant women should avoid overconsumption.

Bok Choy

OTHER NAMES: *Brassica chinensis, xiao bai cai* 小白菜 in Mandarin

Bok choy is one of the many members of the cabbage family, Cruciferae (including broccoli, Chinese cabbage, and mustards), that populate the Asian kitchen, where it offers up its long, crunchy white stems and dark green leaves for stir-fries, wonton fillings, pickling, and soups. There are dozens of varieties of bok choy (including baby bok choy) and the vegetable has become widely available in supermarkets, where it is usually found near red and traditional cabbage, and at gourmet, health, and specialty stores. If you are stir-frying, trim off the base of the vegetable and cook the leaves and stems separately, as the stems need more cooking time. Bok choy offers vitamins A and C, calcium, and fiber, as well as indoles, phytochemicals associated with anticancer properties. From the perspective of traditional Chinese medicine, bok choy is cool and sweet, acting to clear Heat, lubricate the Intestines, quench thirst, and promote digestion.

Bonito Flakes

OTHER NAMES: *katsuobushi* in Japanese

Dried bonito flakes are a staple in Japanese cuisine. These shavings from dried, aged bonito fish, a type of tuna, provide a strong, salty flavor in Japanese soups, salads, and sauces. Look for packages of delicate pinkish-beige bonito flakes in Asian food stores. In the West, fatty fish have been receiving much positive press due to their omega-3 fatty acid content, which has been associated with heart and nervous system health. In terms of traditional East Asian medicine, tuna strengthens the qi and Blood.

Burdock Root

OTHER NAMES: *Arctii lappae Radix*, great burdock, beggar's button, *niu bang gen* 牛蒡根 in Chinese, *gobō* in Japanese, *wu-eong* in Korean

Burdock root is the long, thin root of a plant you may recognize as the abundant producer of the pesky burs that stick to your clothes and cling to your pet's fur. In Japan and other parts of Asia, the plant is cultivated as a food source. The fibrous root adds an earthy and delicate flavor and crunchy texture to stews and other dishes. When shopping for fresh burdock, choose firm and crisp roots (they can be hard to miss among the other vegetables, as these long, brown roots are often more than three feet long). Scrub and peel the roots

if the skin looks tough. Some cooks soak the vegetable in water for 5 to 15 minutes before cooking to eliminate a slightly bitter aftertaste. You may also want to tenderize the root by boiling it in water with baking soda (½ teaspoon to 2 cups of water), then draining before adding to your stew or soup. Burdock root is also sometimes sold dried.

In European herbalism, burdock root oil is applied to the scalp to strengthen and beautify hair, prevent hair loss, and combat dandruff. In the macrobiotic philosophy, burdock root is believed to increase vitality and is recommended as a tea. In China, the seed of the burdock plant (*niu bang zi* 牛蒡子 in Chinese) has been the focus in traditional herbal medicine, but the root, considered pungent, bitter, and cool, is now becoming more popular as a food therapy to clear toxic Heat, reduce inflammation, and promote urination.

Cassia Seeds

OTHER NAMES: *Cassiae Semen*, *jue ming zi* 决明子 in Chinese, *ketsumeishi* in Japanese, *gyeolmyeongja* in Korean

Cassia seeds have been used as a medicinal herb for centuries, first appearing in the *Divine Farmer's Materia Medica*. Ranging from greenish-brown to dark brown, the small seeds can be found in Asian markets and herb shops and are used raw or after being dry-fried. Some studies have suggested that cassia seeds may help prevent heart disease, by lowering blood pressure and cholesterol levels. In traditional Chinese medicine, cassia seeds, considered bitter, sweet, and cool, are used to clear the Liver and the eyes; calm the Liver and anchor yang (addressing symptoms such as headache and dizziness); and moisten the Intestines (treating constipation).

Celery

OTHER NAMES: *Apium graveolens*, *qin cai* 芹菜 in Chinese

Celery is used in cuisines around the world, including those of France, Spain, Greece, Persia, and Russia. The plant has also been used for medicinal purposes by the Romans (who used the seeds to relieve pain) and in homeopathy (where an extract from the seed is used as a diuretic). In China, celery is considered a cool, sweet, and slightly bitter medicinal plant, used to reduce blood pressure, promote urination, cool the Blood, stop bleeding, reduce headaches, and regulate menstruation. In the language of traditional Chinese medicine, celery clears Stomach Heat and Liver Heat, and treats qi stagnation.

Cellophane Noodles

OTHER NAMES: Chinese vermicelli, bean threads, bean thread noodles, glass noodles, *saifun* (from the Cantonese), *fen si* 粉丝 or *dong fen* 冬粉 in Chinese, *harusame* in Japanese, *dangmyeon* in Korean

Cellophane noodles are a noodle made of starch, often from mung beans (especially in China), but sometimes from sweet potatoes, potatoes, or cassava in other parts of Asia. In Asian cuisine, cellophane noodles, which become translucent when cooked, are used in soups, stir-fries, salads, and spring rolls. Cooking times and properties vary according to the starch used (the mung bean variety is easy to work with because it resists dissolving). You can find cellophane noodles, often sold in packages of thin threads wrapped into small bundles like yarn, in an Asian market or in the international section of a well-stocked traditional supermarket. (See also "mung beans," for more information on the properties of mung bean noodles.)

Cherries

OTHER NAMES: several species of the genus *Prunus*, *ying tao* 櫻桃 in Chinese

Cherries, which grow in Europe, Asia, and North America (especially California and Washington), are popular in both the East and West. In the West, cherries have become popular as one of the "superfruits," offering iron, antioxidants, and anthocyanins (responsible for the red pigment in berries). There is interest in using fresh cherries or cherry juice to reduce pain and inflammation, as well as to treat gout, a condition of painful inflammation of the big toe and foot. In traditional Chinese medicine, cherries—sometimes referred to as the "fruit of fire"—are seen as sweet and warm, warming the body and strengthening the Spleen-Stomach to counteract fatigue and generate fluids.

Chestnuts

OTHER NAMES: varieties of *Castanea*, *li zi* 栗子 in Chinese, *kuri* in Japanese, *bam* in Korean

Chestnut trees, which come in various varieties native to Korea and China as well as other temperate regions of the Northern Hemisphere, including the United States and Europe, provide nuts used in many cuisines. Chestnuts are especially popular in Japan, where they are steamed, baked, grilled, cooked in rice, and used to make sweets. In northern China, chestnuts are also favored and used in casseroles and in a famous banquet dessert, Peking Dust, which combines pureed chestnuts, walnuts, brown sugar, and cream. To prepare fresh chestnuts, shell and skin them. To use peeled, dried chestnuts, soak them for 2 to 3 hours and simmer in water for 1 hour. Chestnuts provide vitamin C, thiamine, vitamin

B₆, magnesium, riboflavin, folate, iron, and phosphorus. In traditional Chinese medicine, chestnuts, considered sweet and warm, strengthen the Spleen and Stomach and supplement and warm the Kidney yang, increasing warmth and energy in the body and treating diarrhea.

Chili Peppers (and Related Species)

OTHER NAMES: varieties from the genus *Capsicum*, *la jiao* 辣椒 in Chinese, *tōgarashi* in Japanese, *gochu* in Korean

Peppers, including the spicy varieties, belong to the same nightshade family as two thousand other species, including tomato, potato, eggplant, tobacco, and petunia. Chili peppers, one of the most well known varieties of spicy peppers, originated in Central or South America, and chili peppers, chili paste, and chili oil are now an integral part of the cuisine in some regions of Asia. Hot peppers are not only delicious for those who like spicy food, they are also considered by Chinese traditional medical practitioners as having medicinal qualities. In the West, spicy food is often avoided in cases of stomach distress. But in traditional Chinese medicine, chili peppers, considered pungent and hot, are sometimes prescribed to alleviate abdominal pain or gastric upset if the diagnosis involves too much Cold (for example, in a case when a patient experiences stomach cramping); hot peppers should be avoided during digestive problems involving too much Heat. Scientific studies suggest that chili peppers possess antimicrobial and antiparasitic properties, and that they can relieve some types of stomach problems. (See also "Sichuan peppers.")

Chinese Cabbage

OTHER NAMES: *Brassica rapa*, *bai cai* 白菜 in Mandarin, *napa*, *nappa*, or *hakusai* in Japanese, *baechu* in Korean

Chinese cabbage, a member of the cabbage family that comes in many varieties, is tender, crisp, and mild. Like bok choy in the south of China, Chinese cabbage is one of the most important leafy vegetables in northern China, where it is called the "greater white vegetable" and has been eaten for thousands of years. This vegetable is also a staple in Japanese cooking, and is well known as the main ingredient in the Korean spicy pickle, kimchi. Today, the vegetable is cultivated in the United States as well as Asia, and can be found in many North American supermarkets and health food stores, usually near red and traditional cabbage. Look for tightly packed leaves with firm heads. Chinese cabbage should keep well for several weeks. Chinese cabbage is a good source of fiber, folic acid, vitamin A, potassium, and vitamin C. It also contains phytochemicals that have been associated with anticancer properties. From the perspective of traditional Chinese medicine, this sweet, cool vegetable is thought to strengthen the Stomach, clear Heat, lubricate the Intestines, quench thirst, assist digestion, and promote urination.

Chinese Dates

OTHER NAMES: *Jujubae Fructus*, jujubes, *hong zao* 紅枣 ("red date") or *da zao* 大枣 ("black date") in Chinese, *taisō* in Japanese, *daechu* in Korean, *annab* in Persian

Dried Chinese dates come in red, black, and wild varieties, and have been cultivated for four thousand years in Asia, India, and the Middle East. The taste of this fruit has been compared to that of an apple. They can be eaten fresh or candied as a dessert. Don't be misled by the name—this is a different species than the fruit of the date palm that goes by the common name of "date" in many Western supermarkets. When selecting Chinese dates, look for smaller fruit with firm and deeply wrinkled skin. In Chinese medicine, sweet, warming red dates strengthen the Spleen and Stomach and supplement qi to counteract fatigue, lack of appetite, and shortness of breath; nourish the Blood to treat Blood deficiency (a pattern involving dizziness, blurred vision, pallor, and scanty or absent menstruation); calm the spirit; and harmonize other ingredients in an herbal formula.

Chinese Yam

OTHER NAMES: *Dioscoreae oppositae Rhizoma*, mountain yam, Japanese mountain yam, Korean yam, *shan yao* 山药 or *huai shan* 淮山 in Chinese, *nagaimo* or *yamaimo* in Japanese, *goguma* in Korean

Chinese yam is the starchy root of a plant native to China, Japan, Korea, and Taiwan that is consumed as a food as well as an ancient traditional medicine. The plant consists of a climbing vine with heart-shaped leaves and small, white flowers that smell like cinnamon. The yams are harvested in the winter and can be eaten fresh or dried for later use, in which case the outer bark is removed, the root washed, dried, and stored, then later rehydrated in water and cut into slices. When shopping for fresh Chinese yams, look for relatively unblemished roots that are heavy for their size; be careful not to confuse this beige or light brown-colored vegetable with the darker, more orange or red sweet potato (also often referred to as a "yam"). In its dried, sliced form, Chinese yam

is often sold in packages of chalky white slices about one inch wide and three to four inches long.

This vegetable is commonly used in Japanese cuisine, eaten as a side dish or used as an ingredient in noodles. The root can also be purchased as a powder, or can be ground on request when purchased at an Asian herb store. Scientific studies of Chinese yam have suggested it controls blood sugar and counters diabetes, as well as stimulating intestinal peristalsis. From the perspective of traditional Chinese medicine, the root, which is considered sweet in flavor and neutral in temperature, strengthens the qi and supplements the Spleen, Lungs, and Kidneys. It is often prescribed for diarrhea and is recommended for long-term use to increase vitality, as its effects gently accumulate for those recovering from illness or weakened by old age. Mountain yam also has an important role in traditional prescriptions to manage diabetes, a use supported by scientific studies showing decreased blood glucose levels in mice eating the vegetable.

Chrysanthemum Flower

OTHER NAMES: *Chrysanthemi Flos*, *ju hua* 菊花 in Chinese, *kikuka* in Japanese, *gukhwa* in Korean

Chrysanthemum flowers were cultivated in China as an herb as far back as the fifteenth century BCE, and appear in the name of an ancient Chinese city named Ju-Xian, "chrysanthemum city." In China, the chrysanthemum symbolizes long life. The flower also became important in Japan, where the emperor adopted it as his official seal, and where a Festival of Happiness celebrates the flower. Chrysanthemum tea made from flowers is popular across Asia. Leaves (from plants bred for this purpose) are also part of the cuisine in Japan and China, often parboiled briefly before being served with a light dressing.

In addition to their ornamental uses in Europe and North America, chrysanthemum flowers also appear in Western herbal medicine, where they are boiled into an herbal tea or made into a compress to treat circulatory disorders such as varicose veins and atherosclerosis. In traditional Chinese medicine, the flowers, considered sweet and bitter in flavor and cool in temperature, are used to dispel Wind-Heat, treating some types of common cold; to clear the Liver, benefiting the eyes; to calm the Liver yang, treating hypertension, dizziness, vertigo, and swelling and pain in the head; and to clear Heat and eliminate toxicity, treating various skin disorders.

Cilantro

OTHER NAMES: *Coriandrum sativum*, coriander, Chinese parsley, Mexican parsley, *yan sui* 芫荽 in Chinese

Cilantro leaves are one of the most popular fresh herbs in the world, appearing in dishes and sauces in the Americas, the Middle East, India, Southeast Asia, and China, where the word for the herb means "fragrant plant." An ancient herb related to dill, the plant's seeds have been found in Egyptian tombs, and the Romans are said to have used the seed to help preserve meat. When you're shopping for cilantro, which you will find in the produce section of most supermarkets, look for fresh, leafy plants with thin stems. Cilantro is a good source of vitamins A and C. From the perspective of traditional Chinese medicine, cilantro is a pungent, bitter, and neutral to cooling herb

that moves the qi, acting to remedy lack of appetite, nausea, and indigestion and to promote sweating in the treatment of the common cold.

Cinnamon

OTHER NAMES: *Cinnamomi cassiae Cortex*, *rou gui* 肉桂 in Chinese

Cinnamon, an ancient and aromatic herb from the inner bark of the small evergreen cinnamon tree, is used throughout the world, in dishes from Indian *biryani* to cinnamon-flavored applesauce. Some scientists suggest that this cinnamon can help control blood sugar making it potentially useful in the management of diabetes, and the spice may also have antibacterial activity. In traditional Chinese medicine, cinnamon is considered pungent, sweet, and hot, warming and strengthening the Kidney yang and affecting the Heart, Kidney, Liver, and Spleen channels. It is used to increase vitality, to treat some types of abdominal pain, reduced appetite, and diarrhea, and to alleviate pain.

Cinnamon Twig

OTHER NAMES: *Cinnamomi Ramulus*, *gui zhi* 桂枝 in Chinese, *keishi* in Japanese, *gyepi* ("cinnamon peel") in Korean

Cinnamon twig comes from the same plant that produces the cinnamon in your spice rack, but whereas the cinnamon common in the West comes from the bark of the tree, this herb is made from the tree's twigs. In traditional Chinese medicine, cinnamon twig, considered pungent, sweet, and warm, is used to address an exterior attack of Wind-Cold (a type of common cold that presents with chills, fever, and body aches). The herb is also used to treat problems with the joints and to stimulate the digestive organs.

Clove

OTHER NAMES: *Caryophylli Flos*, *ding xiang* 丁香 in Chinese

The clove is a fragrant herb native to Indonesia now used in cuisines all over the world. The unopened bud of the flower of a tropical tree, in the West cloves are often used to flavor cider, soups, and sauces (such as Worcestershire sauce). Cloves also contribute flavor to many types of curries.

Studies have suggested that cloves promote digestion by increasing gastric acid and bile, inhibit microorganisms such as bacteria and fungi, counteract some toxins, and relieve pain when applied topically. With this in mind, it's no surprise that cloves appear in many herbal traditions: in Europe, cloves have been used as a treatment for gout and as a topical painkiller for dental work; in Ayurvedic medicine, they have targeted respiratory problems and stomach upset; in West Africa, they are infused in water to treat stomach upset, vomiting, and diarrhea. In the tradition of Chinese medicine, cloves, which are considered pungent and warming, can be used to alleviate Cold abdominal pain and gastric upset, as well as to treat conditions such as impotence and weakness associated with Kidney yang deficiency.

Coix

OTHER NAMES: *Coicis lacryma-jobi Semen*, coix seeds, Job's tears, adlay, *yi yi ren* 薏苡仁 in Chinese, *yokuinin* or *hato mugi* in Japanese, *yulmu* in Korean

Coix are sweet, bland seeds that taste similar to barley. Harvested from a tall tropical annual grass native to Asia, these oval, milky white seeds offer more protein than many other grains. In some parts of the world, such as Mexico, the hard, oval covering of the seed is used for jewelry and decoration, as the tear-shaped pods naturally have holes at each end. When shopping in an Asian market, ask for *yi yi ren* (Chinese) or *hato mugi* (Japanese). Coix is an ingredient in soups, and can be cooked together with rice. In traditional Chinese medicine, the sweet, bland, and slightly cold seeds have been used for millennia to promote urination in the treatment of edema (swelling); to resolve Dampness in the treatment of stiff joints associated with Wind-Damp painful obstruction; and to strengthen the Spleen in the treatment of diarrhea, fatigue, and other conditions. Coix also has a reputation for beautifying the complexion by helping to eliminate acne and other blemishes, both when eaten as part of a meal and when applied topically.

Cornsilk

OTHER NAMES: *Maydis Stigma*, *yu mi xu* 玉米须 (literally, "jade rice whiskers") in Chinese, *gyokumaishu* in Japanese, *oksusu teol* (literally, "corn fur") in Korean

Cornsilk, the silky threads that grow between the husk and the golden grains, is part of the Chinese medical pharmacopeia. The silk can be easily harvested from fresh ears of corn in the summer. If necessary, you can also buy dried cornsilk from a Chinese herb shop. In traditional Chinese medicine, cornsilk, which is considered sweet and bland in taste and neutral in temperature, drains Dampness and clears Damp-Heat from the Liver and Gallbladder, reducing water retention and edema, easing painful urination, and counteracting such conditions as diabetes and high blood pressure.

Cucumber

OTHER NAMES: *Cucumis sativus, huang gua* 黄瓜 in Chinese

The cucumber, which probably originated in India, is an ancient vegetable that has been eaten for millennia, such as during the Roman Empire and ancient Mesopotamia. Belonging to the same family as watermelon, squash, and pumpkin, cucumbers offer a crisp, cool flesh commonly used for salads, soups, or pickles. Cucumbers, which are a natural diuretic, contain water, fiber (especially in the skin), vitamin C, and such minerals as silica, potassium, and magnesium. In some parts of the Middle East, cucumber juice is considered good at alleviating skin irritations and is an ingredient in soaps. In terms of traditional Chinese medicine, cucumbers, which are considered sweet and cool, go to the Stomach and Bladder channels to clear Heat, eliminate toxins, treat thirst, and promote urination to reduce edema (swelling). In addition, cucumbers can be applied externally to soothe red, swollen, and dry eyes, regenerate the skin, and heal sunburn.

Cuscuta Seeds

OTHER NAMES: *Cuscutae Semen*, Chinese dodder seeds, *tu si zi* 菟丝子 in Chinese, *toshishi* in Japanese, *tosaja* in Korean

Cuscuta seeds are small brown seeds that come from a vine. Although the vine is often con-

sidered a destructive weed because it grows on other plants, cuscuta seeds have been used in traditional Chinese medicine for thousands of years, often to restore balance, improve vision, or address problems such as impotence, back pain, and incontinence. In the language of Chinese medicine, this herb, which is pungent and sweet in taste and neutral in temperature, strengthens Kidney yin and yang, consolidates Kidney *jing*, and brightens the eyes, among other uses.

Daikon

OTHER NAMES: *Raphanus sativus*, Japanese radish, Chinese radish, Chinese turnip, Korean turnip, *luo bu* 萝卜 in Chinese, *daikon* in Japanese, and *mu* in Korean

Daikon is a light-colored root that has been eaten in Asia for thousands of years. Daikon comes in several varieties, the most common of which is two to three feet long and two to three inches wide. Others are shorter and squatter and can grow up to fifty pounds. Although usually white, the root can sometimes be tinged with green. Related to the more familiar red radish you commonly see in the supermarket, daikon adds a crisp texture and a light, spicy taste to your table. The fall and winter roots offer more flavor but less bite than the hotter, blander roots harvested in the spring. The Japanese serve daikon (literally, "large root") pickled as a side dish, grated as a condiment (often mixed with soy sauce), and raw or boiled as an ingredient for salads. Daikon sprouts and daikon leaves are also part of Japanese cuisine. The Chinese often use daikon root in stews, as potatoes or turnips are used in the West. Before cooking, scrub the skin or remove it with a peeler.

Daikon provides some vitamin C. In macrobiotic cooking, daikon is valued as an aid to digestion, especially of oily foods. In the language of traditional Chinese medicine, daikon, considered pungent in flavor and neutral to cooling in temperature, can address food stagnation and clear phlegm from the Lungs, aiding digestion and easing breathing difficulties.

Dang Gui

OTHER NAMES: *Angelicae sinensis Radix*, dong quai, tang kuei, Chinese angelica root, *dang gui* 当归 in Chinese, *tōki* in Japanese, *danggwi* in Korean

Dang gui (pronounced "dahng gway") is a major herb in traditional Chinese medicine, used for thousands of years and mentioned in the ancient *Divine Farmer's Materia Medica*. *Dang gui* translates literally from the Chinese as "state of return," indicating its central role as a woman's herb in the Chinese pharmacopeia for restoring regular menses. (Do not confuse it with *Angelica arcangelica*, sold in Western groceries, candied, for baking.) The herb, which is considered sweet, pungent, and warm, is also used to nourish the Blood, addressing a pattern of Blood deficiency, and to invigorate the Blood, treating pain or traumatic injury.

Eggplant

OTHER NAMES: *Solanum melongena*, aubergine, *qie zi* 茄子 in Chinese

Eggplant is truly an international vegetable, appearing in the cuisines of Europe, the Middle East, South and East Asia, and North America. Today, China and India are the world's top eggplant producers. Related to the potato, pepper, and tomato, it is part of the Solanaceae (night-shade) family, and grows in climates ranging from tropical to temperate. In addition to the pear-shaped dark purple varieties with which you are probably familiar, eggplants come in many sizes, colors, and shapes, ranging from small and white (more literally resembling an egg) to green and round, to long and lavender.

When shopping for eggplant, select specimens relatively heavy for their size and use them right away if possible. Cook eggplant thoroughly until soft; it is difficult to overcook. Because of its texture and bulk, eggplant can be useful to provide balance to a meal that is light or nonexistent in meat. Eggplant is a good source of fiber, potassium, manganese, copper, thiamine, vitamin B_6, folate, magnesium, and niacin. Some scientific studies have suggested eggplant might be useful in preventing atherosclerosis and heart disease. In the language of traditional Chinese medicine, this cool, sweet vegetable addresses the Large Intestine, Stomach, and Spleen, clears Heat, and invigorates and cools the Blood, addressing such conditions as swelling, pain, hemorrhoids, and breast inflammation (mastitis) or sores.

Enoki

See "mushrooms."

Fennel

OTHER NAMES: *Foeniculi Fructus*, fennel fruit, fennel seed, *xiao hui xiang* 小茴香 in Chinese, *shōuikyō* in Japanese, *sohoehyang* in Korean

Fennel grows wild in many parts of the world today, including North America, Europe, Asia, and Australia. The fennel plant—known to the Greeks and Romans and still figuring prominently in European cuisine—not only produces the seed used as a spice, but also edible roots, stalks, and leaves. The distinctive flavor of fennel comes from a compound known as anethole, which is also found in anise. Fennel has been used medicinally in Europe and the Middle East to address eye problems and to prevent intestinal symptoms such as gas and cramping. In terms of traditional Chinese medicine, the warm, pungent herb is used to disperse Cold, to promote the movement of Liver qi and warm the Kidneys (treating lower abdominal pain), and to regulate the qi and harmonize the Stomach (relieving indigestion).

Five-Spice Powder

OTHER NAMES: *wu xiang fen* 五香粉 in Chinese

Five-spice powder is a mixture of star anise, Sichuan pepper, fennel, cloves, and cinnamon (sometimes also star anise, licorice root, and/or ground ginger). Common in southern China and Vietnam, five-spice powder is often used for roasted meat and poultry. This warming mixture is sometimes put in a bag, and then dropped into a prepared dish for the flavors to blend; the herbs can be easily removed before serving. Five-spice powder is easy to find in the West, sold in most regular grocery stores in the spice section, although you may get a more authentic blend by buying from an Asian food store. Since five-spice powder contains each of the five flavors—sour, bitter, sweet, pungent, and salty—some people have speculated that the ancients were trying to put together a mixture representing all five elements in making the blend.

Fleeceflower

See *"he shou wu."*

Fox Nuts

OTHER NAMES: *Euryales Semen*, makhana, or gorgon nut, *qian shi* 芡实 in Chinese, *kenjitsu* in Japanese, *keomin* in Korean

Fox nuts are pale, oval seeds harvested from a shrub that has floating leaves, like a lotus plant, and a large, purple flower. Fox nuts have been cultivated for millennia in Asia. Try asking for *qian shi* when shopping in a Chinese market. In India, fox nuts are roasted or fried, causing them to pop like popcorn, then eaten seasoned with oil or spices. According to traditional Chinese medicine, fox nuts, which are sweet and astringent in flavor and neutral in temperature, strengthen qi and benefit the Kidneys and Spleen, addressing such conditions as indigestion, diarrhea, and poor bladder control. Fox nuts are also associated with increasing sexual prowess in older men and retarding the effects of aging.

Fritillaria

OTHER NAMES: *Fritillariae cirrhosae Bulbus*, *chuan bei mu* 川贝母 (which translates literally from the Chinese as "shell mother from Sichuan"), *senbaimo* in Japanese, *cheonpaemo* in Korean

Fritillaria grows in China and Nepal and produces a bittersweet white bulb. It is harvested in the summer or fall, and processed. When you buy fritillaria, ask the herb shop to grind it into a powder for you, or use a coffee grinder at home; if the shop only crushes it, you'll need to grind it. There's a wide range of grades (and prices) of this herb; medium-grade is fine for most purposes. In addition to fritillaria's use as a traditional herb to clear Heat and transform phlegm in the Lungs to treat chronic cough, in China this bitter, sweet, and slightly cold herb has a tradition of use against breast and lung cancer. It is considered an especially good herb for the elderly and children. (Caution: If you happen to be in Asia and come upon the plant, note that the unprocessed herb is toxic and should not be ingested.)

Galangal

OTHER NAMES: *Alpiniae officinari Rhizoma*, galanga, *gao liang jiang* 高良姜 in Chinese, *kōryōkyō* in Japanese, *koryanggang* in Korean, *kencur* in Indonesian

Galangal is a member of the ginger family grown both as a spice and as a medicine. Galangal "root" (actually a rhizome resembling ginger) is used extensively in the cooking of Thailand, Indonesia, and other regions of Southeast Asia. It has a spicy, flowery flavor, and can be purchased as a whole root, sliced and frozen, or in powdered form. When buying fresh galangal, look for rock-hard rhizomes (you'll need a sharp knife to cut them) and store them in the refrigerator, wrapped in a paper towel. There are two varieties of galangal, lesser galangal and greater galangal. Lesser galangal (the variety used by traditional Chinese medical practitioners) is sweeter and stronger, and its flesh has a more reddish-brown (rather than yellow-white) hue than does its cousin. Galangal was popular in Europe in the Middle Ages, especially revered by famous herbalist Saint Hildegard of Bingen (1098–1179) as a treatment for such ills as deafness, heart disease, and indigestion. Others in Europe and Asia used the herb as an appetite stimulant and aphrodisiac. The rhizome of lesser galangal, which is native to China, is a traditional herb in Chinese medicine, believed to be pungent and hot, warming the Stomach, dispersing Cold, alleviating pain, and directing qi downward.

Garlic

OTHER NAMES: *Allii sativi Bulbus, da suan* 大蒜 in Chinese, *taisan* in Japanese, *maneul* in Korean

Garlic appears in ancient writings of the Chinese, Egyptians, Babylonians, and Indians, as far back as five thousand years ago. In the West, garlic has captured the popular imagination throughout the ages and has been used to ward off threats from vampires to the plague. In Asia, garlic is a staple in many regions. Traditionally, the Chinese use garlic in cold dishes, both for taste and for health reasons, as it keeps food fresh by killing bacteria. Pickled garlic is especially popular in Korea.

When buying fresh garlic, look for plump, firm bulbs. When you get the garlic home, leave the bulb whole (do not detach cloves until necessary) and store in a cool, dark, and dry location, such as a ceramic jar or mesh bag. If you have a garden, garlic is easy to grow, and it has a reputation for helping to repel insects and other pests.

Today, scientific research supports a view of garlic as a powerful herb with antibacterial and immunity-enhancing properties; it may also help thin blood, dilate blood vessels, and inhibit fat and cholesterol synthesis. In traditional Chinese medicine, this pungent, warming herb is used to reduce swelling, relieve toxicity, kill parasites, and counteract food poisoning by warming the Stomach, strengthening the Spleen, and promoting the movement of qi.

Ginger

OTHER NAMES: *Zingiberis Rhizoma recens, sheng jiang* 生姜, *shōkyō* in Japanese, *saenggang* in Korean

Ginger, the tasty underground stem of the plant *Zingiber officinale,* is a mainstay in Asian cuisine and healing in the Chinese herbal tradition. This tropical plant with fragrant flowers originated in China and spread to Spain around the sixteenth century. Today, ginger is widely grown in the West Indies, Africa, India, and Southeast Asia, and contributes its warm pungent taste to many cuisines. If you have a green thumb, in the United States you can grow the ginger plant in the warm climates of Florida, Hawaii, Southern California, Arizona, New Mexico, and Texas. Ginger is usually planted outdoors in autumn and the "root" (in fact a rhizome) is ready for harvest in the middle of the following summer after the leaves die down.

If you're shopping for fresh ginger, look for plump, firm specimens and avoid those that have begun to dry out around the edges. Most ginger you'll come upon at the market will be "mature" ginger, offering a deep, strong flavor perfect for soups and stews. Sometimes you'll come across "baby" ginger, a lighter, milder, and less fibrous selection that is well matched with seafood dishes or desserts. Don't make the mistake of trying to substitute the pickled variety when you are cooking— although pickled ginger is delightful, it is used primarily as a garnish for Japanese dishes such as sushi. Likewise, candied preserved ginger will be too sweet.

In the West, scientific studies have shown that ginger can be dramatically effective in aiding digestion and helping to alleviate stomach upset in such conditions as motion sickness. In Chinese medicine, fresh ginger, considered pungent and warm, is used to warm the abdomen, treating stomach upset, diarrhea, vomiting, nausea, and suppressed appetite; to treat exterior Wind-Cold syndrome, counteracting some types of the common cold; to warm the Lungs, helping to stop coughing; and to eliminate toxicity, such as from seafood poisoning.

Ginkgo Nuts

OTHER NAMES: *Ginkgo Semen*, gingko seeds, *bai guo* 白果 in Chinese, *ginkyō* in Japanese, *eunhaeng* in Korean

Ginkgo nuts are harvested from the gingko tree (*yin xing* in Chinese), an ancient species of deciduous tree with fan-shaped leaves and yellow flowers. Considered somewhat of a delicacy in China and Japan, ginkgo nuts are eaten roasted or used in soups, stir-fries, and desserts, and can be purchased fresh, in their tan-colored shell, or canned. If you are starting with fresh ginkgo nuts, additional preparation is required, usually shelling, boiling, peeling, and coring. (If you are actually collecting them from a tree, you'll also have to remove the smelly fruit; use rubber gloves to avoid contact dermatitis).

Despite the fact that the memory supplement popular in the West is made from ginkgo biloba leaf, in East Asia the nut is seen as the medicinal part of this ancient plant. According to traditional Chinese medicine, ginkgo nuts, which are considered sweet, bitter, and astringent in taste and neutral in temperature, enter the Kidney and Lung channels to regulate pulmonary activity, ease asthma and wheezing, and help relieve frequent urination. Caution: Ginkgo nuts can be slightly toxic in large quantities (large quantities being more than forty kernels for adults, or seven for children), so avoid overeating and make sure to cook them (ginkgo poisoning symptoms include headache, fever, seizures, and breathing difficulties). One rule of thumb is that you should only eat as many cooked ginkgo seeds as your age—but this only works for children. As a general rule, you need to avoid eating more than a dozen at a time or eating them frequently over the long term.

Ginseng

OTHER NAMES: *Ginseng Radix*, Korean ginseng, Chinese ginseng, Japanese ginseng, Asian ginseng, Oriental ginseng, and a number of other monikers in English, *ren shen* 人参 in Chinese, *ninjin* in Japanese, *insam* in Korean

Ginseng is one of the most well known therapeutic herbs, which you will find in some form—including in supplements, powders, liquid extracts, and teas, as well as the fresh and dried root—in natural food stores, herbal shops, and Asian markets everywhere.

Asian ginseng is the plant native to China and Korea that has been used in traditional East Asian medicine for thousands of years; it was mentioned in the two-thousand-year-old *Divine Farmer's Materia Medica*. The Chinese use Asian ginseng to strengthen the Lungs, Spleen, and Stomach, increasing energy and endurance, improving digestion, and assisting in recovery after an illness. In fact, many traditional Chinese medical practitioners consider the sweet, slightly bitter, slightly warm herb to be so potent that they advise the young and healthy to use it only sparingly, but those who are feeling the effects of illness or aging can draw on its energy-enhancing powers.

The quality of Asian ginseng, a slow growing root that takes six to seven years to reach maturity, is determined by the specimen's age, place of origin, whether wild or cultivated, length, girth, shape, and skin. If you shop for fresh ginseng, look for thick, long, intact roots with a thin body and long branches, and be aware the best specimens can be priced extravagantly.

Both red and white ginseng come from the same plant; the difference is in the preparation method. For red ginseng, the unpeeled root is steamed before it is dried, while for white ginseng the root is peeled and dried. The red variety is considered stronger and most Korean ginseng falls into this category. One trick to storing ginseng root is to keep the root in a jar of rice; the rice absorbs any moisture and keeps the ginseng fresh.

A related species is American ginseng (*Panacis quinquefolii Radix*, *xi yang shen* 西洋参 in Chinese, *seiyōjin* in Japanese, *seoyangsam* in Korean), a plant native to the northern United States and Canada that takes three to six years to mature. American ginseng is also a true ginseng—containing the signature chemical constituent ginsenosides. American ginseng has a history of medicinal use by Native Americans, and also has a place in traditional Chinese medicine—although the plant is used differently than Asian ginseng, so they cannot be used interchangeably.

You may also run across Siberian ginseng (*Acanthopanacis senticosi Radix et Caulis*, *ci wu jia* 刺五加). But beware. Although Siberian ginseng can be a useful herb, this is an entirely different species of plant, lacking ginsenosides and most likely dubbed "ginseng" for marketing purposes. Avoid roots or powders labeled "Siberian ginseng" when looking for true ginseng.

Goji Berries

OTHER NAMES: *Lycii Fructus*, lycium fruit, wolf-berries, matrimony vine fruit, *gou qi zi* 枸杞子 in Chinese, *kukoshi* in Japanese, or *gugija* in Korean

Goji berries, used in Chinese cooking and herbal medicine for thousands of years, are sweet red berries that grow on a wild bush that blooms between April and October. Similar to raisins, goji berries can be cooked, eaten raw, or brewed into a tea. Goji berries are now widely available not only at Asian markets, but also at natural food stores and even the health food aisles of some regular supermarkets. When shopping, look for dried fruit that still looks plump and avoid any produce that is bright orange-red, which might be an indication of artificial coloring. The fruit is rich in nutrients, such as beta-carotene, thiamine, riboflavin, and vitamin C, as well as other vitamins, minerals, antioxidants, and amino acids. Studies have suggested that an element of goji berries can prevent macular degeneration, deter tumors, enhance the immune system, and protect the liver. In traditional Chinese medicine, this herb, which is considered sweet in taste and neutral in temperature, nourishes the Blood and the yin, increases the essence, and improves vision.

Grapes (and Raisins)

OTHER NAMES: varieties of the genus *Vitus*, *pu tao* 葡萄 (fresh) or *pu tao gan* 葡萄干 (dried) in Chinese

Grapes have been consumed for millennia not only as fresh fruit, but also as raisins (dried grapes), juice, wine, vinegar, jams and jellies, and grape seed oil. Different varieties are cultivated around the world, from Italy to China, and the United States to Argentina. Grapes made the news in recent years as an excellent source of the phytochemical resveratrol, which has been linked to such beneficial health effects as increased resistance to cancer, heart disease, and inflammation. From the viewpoint of traditional Chinese medicine, raisins or grapes (considered sweet and slightly sour in flavor and neutral in temperature) enter the Liver, Kidney, and Stomach channels, supplementing the qi and Blood to address weakness. Grapes also generate fluids, counteracting dry mouth and thirst, and promote urination, reducing edema (swelling).

Green Onion

OTHER NAMES: *Allii fistulosi*, scallion, spring onion, bunching onion, Chinese onion, *cong* 葱 in Chinese, *sōhaku* or *negi* in Japanese, *pa* in Korean

The young shoot of a bulb onion, the green onion has been a popular remedy in Asian folk medicine for thousands of years, having been first described about two thousand years ago in the Chinese herbal classic *Divine Farmer's Materia Medica*. In Asian cooking, green onions are used both raw and cooked; they are widely available in most supermarkets. Although the green onion's fresh bulb, called *cong bai* 葱白 by Chinese herbalists, is used to treat the common cold and fight parasitic infections, the entire plant is believed to have medicinal properties. In traditional Chinese medicine, green onion, considered pungent and warming, is often used in conjunction with ginger (see page 33), to cause sweating in the treatment of an attack of exterior Wind-Cold.

Hawthorn Berries

OTHER NAMES: *Crataegi Fructus*, hawthorn fruit, *shan zha* 山楂 in Chinese, *sansa* in Japanese and Korean

Hawthorn berries, which are produced by a tree native to Europe, Asia, and North America, are a tart, bright red fruit used in sweets (such as haw flakes), jams, jellies, juices, and other products. In European herbalism, hawthorn berries have been associated with improving cardiovascular function, an effect supported by a number of scientific studies. In traditional Chinese medicine, hawthorn berries, which are considered sour, sweet, and slightly warm, are used to promote digestion, reduce food stagnation, invigorate Blood, and transform Blood stasis. Caution: If you are pregnant, large doses of this herb should be avoided; check with your doctor or health-care practitioner.

He Shou Wu

OTHER NAMES: *Polygoni multiflori Radix*, fleeceflower, Chinese knotweed, fo ti, *he shou wu* 何首乌 in Chinese, *kashuu* in Japanese, *hasuo* in Korean; we call the herb *he shou wu* here because "fleeceflower" and "knotweed" also refer to a variety of other plants, and its designation as "fo ti" is a misnomer

He shou wu (pronounced "huh show woo") is a root that comes from a perennial flowering vine native to southwestern China, Japan, and Taiwan. You can purchase this herb whole or sliced. Older, larger, and darker roots are considered the highest grade. You may also see the herb in tablet form. *He shou wu* contains lecithin, which aids in fat metabolism and helps lower cholesterol, and a flavonoid called catechin (also in green tea), which has been associated with lowering the risk for stroke, heart failure, cancer, and diabetes. Some studies have suggested that it has antitumor and antibacterial properties, lowers blood pressure, and increases circulation. In traditional Chinese

medicine, *he shou wu*, considered bitter, sweet, and astringent in taste and slightly warm in temperature, nourishes the Blood and augments *jing* essence, counteracting some types of dizziness, blurred vision, gray hair, and other signs of aging; relieving sores and swellings; treating symptoms of malaria; relieving some types of constipation; and treating cardiovascular disorders.

Hijiki

See "seaweed."

Honey

OTHER NAMES: *Mel*, *feng mi* 蜂蜜 in Chinese

Honey is a familiar item in both the West and the East, adding a delicious sweetness to many a dish. This golden substance has been used in traditional folk medicine around the world for thousands of years. In traditional Chinese medicine, honey, which is considered neutral in temperature, moistens the Lungs to calm coughing, strengthens the Spleen and Stomach to aid digestion and alleviate pain, and moistens the Intestines to relieve constipation. Modern research supports the view that honey is an effective antiseptic (due to its low water activity), and a spoonful can effectively soothe coughs as effectively as many commercial cough remedies. Caution: Avoid feeding honey to infants, as it can be dangerous for immature intestinal tracts.

Honeysuckle Flowers

OTHER NAMES: *Lonicerae Flos*, *jin yin hua* 金银花 (literally, "golden silver flower") in Chinese, *kinginka* in Japanese, and *keumeunhwa* in Korean

Honeysuckle flowers come from a vine that blossoms with sweetly scented flowers in the summer and late fall, with petals that change color from white to yellow in a season. The largest number of honeysuckle varieties grow in China, but the plant also appears in Europe and North America. The flowers can be eaten by removing the blossom by hand to suck at the sweet nectar in the center. The flowers have also been used as an ingredient in homeopathic medicine for treating asthma and syphilis. In traditional Chinese medicine, the honeysuckle flower, considered sweet and cold, is used to treat an attack of Wind-Heat with sore throat, and to clear Heat and toxicity in disorders with fever, sores, or diarrhea.

Kiwi Fruit

OTHER NAMES: *Actinidia chinensis/Actinidia deliciosa*, formerly known in English as Chinese gooseberry, melonette, *yang tao* ("sunny peach") or *mihou tao* 獼猴桃 (also known as *qi yi guo* 奇异果 in Chinese) before it was renamed "kiwifruit" or "kiwi fruit" in the 1950s as a New Zealand export

Kiwi fruit is native to southern China, where it was virtually unknown to the West until the early twentieth century. Today, the egg-shaped fruit with a brown skin and sweet green interior is also grown in such countries as Italy, Japan, and the United States. Kiwis are a rich source of vitamins C, A, E, potassium, and fiber, as well as alpha-linoleic acid (an omega-3 essential fatty acid). In the West, kiwis have been linked to such health benefits as reducing the risk of blood clots, warding off asthma, protecting against cancer, and helping to prevent macular degeneration. In traditional Chinese medicine, kiwi fruit, which is considered

sweet and sour in flavor and cold in temperature, clears Heat, generates body fluids, counteracts indigestion, and promotes urination.

Kombu

See "seaweed."

Kudzu Root

OTHER NAMES: *Puerariae Radix*, Japanese arrowroot, *ge gen* 葛根 in Chinese, *kakkon* or *kuzuko* (the powdered starch) in Japanese, *chilg* or *kalgeun* in Korean

Kudzu is a plant native to East Asia. A climbing perennial vine, it is noted for its rapid growth in particular climates, especially in the Southern United States, where it has become a monumental pest that can grow some twelve inches a day. Various parts of the plant are edible, including its leaves, flowers, and roots. The white root, which is sold in a powdered form in many Asian markets (try asking for "*kuzuko* powder") and natural food stores, is commonly used as a thickener for cooking. The root is also sold dried as an herb in Chinese herb shops. Studies in the West have suggested kudzu may evoke an aversion to alcohol that may be helpful in the treatment of alcohol addiction. Kudzu has also been linked to control of hypertension. In traditional Chinese medicine, the sweet, pungent, cooling root—mentioned as far back as the ancient text, *Divine Farmer's Materia Medica*—is thought to affect the Spleen and Stomach channels, and is used to treat such ailments as headache, fever, stiffness or pain in the neck and shoulders, certain types of diarrhea, and hypertension. In the language of traditional

Chinese medicine, the root dispels Wind from the exterior, releases muscles, clears Heat, and generates fluids.

Lemon and Lemon Juice

OTHER NAMES: *Citrus limonum*, *ning meng* 柠檬 in Chinese

Citrus is native to Southeast Asia, and lemons, oranges, and related plants are an important part of Asian cuisine as well as a now well-loved source of produce and flavoring in the West. In addition to their distinctive zing, lemons provide vitamin C, citric acid, malic acid, thiamine, riboflavin, calcium, phosphorus, and potassium. In traditional Chinese medicine, lemon, considered slightly cold and very sour, is thought to enter the Stomach, Liver, and Lung channels to clear Heat, quench thirst, harmonize the Stomach, and relieve coughing.

Licorice Root

OTHER NAMES: *Glycyrrhizae Radix*, liquorice, *gan cao* 甘草 ("sweet herb") in Chinese, *kanzō* in Japanese, *gamcho* in Korean

Licorice root, which you probably know as a flavoring for candy and liqueur, is native both to southern Europe and parts of Asia. In addition to its role in Asian cuisine as a flavoring for foods and broths, in traditional Chinese medicine licorice (the herb, not the candy) often plays a harmonizing role in multiherb formulas, helping the other herbs work well together. In the language of traditional Chinese medicine, licorice, which is considered sweet in flavor and neutral in temperature (but warming when dry-fried or honey-fried), enters all 12 channels, strengthening the Spleen and supplementing qi, moistening the Lungs, clearing Heat, and relieving pain and spasms; licorice root is also used as an antidote for a number of toxic substances. The herb also plays a role in Ayurvedic medicine.

Lily Bulb

OTHER NAMES: *Lilii Bulbus*, *bai he* 百合 in Chinese, *yurine* or *byakugō* in Japanese, *baekhap* in Korean

Lily bulb, a starchy root vegetable, offers a delicious and delicate flavor and has been used in herbal preparations and medicines for centuries—as far back as the second century BCE. Lily bulbs—which look somewhat like milky-white flower petals when dried—are grown on a large scale in China. There, they are traditionally gathered in the autumn, cleaned, boiled or steamed, then lightly baked, fried with honey, or dried in the sun. The dried form is reconstituted for use in stir-fries, grated and used to thicken soups, and processed to extract starch. In addition to proteins and starches, lily bulbs offer calcium, iron, phosphorus, thiamine, riboflavin, and vitamin C. In traditional Chinese medicine, lily bulb, which is considered sweet, slightly bitter, and slightly cold, is used as an herb to moisten the Lung, soothe coughs, clear Heat, and calm the spirit.

Longan Fruit

OTHER NAMES: *Longan Arillus*, *long yan rou* 龙眼肉 (literally, "flesh of the dragon's eye") in Chinese, *ry ganniku* in Japanese, *yonganyuk* in Korean

Longan fruit—similar to lychee nuts, but smaller, smoother, and darker in color—are harvested from the tree by hand and sold in bunches when fresh, and are also available dried and sliced, which is usually how you'll find them in the West. Longan fruit, which is reputed to add luster to the skin, is traditionally eaten raw or cooked, sometimes as a dessert. Both longan flowers and the sweet, aromatic fruit are used in herbal preparations, but the fruit is used more often, sometimes brewed into a single-ingredient tea. From the perspective of traditional East Asian medicine, the longan fruit, considered sweet and warming, is thought to act on the Spleen and Heart, nourishing the Blood and calming the spirit.

Loquat

OTHER NAMES: *Eriobotrya japonica*, Japanese medlar, Japanese plum, May apple, *pipa* 枇杷 or *luju* in Chinese, *biwa* in Japanese, *mogua* in Korean

The loquat is an orange or cream-colored oval fruit related to apples, pears, and quinces. Native to China and cultivated in Japan for a millennium, it now also grows in parts of the United States (California, Florida, and Hawaii), Mexico, Spain, India, South America, South Africa, and the Middle East. Loquats can be eaten fresh, poached in light syrup with a cinnamon stick, or used in fruit salads, jams, jellies, and chutneys. Depending on your location, in the Northern Hemisphere loquats are in season some time between March and August. Loquats are fragile and bruise easily and because of this can be difficult to find fresh. In season, look for fresh loquats, which resemble small apricots, at your local farmers' market, Asian food store, or your neighbor's tree (or buy your own tree) if you live in the right part of the country; you may also have luck buying

fresh fruit online. Loquats are also available canned (sometimes from Mexican groceries as well as Asian food stores). High in potassium and vitamin A, the fruit is used to make a cough syrup popular in Asia and is reported to have a sedative effect. Loquat leaves, which can be used to make a tea, are considered a classic herb in traditional Chinese medicine. Caution: Like other members of this fruit family, the seeds of the loquat are slightly toxic, so avoid eating them. From the Chinese perspective, loquat fruit clears Lung Heat, redirects Lung qi downward to stop coughing, moistens the Lungs, treats thirst, and regulates the Stomach to treat nausea and vomiting.

Lotus Leaf

OTHER NAMES: *Nelumbinis Folium*, *he ye* 荷叶 in Chinese, *kayō* in Japanese, *yeon ip* in Korean

Lotus leaf is harvested June through September in China from the famed lotus plant, which in many Asian traditions symbolizes immortality, purity, and enlightenment. The Buddha is often depicted sitting on a lotus leaf, and lotus flowers were said to bloom wherever he walked. Although usually sold dried, fresh lotus leaves are available seasonally, in the summer, from Asian grocery stores. Lotus leaf is available from Chinese herb stores in its dried form, in which the broad leaves become beige and papery. In traditional Chinese medicine, the lotus leaf, considered bitter and slightly sweet in flavor and neutral in temperature, is used to treat symptoms of Summer Heat, such as fever, irritability, and excess sweating, and to raise the clear yang of the Spleen to treat diarrhea. Lotus leaf can also be used externally as a compress to help stop bleeding.

Lotus Root

OTHER NAMES: the root of *Nelumbo nucifera*, *ou* 藕 in Chinese, *renkon* in Japanese, *yeon ppuri* in Korean

Lotus root is common throughout Asia. Edible rhizomes lie underneath the surface of lakes and ponds where lotus flowers float. These gray-brown lotus "roots" (actually rhizomes) are often eaten as a starchy vegetable. Lotus root resembles links of sweet potatoes with a lacy interior, growing in strings up to a yard long. Young specimens are sometimes peeled and eaten fresh in salads. More mature roots can be stir-fried, stuffed, and deep-fried or simmered in soup, or made into a starchy paste (used as a thickener) or a beverage. When shopping for fresh root, look for those with a lighter beige peel, which indicates a fresher vegetable than the darker brown pieces. You may also encounter lotus root vacuum packed or canned. Lotus root offers dietary fiber, vitamin C, potassium, thiamine, riboflavin, vitamin B_6, phosphorus, copper, and manganese. Studies have suggested that lotus root may be helpful for managing high cholesterol and hypertension. In macrobiotics, lotus root is considered good for the respiratory organs. In the Chinese tradition, fresh lotus root, considered sweet and cooling, is used to counteract summer Dryness, clear Heat, and harmonize the Spleen and Stomach.

Lotus Seeds

OTHER NAMES: *Nelumbinis Semen*, *lian zi* 蓮子 in Chinese, *renshi* in Japanese, and *yeonja* in Korean

Lotus seeds are rich, nutritious seeds common in East Asian cuisine. The off-white, oval seeds are harvested in the autumn from the lotus plant, which also provides us with lotus root (used in soups, stews, and other dishes), lotus leaves (used as a wrapper for cooking and as a medicinal herb) and lotus stamens (sometimes used to make tea), not to mention lovely pink or white lotus blossoms. Lotus seeds can be eaten raw, or cooked into a soup, crystallized with sugar to make sweets, or made into a sweet paste used to fill Chinese moon cakes. Lotus seeds are available in Asian groceries dried (sometimes called "lotus nuts" in this form) or canned. In traditional Chinese medicine, lotus seeds, considered sweet and astringent in flavor and neutral in temperature, are believed to act on the Heart, Kidney, and Spleen channels, calming the spirit, counteracting insomnia, treating loss of appetite, and addressing such problems as diarrhea and excessive urination.

Maitakes

See "mushrooms."

Miso

OTHER NAMES: *miso* in Japanese, including *shiromiso* (white miso) and *akamiso* (red miso)

Miso is a fermented paste made from soybeans, and usually also such grains as rice, barley, wheat, and/or buckwheat. Although there is some debate about whether miso originated in China or Japan, today miso is a key part of Japanese cuisine, used in soups, stews, pickles, vegetables, marinades, and various sauces. China, Korea, and other countries in Asia also have their own varieties of fermented bean paste, although miso is probably easiest to find in the West. Since miso contains healthy microorganisms (similar to those in yogurt), it is often added as one of the final ingredients in a dish to maximize its probiotic benefits.

For this reason, avoid boiling soup or stew after adding miso—too much heat will kill the precious microorganisms.

When shopping for miso, you may be faced with an array of choices. One of the most common distinctions is between white and red. The white miso is milder, often used in dressings, whereas the red variety offers a stronger flavor and is often used in stews. Don't be afraid to experiment to find out what you like, as the flavors range from quite pungent and salty to sweeter and more earthy, depending on each kind's ingredients and preparation method. Avoid any miso labeled "pasteurized," as it will not offer the same probiotic benefits as less-processed types. Refrigerate miso in an airtight container after opening.

The Japanese view miso as a health food and use it as a home remedy for digestive problems, cancer, low libido, and tobacco poisoning. Some scientists have suggested miso helps counteract radiation poisoning and cancer. A staple in Japan and much used in macrobiotic cooking, miso is a good source of calcium and protein, and also offers iron, potassium, and a variety of B vitamins. Because of the fermentation process, the protein in miso can be easily absorbed by the digestive system. In traditional East Asian medicine, miso, which is considered salty in flavor and neutral to cooling in temperature, is seen as harmonizing the digestion.

Mulberry Fruit

OTHER NAMES: *Mori Fructus, sang shen* 桑椹 in Chinese, *sōjin* in Japanese, *odi* in Korean

The mulberry tree, especially the white mulberry, has a long history in China. Almost all parts of the tree—from fruit to leaves and twigs—play a role in traditional Chinese medicine. As the plant's leaves are the sole food source of the silkworm, used to make silk thread, the tree has also played a major role in economics and trade. The fruit is known to contain significant amounts of resveratrol, a substance that has recently received a lot of press about its health benefits, especially through consumption of red wine. Scientific studies have also suggested that mulberry may help to control blood sugar. In traditional Chinese medicine, the fruit is believed to be sweet and cold, and is used to nourish the Blood and yin, treating symptoms such as dizziness, blurry vision, prematurely gray hair, tinnitus, and insomnia, as well as to generate body fluids and to lubricate the Intestines. Mulberry leaves (*Mori Folium, sang ye* 桑葉 in Chinese, *sōyō* in Japanese, and *sangyeop* in Korean), which are considered bitter, sweet, and cold, relieve coughs, dizziness, and headache, as well as red, dry, and sore eyes. Mulberry also plays a role in the traditional medicine of Azerbaijan.

Mung Beans

OTHER NAMES: *Phaseoli radiati Semen*, mung, moong, mash bean, munggo, green gram, green soy, *lu dou* 绿豆 in Chinese (literally, "green bean"), *ryokuzu* in Japanese, *noktu* in Korean

Mung beans are small, soft, green beans with a yellow interior that serve as a staple throughout much of Asia. They make a variety of tasty contributions to the kitchen—as a whole bean, as a sprout (most sprouts found in stores are grown from mung beans), as a paste (the filling in Chinese sweets, such as steamed buns), as noodles (known as bean thread noodles, cellophane noodles, glass noodles, and spring rain noodles), and as a tea (popular across Asia). Unlike many other types of beans, they are easy to digest but still offer protein as well as such nutrients as calcium, iron, phosphorus, thiamine, and riboflavin. In traditional Chinese medicine, mung beans, considered sweet and cold, are used to clear Heat from the exterior of the body, targeting some skin disorders and relieving toxicity. They are also used to dispel Summer Heat, and alleviate thirst and restlessness.

Mushrooms

OTHER NAMES: a loose classification in the fungi kingdom, comprising plants in the order *Agaricales* and *Agaricomycetes*, *jun* 菌 or *mo gu* 蘑菇 in Chinese, *kinoko* or *take* in Japanese, *beoseot* in Korean

Mushrooms, which come in hundreds of varieties, have a long history of use in traditional medicine in addition to their mouthwatering contributions to dishes around the globe. In Asia, they are an important ingredient in traditional vegetarian dishes, adding depth and body to the flavor. Although mushrooms are commonly thought to contain little nutrition, in fact they offer such vitamins as thiamine, riboflavin, niacin, and biotin, and such minerals as iron, selenium, potassium, and phosphorous. Scientists are also investigating several species for potential anticancer, antiviral, and immunity-enhancing properties. In Asia, mushrooms have been believed to be good for health for centuries. Some noteworthy varieties of mushrooms and related fungi include:

● BUTTON mushrooms (*Agaricus bisporus*), native to North America and Europe, are the most widely cultivated mushrooms in North America. Their light forms with round heads present a familiar sight in most supermarkets. While grown as "button mushrooms" for sale in their immature, unopened form, this species graduates to cremini or baby bella mushrooms when grown to a more mature stage, and then to portobello, when assuming its mature large, brown, and more meaty appearance. This species is considered sweet and cooling, according to the Chinese system, strengthening the Spleen, increasing the qi, and moistening dryness.

● ENOKI mushrooms (a.k.a. *Flammulina velutipes*, golden needle mushroom, velvet shank, *jin zhen gu* 金针菇 in Chinese, *enoki-take* in Japanese, *pengi beoseot* in Korean), which appear often in Asian dishes, can be recognized by their long, slender stems and tiny caps. In the wild, enokis tend to grow on the stumps of trees such as the Chinese Hackberry, mulberry, or persimmon. Both wild and cultivated varieties have a mild, delicate flavor. When shopping, look for mushrooms with firm, white, shiny caps and avoid those with slimy or brownish stalks. Before cooking, rinse the mushrooms and cut off the roots at the base of the cluster.

● MAITAKE, which translates to "dancing mushroom" in Japanese (a.k.a. *Grifola frondosa*, Sheep's Head, Ram's Head, and Hen of the Woods, *sae beoseot* in Korean) is native to parts of Japan and North America, where it tends to grow at the base of trees. In East Asia, the mushroom and the underground tuber from which it grows are highly prized for balancing the body and enhancing immunity. Studies have suggested that maitakes help regulate blood pressure, blood sugar, and cholesterol levels.

● OYSTER mushrooms (*Pleurotus ostreatus, xing bao gu* 杏鲍菇 [literally, "flat mushroom"] in Chinese, *hiratake* in Japanese [also sold under *eryngii* in Japanese stores], *neutari beoseot* in Korean) have been cultivated in Asia for centuries, and are now a popular variety around the world both fresh and dried. The shape of these light mushrooms indeed hearken back to the shelled sea creature and some people think the taste does, too. Studies have suggested that oyster mushrooms contain natural statins, which lower cholesterol levels. In traditional Chinese medicine, oyster mushrooms, considered sweet and slightly warm, strengthen the Spleen, drain Dampness, and treat painful obstruction (*bi* syndrome).

● REISHI mushrooms (*Ganoderma lucidum, ling zhi* 灵芝 [literally, "herb of spiritual potency"] in Chinese, *reishi* from the Japanese, *yeongji* in Korean) grow on trees and are among the oldest mushrooms known to have been used in medicine. In China, reishis are sometimes referred to as the "mushroom of immortality," and the ancient *Divine Farmer's Materia Medica* (ca. 250 CE) tells us that this mushroom belongs in the highest class of herbs, a class that makes the body light, strengthens the qi, and prolongs life without aging. Traditional Chinese medicine practitioners still recommend this mushroom, usually prepared by simmering in hot water to release its healing properties, to augment the qi, nourish the Blood, and calm the spirit.

● SHIITAKES (a.k.a. *Lentinus edodes*, black mushroom, black winter mushroom, black forest mushroom, *dong gu* 冬菇 or *xiang gu* 香菇 in Chinese, *shiitake* [literally, "oak mushroom"] in Japanese, *pyogo* in Korean) are native to East Asia and have been cultivated there for thousands of years. These dark, tasty specimens grow on fallen chestnuts and oaks and are widely available dried and fresh in Asian and natural food stores. Shiitake mushrooms are one of the leading foods recommended in traditional East Asian medicine for enhancing immunity. In Chinese medicine, they are used to strengthen the Spleen and Stomach and augment qi. In macrobiotic cooking, they are valued for helping the body rid itself of excess animal fats and salt.

● STRAW mushrooms (*Volvariella volvacea*, paddy straw mushroom, *cao gu* 草菇 in Chinese), named after the rice straw they are grown on, are frequently used in Asian cuisine. Commonly available canned or dried in the West (and fresh in Asia), these dark vegetables add an earthy flavor to soups and stir-fries.

● WOOD EAR (*Tremella fuciformis*) is a variety of tree fungus (not quite a mushroom since it doesn't grow in the classic mushroom shape with a cap, stem, and gills) that offers a neutral flavor and crunchy texture, as well as a long history of use in traditional Chinese medicine. See "black wood ear" and "white wood ear." Cloud ear (*Auricularia polytricha*) is a closely related but more expensive variety that can be substituted when cooking.

Nori

See "seaweed."

Nutmeg

OTHER NAMES: *Myristicae Semen, rou dou kou* 肉豆蔻 in Chinese

Nutmeg is used in both Eastern and Western cuisine, from Japan to Holland. Nutmeg is made from the tree's seed; a related spice, mace, is made from the reddish covering of the seed. Nutmeg lends its sweet flavor to puddings, eggnog, vegetables, soups, and sauces in the West, and to dishes such as curries and soups in the East. In traditional Chinese medicine, nutmeg, considered pungent and warming, is thought to enter the Spleen, Stomach, and Large Intestine channels and is an important herb for treating deficiency diarrhea. Caution: Use only in small quantities, as nutmeg seed is toxic in an unprocessed form; roasting, however, reduces the toxicity. Nutmeg has been used safely in small quantities for centuries.

Ophiopogon Tuber

OTHER NAMES: *Ophiopogonis Radix, mai men dong* 麦门冬 (literally, "lush winter wheat") in Chinese, *bakumondō* in Japanese, *maekmundong* in Korean

Ophiopogon tuber comes from a perennial plant native to Japan. Harvested in the summer, the sweet, slightly bitter, slightly cold root is used in traditional Chinese medicine to moisten the Lungs and stop coughing, augment the Stomach yin and generate fluids, treat irritability due to Heat, and moisten the Intestine. Look for thick, soft, fragrant, and light yellow-white specimens.

Oranges

OTHER NAMES: *Citrus sinensis, cheng* 橙 in Chinese

Oranges, which originated in Southeast Asia, are now enjoyed around the world and cultivated in such countries as Brazil, the United States, Mexico, India, China, Spain, Italy, and Iran. Oranges, which are high in vitamin C, are typically eaten fresh or made into juice, salads, or marmalade. In Chinese culture, oranges often symbolize happiness and prosperity, and are given to friends and relatives during the Chinese New Year. In traditional Chinese medicine, the orange is considered sweet and sour in flavor, and cool to cold in temperature; it enters the Lung and Stomach channels, generating fluids, treating thirst, calming restlessness, and countering some types of nausea and vomiting.

Peaches

OTHER NAMES: *Prunus persica, tao zi* 桃子 in Chinese

Peaches, which grow on a tree native to China, are now also cultivated in the United States, Italy, and Greece, regions with warm summers and a winter season. Although the delightful, sweet fruit is enjoyed by all, in Asia the peach has special status as a symbol of hope, long life, and immortality, and is reputed to have been a favorite of ancient Chinese emperors. Peaches, which are in season sometime between late May and August, are high in vitamin C and beta-carotene. From the viewpoint of traditional Chinese medicine, the peach, which is considered sweet, sour, and warming, can help generate body fluids and move the Blood, alleviating thirst, dry throat, constipation, and painful menstruation. The seed is also used as a medicinal herb.

Peanuts

OTHER NAMES: *Arachis hypogaea* or groundnut, *hua sheng* 花生 in Chinese

Peanuts, which are native to Central and South America, are now popular around the world, especially in the United States. Peanuts were a relatively late introduction to China, arriving by way of Portuguese traders in the 1600s and American missionaries in the 1800s. Also popular in Thai, Vietnamese, and Philippine cuisine, peanuts are now featured, often boiled, in Chinese cuisine. They are a good source of protein, B vitamins, magnesium, phosphorus, and zinc. They also contain the phytochemical resveratrol, which has been linked to longevity and reduced risk of cardiovascular disease and cancer. However, make sure to use fresh peanuts, preferably grown in a dry climate such as New Mexico's or Arizona's (try looking for the Valencia or Spanish varieties), to avoid contact with a toxic mold. Store in a cool, dry place, such as the freezer. From the perspective of Chinese medicine, peanuts are considered sweet in flavor and neutral in temperature (although more cooling when raw and warming when roasted or boiled), and can be used to strengthen the Spleen to help increase strength and appetite, moisten the Lungs to treat a dry cough and dry throat, moisten the Large Intestine to help relieve constipation, and address qi and Blood deficiency to help promote lactation.

Pears

OTHER NAMES: *Pyrus*, *li* 梨 in Chinese

Pears grow in many varieties in temperate regions around the world. In Asia, pears, pear juice, and pear syrup are widespread, and the many Chinese words for this fruit—including *kuai go* ("happy fruit"), *guo zong* ("fruit ancestor"), *yu ru* ("jade milk"), or *mi fu* ("honey father")—reflect its popularity. Pears provide vitamin C, riboflavin, vitamin B_6, potassium, magnesium, and other nutrients. In Asia, pears are known not only for their sweet taste, but also for their medicinal properties that address dry cough and constipation, as well as restlessness. In the language of traditional Chinese medicine, pears, which are considered sweet and cooling, enter the Lung and Stomach channels, clearing Heat, moistening dryness, generating body fluids, and transforming phlegm.

Pepper (Black and White)

OTHER NAMES: *Piper nigrum*; look for white pepper under *hu jiao* 胡椒 in Chinese, *koshō* in Japanese, *huchu, hoochoo* in Korean

Pepper was first harvested in India and later spread across Asia, although it never reached the same height of popularity that it now boasts in the West. Black pepper is the type you'll find on Western dining room tables. To create black pepper, the immature fruit is harvested and then dried with the hull intact (called a peppercorn before it is ground). In China, white pepper is more common, giving such dishes as hot and sour soup their characteristic zing. White pepper comes from the same plant species as black pepper, but the fruit is fully ripened and then removed. Most local supermarkets and natural food stores stock white pepper; if you can't find it there, look in Asian markets, where this type of pepper is available both ground and whole. In traditional Chinese medicine, this pungent, hot spice is thought to warm the Spleen, Stomach, and Large Intestine, relieving pain from excess Cold and addressing some cases of lack of appetite, indigestion, and bloating.

Peppermint

OTHER NAMES: *Menthae haplocalycis Herba, bo he* 薄荷 in Chinese

Peppermint is a member of the large mint family, which not only includes spearmint (*Menta spicata*), but also sage, hyssop, thyme, lavender, marjoram, pennyroyal, savory, perilla, and catnip. Peppermint and spearmint are hardy plants found throughout many parts of the world, offering leaves with a clean, uplifting taste that has become a staple in many cuisines—for example, as mint sauce in Britain and as an ingredient in Touareg tea, a popular beverage in North African and Arabian countries. The Romans used mint as a healing herb. Scientific studies have suggested that peppermint relaxes some of the involuntary muscles in the digestive tract, helping with some types of indigestion, gas, and bloating (although if you have acid reflux, this herb might not be right for you). The Chinese like peppermint in the summer for its cooling effects, and also use it in traditional medicine as a pungent and cooling herb to treat an external attack of Wind-Heat (the common cold presenting with symptoms of fever, headache, sore throat, and cough), to soothe rashes, and to address some types of stomach distress.

Perilla Leaf

OTHER NAMES: *Perillae frutescentis Folium*, beefsteak leaf, *zi su ye* 紫苏叶 in Chinese, *shiso*—more specifically, *akajisō* for purple perilla, or *aojiso*, *aoba*, or *ōba* for green perilla—in Japanese, *bu chu* or *jasoyeop* in Korean

Perilla leaf is a member of the mint family with both purple and green varieties. Its delicious and distinctive taste flavors many Japanese dishes, including *umeboshi*, a popular pickled plum, where it also produces a distinctive reddish color; you may recognize the leaf as a garnish for sushi. Perilla is also used in the cuisines of Vietnam, Korea, India, Indonesia, and the Hunan province of China, and oil from the seeds is sometimes used in cooking. To buy fresh leaves, look in the produce section of an Asian food store. Chinese herb stores can supply perilla leaves in dried form. If you come across perilla in a can, note that it is probably seasoned with soy sauce, hot pepper, and other spices (delicious with rice, but not so good for cooking). In addition to its vitamins and minerals, perilla leaf has anti-inflammatory properties and is believed to help preserve and sterilize other foods. In traditional Chinese medicine, perilla leaf is seen as pungent and warm, entering the Lungs and Spleen, treating some types of common cold (exterior Wind-Cold syndrome) regulating qi, alleviating nausea and vomiting, calming morning sickness, and counteracting seafood poisoning.

Persimmon

OTHER NAMES: *Diospyros kaki*, *shi zi* 柿子 in Chinese, *kaki* in Japanese, *gam* in Korean

The fruit of the persimmon tree is light yellow-orange to dark orange-red. Specimens can be found fresh in the fall in some parts of North America, such as California, and dried in most Asian markets year round. When buying fresh persimmons, be aware of the important distinction between the astringent varieties (such as the Hachiya) and nonastringent varieties (such as the fuyu). The nonastringent fruit can be eaten firm and crunchy, whereas the astringent fruit needs to ripen until the center is soft like jelly (light and cold will also help remove the astringency; one trick is to put the fruit in the freezer overnight before using). The astringent variety can also be dried for a delicious treat, as is traditional in Korea. Persimmons contain tannin and lycopene, substances that have been linked to reducing the risk of cancer. A tea can be made from the leaves of the persimmon tree. Persimmons are a good source of fiber, beta-carotene, and potassium. In traditional Chinese medicine, the persimmon, which is considered sweet and cold, is seen as moistening the Lungs to alleviate dry cough, generating fluids to relieve thirst and dry mouth, and astringing the Intestines to treat diarrhea or hemorrhoids.

Pine Nuts

OTHER NAMES: *Pinus koraiensis*, pine kernel, pignolia, *song zi* 松子 in Chinese, *jat* in Korean

Pine nuts, true to their name, are buttery-tasting seeds harvested from pine trees. These seeds have been eaten by peoples from Europe to Asia to North America from time immemorial, and are used in dishes from Italian pesto to Middle Eastern baklava. In China, pine nuts have been associated with long life. In traditional Chinese medicine, pine nuts, which are considered sweet in flavor and slightly warm in temperature, are used to moisten the Lungs to treat dry cough and act on the Large Intestine to treat constipation. After you buy pine nuts, store them in a cool, dry place such as the refrigerator, preferably in an airtight container. Like other nuts, pine nuts can become rancid once taken out of their shell.

Poria

OTHER NAMES: *Poria*, hoelen, Indian bread, tuckahoe, China root, *fu ling* 茯苓 in Chinese, *bukuryō* in Japanese, *bokryeong* in Korean

Poria is a type of oval, light-colored fungus that grows, both wild and cultivated, on pine tree roots. Poria is sold in Asian markets sliced and dried, sometimes as part of an herbal mixture, or in powdered form. In traditional Chinese medicine, poria, which is considered sweet and bland in taste and neutral in temperature, is used to promote urination and resolve Dampness, strengthen the Spleen, and calm the spirit.

Pumpkin and Winter Squash

OTHER NAMES: *Cucurbita maxima, Cucurbita moschata*, or *Cucurbita pepo, nan gua* 南瓜 in Chinese

Different varieties of pumpkin and winter squash are enjoyed not only in the United States and Canada, but also in Australia, Italy, India, New Zealand, Mexico, Thailand, Japan, and China. Used in dishes from tempura to roasted vegetables, these members of the squash family are a good source of beta-carotene, fiber, B vitamins, vitamin C, vitamin E, iron, and potassium. The term *winter squash*, which is often used interchangeably with the term *pumpkin*, encompasses members of the squash family that have a tough outer rind surrounding a sweet, often orange flesh. In contrast, summer squash, such as yellow squash and zucchini, have a softer, thinner outer layer. Ongoing scientific research suggests that a compound in Asian pumpkins improves insulin levels and lowers blood sugar. This dovetails with the Chinese tradition, in which pumpkin is considered especially good for people with diabetes; pumpkin is described as sweet and neutral to warming, entering the Spleen and Stomach to strengthen the qi.

Rice

OTHER NAMES: thousands of varieties within the genus *Oryza*, *mi* 米 in Chinese, *gohan* in Japanese, *bap* (cooked) or *ssal* (raw) in Korean

The staple food of literally billions of people on the planet, rice has been enjoyed since the dawn of recorded history, with some evidence suggesting cultivation as far back as 4000 BCE. Perhaps not surprisingly given the central role of rice in diet and culture around the world, strong preferences exist for specific varieties and cooking techniques (including adding salt or not), depending on the region. Famous rice dishes include the Italian risotto, Spanish paella, British rice pudding, U.S. Creole and Cajun jambalaya, Central and South American and Caribbean rice and beans, West African *joloff* rice, Middle Eastern rice pilaf, and Indian and Pakistani *biryani*, in addition to Asian rice bowls, rice cakes, porridges, soups, and sweets. Rice is also frequently transformed into other ingredients used in the kitchen, such as flour (used in noodles, dumpling wrappers, and crackers), vinegar, and wine.

Here's some vocabulary to help you navigate the wonderful world of rice when you're shopping:

- BASMATI. This aromatic, long-grain rice is especially popular in India.
- BLACK RICE. This specialty rice, popular in Indonesia and Philippines, has a nutty flavor and deep purple color. Black rice includes "forbidden rice," purported to have been enjoyed by Chinese royalty and shared only at the emperor's discretion.
- BROWN RICE. Brown rice refers to any variety of rice that has been processed so it retains the bran and germ of the grain (unlike white rice), while still removing the inedible hull. Brown rice contains more fiber and natural vitamins than white rice.
- ENRICHED. The term *enriched* refers to white rice that has had some of the vitamins and minerals that were removed during polishing added back in. Depending on the way this supplementation is accomplished, the added vitamins may wash away if you rinse the rice.
- JASMINE. This long-grain variety, which originated in Thailand, offers a fragrant flavor and is a popular specialty rice.
- LONG-GRAIN. Long-grain varieties encompass many strains of rice, including basmati, jasmine, wild pecan, as well as rice sold as "all-purpose." Long-grain rice is the most common type found in Chinese cooking.
- MEDIUM-GRAIN. You guessed it—medium-grain rice grains have a length in between short and long varieties. Medium-grain varieties are preferred for such dishes as paella and risotto.
- PARBOILED. This term refers to a type of processing, first developed several thousand years ago, in which the grain is boiled after harvesting, making the outer husk easier to remove by hand (although sometimes more difficult to process by machine). Some of the nutrients in the bran are absorbed by the grain during parboiling, making this type of rice more nutritious than unfortified white rice, as well as giving it a harder and glassier form.
- RED RICE (*hong mi* 红米). A staple in some parts of the Himalayas, red rice, also known as Bhutanese red rice, is a reddish grain with a strong nutty flavor. Don't confuse

this rice with red rice yeast, however, which is made by the cultivation of a red mold, *Monascus purpureus*, on white rice.

- SHORT-GRAIN. Also known as round-grain or pearl rice, short-grain rice is the type most popular in Japan. Short-grain varieties, including sushi rice, are somewhat sticky (but not all are as sticky as sticky rice, below).
- STICKY RICE (*zhan mi* 粘米 or *nuo min* 糯米). Also known as sweet rice and glutinous rice (although containing no gluten), sticky rice is a short-grain variety that lives up to its name, making it preferred in a number of dishes, including many desserts.
- WILD RICE (*ye sheng mi* 野生米). Wild rice is not technically a rice (although still delicious and nutritious), but the seed of a wild aquatic grass, *Zizania aquatica*, which provided a staple food for some Native American groups.
- WHITE RICE (*bai mi* 白米). This term refers to any variety of rice that has had the bran and germ removed by polishing.

When you are shopping and cooking, you will be often be faced with the question of white versus brown rice. Before machine milling was introduced a few hundred years ago, rice processing was much less efficient, blurring the distinction between the two. Even the whitest rice polished by hand retained some of the vitamins and fiber provided by the bran, the dark layer covering each grain, and germ, the vitamin-rich inner core, while removing the tough and inedible outer husk. Today, however, the efficiencies of mass production enable the total separation of the grain from its bran and germ, posing the dilemma of choosing white or brown rice, or mixing the two.

Brown rice has numerous benefits. Compared with unfortified white rice, brown rice offers much higher levels of essential vitamins and minerals, particularly vitamins B_3 (niacin) and B_1 (thiamine), magnesium, and iron. Brown rice also has a lower glycemic index because of its high fiber content, leading to a steadier and more sustained effect on energy levels. When machine-polished white rice spread across Asia, for the first time people started coming down with a strange condition in which they suffered from dizziness, emotional distress, weakness and pain in the limbs, swelling, and irregular heart rate. It was later identified as beriberi, caused by a lack of vitamin B_1. (The discovery is credited to Dutch physician Christiaan Eijkman, who noticed that chickens fed white rice experienced symptoms similar to this epidemic, while the birds fed brown rice were spared. The work led to the discovery of vitamins and the 1929 Nobel Prize in Physiology or Medicine, shared with Sir Frederick Hopkins.)

Despite the powerful nutritional profile of brown rice, white rice has something to offer in some situations. The feature that probably propelled its widespread adoption across Asia is a long shelf life. Although brown rice can spoil in six months, especially if not sealed in an airtight container or kept in a cool place, white rice will wait almost indefinitely for you. In addition, white rice requires less cooking time. Today, white rice is usually fortified with some of the vitamins and minerals removed by processing, namely vitamins B_1, B_3, and iron (although depending on the method of supplementation, these may wash away with rinsing, as noted above). White and brown rice both provide protein, carbohydrates, and calories. In contrast to brown rice, these nutrients are available without the grains needing to be chewed well, which can be a challenge for the very young, the very old, and the very ill.

In traditional Chinese medicine, rice is thought to supplement the qi, harmonize the Stomach, strengthen the Spleen, and address symptoms of Heat, such as dry mouth, thirst, and insomnia. Brown rice is seen as especially good for the Spleen and Kidneys, while white rice focuses on the Spleen and Stomach.

Rock Sugar

OTHER NAMES: Chinese sugar, yellow or clear lump sugar, rock candy, *bing tang* 冰糖 in Chinese

Rock sugar is clear, hardened cane sugar formed into large crystals. Rock sugar is less sweet than regular sugar since it is composed of about one part water to two parts sugar, without the hint of caramel flavor found in many other types of sugar. You may recognize rock sugar crystallized on a stick, which is sometimes sold as a candy. In Asia, rock sugar is used to flavor teas, dessert soups, marinades, and sauces, and can be purchased in bags from Asian food stores. A smaller amount of granulated sugar or other natural sweetener can be substituted if necessary, although in terms of traditional Chinese medicine, granulated white sugar is to be used only with caution because it may injure the Spleen and Stomach. From the perspective of Chinese medicine, rock sugar enters the Lung, Spleen, and Stomach channels, where it moistens the Lungs, strengthens the qi of the Middle Burner, and generates body fluids.

Schisandra Berries

OTHER NAMES: *Schisandrae chinensis Fructus* (sometimes *Schisandrae sphenantherae Fructus*), magnolia vine fruit, *wu wei zi* 五味子 (literally, "five-flavored seed") in Chinese, *gomishi* in Japanese, *omija* in Korean

Schisandra berries are the berries of a climbing plant native to East Asia that also now grows in the eastern United States. The pinkish berries, which become ripe in the fall, are thought to possess all five of the flavors recognized in traditional Chinese medicine: sweet, salty, bitter, spicy, and especially sour. These berries can be found dried and packaged in most Asian markets. Scientific research has suggested that schisandra berries contain biologically active ingredients that may quicken reflexes, protect against liver damage (as in hepatitis), and regulate other systems in the body. Rumor has it that the berry has been fed to race horses in the United States before events to improve their performance. In East Asia, schisandra is used to treat coughs, night sweats, insomnia, and physical exhaustion; in the language of traditional Chinese medicine, it contains leakage of Lung qi, strengthens the Kidneys, quiets the spirit, and stops sweating.

Seaweed

OTHER NAMES: *hai dai* 海带 or *hai zao* 海藻 in Chinese, *kaiso* in Japanese, *myeok* (kelp) in Korean

Seaweed, probably most familiar to Americans as the delicate wrapper of sushi rolls, offers a complex, salty flavor and contains a wealth of minerals—including iodine, calcium, iron, zinc, copper, selenium, molybdenum, fluoride, and manganese—from its rich ocean environment. In traditional Chinese medicine, seaweed, which is considered salty and cold, is used to soften hard masses (goiter, ovarian cysts, breast lumps, and lymph node swelling) and to drain Dampness. Seaweed is so popular in Japan that many delicious varieties of seaweed are known in the West by hijiki, their Japanese names, such as nori, arame, kombu, and wakame.

Types of seaweed include:

* ARAME. A type of kelp with a mild flavor that blends well with other ingredients. Arame is often added to soups, stews, salads, and stir-fries. If not using arame in a soup, soak these pencil-size strips prior to use.
* DULSE. Commonly used in Northern Ireland, Atlantic Canada (as "sea parsley"), and Iceland, this red-to-purple plant is slightly spicy in taste. Dulse can be added to salads and soups, or dry roasted and crushed to sprinkle on other dishes. This seaweed does not need to be soaked prior to use.
* HIJIKI. A brown sea vegetable growing wild along the coasts of Japan, Korea, and China. Part of the traditional diet of these countries, hijiki (sometimes known as *hiziki*) can be added to brown rice or soups (cook with them for at least 30 minutes), or soak for 20 minutes before adding to salad or stir-fries (it will expand to roughly four times its size, so a little goes a long way).
* KOMBU. A kelp widely used in Japanese cuisine, kombu is sold in sheets or strips, and is used as one of the three main ingredients to make the traditional soup stock *dashi*. The Japanese also cook kombu with beans to make them softer and more digestible. Many recipes call for soaking for 20 min-

utes or more, then cooking for at least 45 minutes. Most Japanese kombu is cultivated and harvested around Hokkaido.

* NORI. Most recognizable in the West as the delicate wrapper on sushi rolls, nori is often sold in thin sheets, and can be eaten raw or straight after being toasted gently over a burner. You will also find nori in rice dishes or stews, and it is available packaged in flakes, sometimes mixed with sesame seeds and other ingredients, which can be sprinkled on soups, salads, stir-fries, and other dishes.
* WAKAME. A type of kelp that can be added to miso soup, tofu salad, or stir-fry dishes. Wakame, which has a slightly sweet flavor, requires only 5 minutes of soaking. Look for pre-cut wakame, or be prepared to cut the long strips into small pieces about ¼ inch long. In Chinese, this variety of seaweed is called *qun dai cai*. In Japan, traditional uses include purifying a mother's blood after childbirth.

In addition, a translucent white seaweed extract called agar-agar (a.k.a. agar, agar agar, *hai zao qiong zhi* 海藻瓊脂 or *dong fen* 凍粉 in Chinese, *kanten* in Japanese, *hancheon* in Korean), is sold in several different forms—in flakes, strands, or powder as well as bars. Agar-agar is used in a number of traditional gelatin-type desserts popular in Japan and other parts of Asia. In terms of traditional Chinese medicine, agar-agar, considered sweet, salty, and cold, moistens Lung Dryness, transforms phlegm and clears Heat in the Lungs, and treats Dry constipation.

Sesame Seeds

OTHER NAMES: *Sesami indici Semen*, *zhi ma* 芝麻 in Chinese, *goma* in Japanese, *kkae* in Korean; look for black sesame seeds under *hei zhi ma* 黑芝麻 in Chinese, *kuro goma* or *kokushima* in Japanese, and *heukjima* in Korean

Sesame seeds, one of the world's first spices, are commonly used throughout Asia and parts of Europe and Africa. The seeds are usually harvested in early autumn, after the fruit has ripened, and dried in the sun. Sesame seeds are ubiquitous in Asian cuisine, especially in Japan and Korea, where they are typically toasted and lightly ground with a special mortar and pestle for a garnish, or used in cooking in the form of sesame paste or sesame oil. Both black and brown sesame seeds are available at Asian markets, herbal shops, and some natural food stores; avoid the white hulled seeds if possible. Like many other seeds and nuts, sesame seeds do age, so when you are shopping, select a batch that looks and smells fresh and sweet.

Both the brown and black varieties of sesame seed provide calcium, protein, phosphorous, iron, and magnesium. Some scientific studies have suggested that sesame seeds may help regulate glucose levels in the body. Other studies indicate that sesame seeds lower cholesterol, inhibiting its production and absorption. In traditional Chinese medicine, sesame seeds, sweet in flavor and neutral in temperature, are considered a longevity herb that is used to nourish the yin for the treatment of yin deficiency with signs of dizziness, blurred vision, and ringing in the ears; to nourish the Blood and extinguish Wind that might cause headache, dizziness, or numbness; and to moisten the Intestines to counteract dry constipation. Black sesame seeds are also thought to darken gray hair caused by Liver, Blood, and Kidney essence deficiencies, whereas brown sesame seeds nourish the Lungs.

Shiitakes

See "mushrooms."

Sichuan Peppercorns

OTHER NAMES: *Zanthoxyli Pericarpium*, Chinese pepper, Japanese pepper, zanthoxylum, wild pepper, Chinese prickly-ash, *hua jiao* (花椒 literally, "flower pepper") or *shan jiao* (山椒 "mountain pepper") in Chinese, *sanshō* in Japanese and Korean

Sichuan peppercorns are used to give a spicy flavor to dishes in many parts of Asia, including China, Japan, Tibet, and Nepal. Harvested from a different species of plant than black peppercorns or chili peppers, the hull (fruit) is used for cooking, but the seed is discarded. Sichuan peppercorns are used to season roasted meats and poultry, and they contribute their distinctive flavor to Chinese five-spice powder and the Japanese seven-spice mixture *shichimi*. Sichuan peppercorns are sold in packages at Asian markets, and are often used to make Sichuan pepper-flavored oil. They are easy to crush into a powder. In traditional Chinese medicine, pungent, hot Sichuan pepper is thought to warm the Spleen and Stomach, relieving pain and diarrhea from too much Cold and combating intestinal parasites.

Soba Noodles

OTHER NAMES: *soba* in Japanese, *qiao mai* 蕎麦 in Chinese, *meomil guksu* in Korean

A common offering in Japanese cuisine, where noodles are popular, soba noodles are made in part or in whole from buckwheat. They are served cold in the summer, warm in the winter, and are a traditional evening meal on New Year's Eve, when they are called *toshikoshi soba* ("year-bringing soba"), symbolizing longevity. Buckwheat (which is actually a seed rather than a grain) contains a significant amount of protein, as well as iron, phosphorus, copper, magnesium, thiamine, and riboflavin. Buckwheat also contains compounds that have been linked to lowering cholesterol levels, reducing high blood pressure, and controlling blood sugar. In traditional Chinese medicine, buckwheat is considered sweet and cool, supplementing the Spleen, dispelling Dampness, and treating food stagnation.

Sour Date Seeds

OTHER NAMES: *Ziziphi spinosae Semen*, sour jujube seeds, spine date seeds, zizyphus, zizyphus seeds, *suan zao ren* 酸枣仁 in Chinese, *sansō nin* in Japanese, *sanjoin* in Korean

Sour date seeds are small, reddish-brown seeds from a fruit tree native to China, cultivated for over four thousand years. Sour date seeds are one of the most commonly used herbs in East Asian medicine, availed for their calming properties. In the language of traditional Chinese medicine, sour date seeds, which are sweet and sour in flavor and neutral in temperature, act on the Heart, Liver, Gallbladder, and Spleen channels and are commonly used as a chief herb in classic formulas to treat insomnia. Laboratory research has supported the idea that the seeds possess sedative and antianxiety properties.

Soybeans

OTHER NAMES: *Glycine max*, *huang dou* 黄豆 in Chinese, *daizu* in Japanese, *maeju kong* ("miso bean") in Korean

Soybeans, which come in black or green varieties, are native to East Asia, and became an important crop in other parts of the world about one hundred years ago. Soybeans are made into a variety of products—tofu, soy sauce, soy oil, tempeh, miso, tofu skin (yuba, tofu sheets, or dried bean curd), soy milk, and now a variety of dairy substitutes, including soy cheese, soy ice cream, and soy yogurt. Soybeans, a good source of protein, vitamins K and C, and other nutrients, have generated interest in the West for their potential health benefits, including lowering LDL "bad" cholesterol and reducing hot flashes in menopausal women, although some people caution against excessive consumption. From the perspective of traditional Chinese medicine, black soybeans, considered sweet in flavor and neutral in temperature, strengthen the Spleen, nourish the Kidney yin, resolve Dampness, and treat toxicity; green soybeans (which are yellow when dried) are considered sweet in flavor and neutral in temperature and are used to strengthen the Spleen and resolve Dampness.

Soy Sauce

OTHER NAMES: *jiang you* 酱油 in Chinese, *shōyu* in Japanese, *ganjang* in Korean

Soy sauce, now at least glancingly familiar to most Westerners, is ubiquitous in China, Japan, and Korea as a salty condiment at hand to flavor rice, soups, sushi, sauces, and entrées. Originally used to help preserve food, soy sauce is a fermented product typically made with soybeans, a lightly ground grain (often wheat), water, salt, and a yeast starter. Soy sauce can vary greatly from one type to another, depending on the region it is from and the grade of the product. Some types are subtle and delicious, and have taken years to age to perfection; others contain undesirable ingredients such as hydrolyzed soy protein, caramel coloring,

MSG, or sugar. Look for naturally fermented brands and don't forget to read the list of ingredients. Low-sodium ("lite") and wheat-free (tamari) varieties are available. From the perspective of traditional Chinese medicine, soy sauce is considered sweet, salty, and neutral, strengthening and harmonizing the Spleen-Stomach to aid digestion and treat a loss of appetite.

Star Anise

OTHER NAMES: *Anisi stellati Fructus*, Chinese star anise, *da hui xiang* 大茴香 or *ba jiao hui xiang* in Chinese, *but sun* in Korean

Star anise is cultivated from an evergreen tree native to China. This fragrant spice, which is attractively shaped like an eight-pointed star, is often used in Chinese, Indian, Malay, and Indonesian cuisine. Look for star anise in Asian markets, where it is sold whole (most commonly) or ground. You can grind your own, if necessary, by putting whole pieces in a coffee mill or crushing them between two clean sheets of paper with a hammer. Star anise keeps well in an airtight container stored in a cool, dark place. Interestingly, while star anise is unrelated botanically to anise, it has the same compound, anethole, that lends it its distinctive flavor. If you don't have star anise on hand, anise can be substituted. Don't confuse regular star anise with Japanese star anise (botanically *Illicium anisatum* rather than *Illicium verum*), which is toxic to eat. In addition to its use as a spice, star anise is used for its fragrance in such products as toothpaste, soaps, and cosmetics. It is also the source of the key ingredient, shikimic acid, of the prescription medication Tamiflu (oseltamivir phosphate) for flu treatment and prevention. According to traditional Chinese medicine, star anise, which

is considered pungent, sweet, and warm, disperses Cold, warms the Liver and Kidneys, relieves pain, regulates the qi, and improves appetite.

Star Fruit

OTHER NAMES: *Averrhoa carambola*, carambola, *yang tao* 杨桃 in Chinese (not to be confused with kiwi, whose transliteration is the same)

Star fruit might have caught your eye as you passed it in the specialty section of the supermarket or in a bin in front of an Asian grocery store, due to its one-of-a-kind five-angled form and glossy yellow (sometimes white) color. This juicy fruit, an important crop in Asia, keeps well and does not require peeling or seeding. Available in both sweet and sour varieties, the fruit is served on fish and other seafood, is used as a garnish on salads, or can be eaten by itself after simply rinsing and slicing. Look for a bright, firm, fragrant fruit with juicy-looking ribs. Star fruit offers alpha- and beta-carotene, vitamin C, potassium, and fiber. In traditional Chinese medicine, star fruit, considered sweet and sour in flavor and cool in temperature, is thought to soothe dry or sore throats, generate body fluids, promote urination, quench thirst, relieve coughs and hiccoughs, and reduce internal Heat; for these purposes, the star fruit can be juiced, or boiled with water and honey.

Tangerine Peel

OTHER NAMES: *Citri reticulatae Pericarpium*, *chen pi* 陈皮 in Chinese, *chinpi* in Japanese, *jinpi* in Korean

Tangerine peel gives a citrus flavor to any dish. In Western cuisine, orange or tangerine peel, known as zest, is usually used fresh and grated as a tangy ingredient. For Chinese cuisine, tangerine peel can be bought in small packages of dried strips at Asian food stores (but fresh, grated tangerine or orange peel can be substituted). Look especially for thin, shiny, red, and aged pieces. You can also dry your own under the sun or in the oven after scraping off the white pith, then store the dried peel in an airtight container until you need it. In traditional Chinese medicine, tangerine peel is considered a pungent, bitter, and warm herb that can regulate qi in the Lungs and Spleen-Stomach, helping to clear phlegm from the Lungs and treat digestive problems.

Tea

OTHER NAMES: *Camelliae sinensis Folium, cha* 茶 in Chinese, Japanese, and Korean

Known as the "liquid of health," in East Asia tea is not only a beverage, but part of the fabric of everyday life among the rich and the poor. True tea (as opposed to herbal infusions technically called tisanes, brewed from other plants such as mint and ginger) comes from a single plant, *Camellia sinensis*. This plant, a hardy evergreen related to the rose that can live more than one hundred years, grows in well-drained soil of tropical to subtropical climates in China, Japan, India, Sri Lanka, Korea, and some parts of Africa. In some regions tea is harvested year-round, whereas in others the harvesting season is more limited and plants are allowed to rest in the winter months. Leaves harvested in the spring tend to be the highest quality.

Although there are thousands of varieties of teas, most fall into a few distinct categories largely depending on how the leaves are processed:

- **GREEN TEA** (*lu cha* 绿茶). Once tea leaves are picked, they quickly begin to oxidize and turn a darker shade. For green tea, oxidation is halted soon after the leaves are picked by applying heat, either by steaming (typical for Japanese teas) or dry cooking in pans or baskets (typical for Chinese teas).
- **BLACK TEA** (*hong cha* 红茶). For black tea, the type popular in Great Britain, tea leaves are allowed to oxidize completely while drying. This tea type is commonly referred to as "red tea" in Asia.
- **OOLONG TEA** (*wu long cha* 乌龙茶). Oolong tea falls somewhere in between the processing of green and black tea, as the leaves are allowed to oxidize, but only up to a point.
- **WHITE TEA** (*bai cha* 白茶). White tea, a rarer tea type that offers a lighter flavor than the other varieties, is similar to green tea in its minimal processing, but consists of early spring buds, which are still covered by fine white hair, and young leaves before they open fully.
- **PU-ERH TEA** (*puer cha* 普洱茶). Pu-erh tea, which is sometimes classified as a green or black tea depending on its preparation method, is traditionally made from leaves from old, wild tea trees, especially the "broad leaf" variety. Unlike other teas, which are best consumed fresh, pu-erh tea can be consumed fresh or aged like a fine wine.

All of these types of tea contain thousands of chemical compounds, including flavonoids (such as epigallocatechin gallate or EGCG), fluoride, vitamins (such as A, B_2, and C), and minerals (calcium, potassium, sodium, zinc, copper, iron, and manganese). The National Institutes of Health (NIH) National Center for Complementary and Alternative Medicine lists green tea as one of its herbs of interest, supporting studies to learn more about the components in green tea and their effects on conditions such as cancer, diabetes, and heart disease. To date, some laboratory studies have suggested that green tea may help protect against or slow the growth of certain cancers. Additional studies have suggested green tea improves mental alertness, possibly because it contains caffeine. Tea has also been associated with aiding weight loss, lowering blood cholesterol levels, inhibiting the absorption of fatty foods, and protecting the skin from sun damage, although the NIH finds current data on these uses inconclusive. Chinese medical practitioners believe green tea, classified as bitter, sweet, and cool, helps harmonize the Stomach, direct rebellious Stomach qi downward, promote urination, and assist in clear thinking.

Thyme

OTHER NAMES: members of the genus *Thymus*, *bai li xiang* 百里香 ("one hundred mile fragrance") or *po xiao de tian tang* ("heaven's sun rise") in Chinese

You may associate thyme, a member of the mint family, with European or Middle Eastern cooking, but this herb is also found in China. In addition to its use in cooking there, this plant with small, fragrant leaves is made into incense and tinctures. Easily found in its dried form in the herb section of most Western supermarkets, thyme also has a reputation for being simple to grow, its leaves at their sweetest just after the small bluish-purple flowers appear. One fresh sprig equals about ½ teaspoon of dried thyme; crush fresh leaves in your

hands before adding to a dish to bring out the flavor. Don't overcook the fresh or dried herb, so that the sweet scent stays intact.

Thyme—which contains volatile oil components and is high in vitamin K, iron, and manganese—has a long medicinal tradition in Europe, where the herb has been used as an antiseptic in topical applications and mouthwashes, and as a preservative, antispasmodic, digestive aid, and cough remedy. It is still used today as an ingredient in commercial mouthwashes and other preparations. In the Chinese herbal tradition, thyme plays a less prominent role, but is considered pungent and warming, entering the Lung and Stomach channels to release exterior Wind-Cold (a type of common cold), stop cough, and treat nausea, vomiting, and indigestion.

Tofu

OTHER NAMES: bean curd, *dou fu* 豆腐 in Mandarin, *tofu* in Japanese, or *dubu* in Korean

Tofu, a word of Japanese origin, has been a common ingredient in Chinese cuisine for some two thousand years. Its invention is often attributed to Chinese ruler Liu An of Huai Nan during the second century BCE. Tofu is made by curdling fresh hot soy milk then pressing the curds into blocks, similar to the technique used for making cheese. In fact, in China most families make their own, starting with grinding their own beans, then adding gypsum to curdle the mixture. Some of the best tofu dishes can be found in temple restaurants, as Buddhist monks, who are vegetarians, have developed a wide variety of tofu preparations. When you use tofu, don't forget that it is perishable—check the expiration date, refrigerate after opening, and change the water in the container daily. From the perspective of East Asian medicine, tofu is sweet and cool, supplementing the Spleen qi, generating fluids, clearing Heat, and moistening Dryness.

Triticum

OTHER NAMES: *Tritici Fructus levis*, light wheat grain, *fu xiao mai* 浮小麦 in Chinese, *fushōbaku* in Japanese, *pusmaek* in Korean

Triticum is a kind of wheat common throughout China. Used in its whole grain form, the wheat is harvested in the late summer to autumn just before it becomes fully ripe. Look for glossy, evenly sized grains. They should float to the top when added to water. In traditional Chinese medicine, triticum, considered sweet, slightly salty, and cool, stops excessive sweating due to qi or yin deficiency, nourishes the Heart, and calms the spirit.

Turmeric

OTHER NAMES: *Curcumae longae Rhizoma*, mango ginger, Indian ginger, *jiang huang* 姜黄 in Chinese (literally, "yellow ginger"), *kyōō* in Japanese, *kanghwang* in Korean

Turmeric, a member of the ginger family native to tropical South Asia, is used widely as a spice and colorant; this plant lends most curries and curry powders their distinctive taste and yellowish hue. Turmeric is prepared as a spice from the plants' rhizomes, which are harvested, boiled for several hours, dried, then ground into a powder. In some parts of Asia turmeric rhizomes are used fresh, similar to ginger; in Okinawa, Japan, for example, they are boiled to make tea.

Interest in the health-promoting properties of turmeric has recently exploded in the West, as some scientific studies have suggested the active ingredient of turmeric, curcumin, may counteract such conditions as inflammation, cancer, pain, Alzheimer's disease, and diabetes. The healing properties of turmeric have long been exploited in traditional Ayurvedic medicine. In traditional Chinese medicine, turmeric is considered pungent, bitter, and warm and is used to invigorate the Blood, aid digestion, relieve pain, and reduce swelling.

Umeboshi Plum

OTHER NAMES: *suan mei zi* 酸梅子 (literally, "sour mei fruits") in Chinese, *maesil* in Korean

Umeboshi is a pickled fruit of the *ume* tree (*Prunus mume*), which is native to China and later spread to Korea and Japan. Although often translated as "plum," the species is more closely related to apricot. *Umeboshi*, made from green, immature *ume* fruit pickled with red perilla leaf, is a traditional food of Japan that can be served as a mouth-puckering and head-clearing accompaniment to rice (often eaten for breakfast), in salad dressings or other sauces, or as *ume-su* (*ume* vinegar). It is also available as a paste. The Japanese believe *umeboshi* helps prevent and treat a variety of illnesses, including digestive problems, infections, hangovers, and colds. As a home remedy, sometimes it is consumed as a single-ingredient tea. In addition to the pickled *ume*, Chinese foods and beverages made with the *ume* fruit include plum juice, plum sauce, and plum wine. Interestingly, the Chinese pharmacopoeia features smoked, dried *ume* fruit (*wu mei* 乌梅), considered sour, astringent, and warm, to treat a chronic cough, counteract diarrhea or dysentery, generate fluids, expel parasites, and stop intestinal or uterine bleeding.

Vinegar

OTHER NAMES: *cu* 醋 in Chinese, *su* (*komezu* or *yonezu* is rice vinegar) in Japanese, *shikcho* in Korean

Vinegars, which have been made for thousands of years in China and other parts of the world using a natural fermentation process, come in many wonderful varieties. Here we recommend rice vinegar, as it is an easy-to-find staple of traditional East Asian cuisine. However, other vinegars can easily be substituted. In China, choices include black vinegar, a smoky, aged variety that can be made from rice, wheat, millet or sorghum; red vinegar, made from red rice, barley, and sorghum, and popular for dipping sauces; as well as vinegars made using fruit. The Western, grape- or apple-cider-based varieties are fine as well.

Vinegar has been linked to health benefits in many traditions, including those of ancient Greece. In China, vinegar is commonly believed to prevent the spread of infectious diseases; when the flu or another epidemic is going around, people will boil vinegar in the house with the windows closed in an effort to kill viruses. Vinegar is also considered helpful in treating cardiovascular disease and preventing seafood poisoning. In the vocabulary of traditional Chinese medicine, vinegar, which is considered sour and warm to neutral, enters the Stomach and Liver to invigorate the Blood, stop bleeding, and improve digestion.

Wakame

See "seaweed."

Walnuts

OTHER NAMES: *Juglandis Semen*, *he tao ren* 核桃仁 in Chinese

You might associate walnuts with the bowl of nuts that appears around the holidays, but walnuts have a host of health benefits year round, according to both the Eastern and Western perspectives. Walnuts are an excellent source of omega-3 fatty acids and are now being studied in the West for their potential for reducing the damage of unhealthy fats and for counteracting Alzheimer's disease. The nuts are best stored in an airtight container in the fridge. The Chinese, who eat walnuts whole or as a tasty ingredient in stir-fries, stuffing, and other dishes, call walnuts "longevity fruit" (*chang cheng guo* 长生果), both because walnut trees live hundreds of years and because walnuts impart health to those who eat them. According to traditional East Asian medicine, these sweet, warm nuts enter the Lungs and Kidneys to ease coughing and wheezing, counteract fatigue, increase sexual potency in men, and treat frequent urination; they also moisten the Intestines to relieve constipation. To preserve freshness, keep walnuts dry and cool.

Wasabi

OTHER NAMES: *Wasabia japonica*, Japanese horseradish, wasabi root, *jie mo* 芥末 ("mountain sunflower") in Chinese, *gyoja* in Korean

If you are a connoisseur of sushi, you have no doubt encountered wasabi—the innocent-looking green relative of mustard and cabbage that can travel to your sinuses and make your eyes water in an instant if you happen to take too big a bite, but which can add a pleasing zing to your meal if you don't overdo it. Wasabi is a rhizome that is sold fresh in Japan, where it is grated finely before use, or as a paste or powder, forms that are easier to locate in the West, where they have made their way into many regular grocery stores and health food stores. Scientific studies have suggested that wasabi could possess anticancer, antibiotic, anticoagulant, anti-inflammatory, and bone-building properties. From the perspective of traditional Chinese medicine, wasabi, which is pungent and hot, clears phlegm in the Lungs and Stomach, promoting appetite and easing pain such as from arthritis.

Watermelon

OTHER NAMES: *Citrulli Fructus*, *Citrullus lanatus*, *xi gua* 西瓜 in Chinese

Watermelon, which originated in Africa and is now a popular fruit in North America, has been in Asia for a millennium. Rich in vitamin C and beta-carotene, it is composed of mostly water by weight but also contains the phytochemicals lycopene and citrulline. Lycopene, also found in tomatoes and mangoes, has been linked to a reduction in the risk of cancer, cardiovascular disease, and macular degeneration. Citrulline has been associated with increased flexibility of the arteries. Watermelon plays an official part in traditional Chinese medicine, where it is known as the single-herb version of the famous herbal formula White Tiger Decoction (*bai hu tang* 白虎汤). Considered sweet and cold, watermelon is used to clear Summer Heat, relieve thirst, and promote urination.

White Peony Root

OTHER NAMES: *Paeoniae Radix alba*, *bai shao* 白芍 in Chinese, *byakushaku* in Japanese, *baekjak* in Korean

The root of the peony plant, which comes from the same botanical family as the buttercup (*Ranunculaceae*), is one of the oldest remedies in Chinese medicine, mentioned in the ancient text *Collection of Commentaries on the Materia Medica*. In traditional East Asian medicine, the peony root, which is harvested in the summer or autumn from a three- to four-year-old plant and then dried, is highly prized to nourish the Blood and alleviate cramping or spasms anywhere in the body. The best quality root is thick, firm, and straight, without cracks. For women, the herb is traditionally used to help regulate the hormonal cycle, relieving menstrual cramps, addressing complaints of menopause, and enhancing beauty. According to a Chinese proverb, a woman who consumes peony root regularly becomes as beautiful as the peony flower. For men, peony root is reputed to have anti-aging effects. In the language of traditional Chinese medicine, the bitter, sour, and mildly cold herb is thought to nourish the Blood and preserve yin, nourish the Liver to calm Liver yang and Liver Wind, and alleviate pain and spasms.

White Wood Ear

OTHER NAMES: *Tremella fuciformis*, white fungus, silver fungus, white tree ear, white jelly fungus, tremella, *bai mu er* 白木耳 or *yin er* 银耳 in Chinese, *hakumokuji* or *shiro kikurage* in Japanese, *baekmoki* in Korean

White wood ear is closely related to black wood ear, and is similarly a mushroomlike fungus whose neutral taste absorbs the flavor of a dish, and whose texture offers a pleasant crunch. White wood ear is slightly less common than the black variety, but you should be able to find it dried in Asian grocery stores or Chinese herb shops. Soak the wood ear in warm water for 15 to 30 minutes before cooking. White wood ear is often used for warm or cold sweetened dessert soups, which are made by simmering the wood ear with rock sugar.

In China, white wood ear is prized as a food to extend life. In traditional Chinese medicine, white wood ear, considered sweet and bland in flavor and neutral in temperature, is seen as nourishing the Stomach yin and generating body fluids, nourishing the Lung yin and moistening dryness to improve dry coughs, and moistening and beautifying the skin by keeping tissues supple.

Winter Melon

OTHER NAMES: *Benincasa hispida*, wax gourd, white gourd, *dong gua* 冬瓜 in Chinese, *tōgan* in Japanese, *donggwa* in Korean

Winter melon is a fast-growing vegetable with greenish-gray and white skin, cultivated in the warm climates of East and South Asia. Used by the Chinese for thousands of years, the melon—actually a kind of large squash tasting somewhat like a zucchini—was mentioned in the *Divine Farmer's Materia Medica*, compiled about two thousand years ago. The plant produces fruit on vines (similar to pumpkins), which can stay fresh for months when stored in a cool place. Winter melon is available fresh—in slices or whole—or canned. According to Shiu-ying Hu's *Food Plants of China*, winter melon contains protein, polysaccharides, fiber, sulfur, phosphorous, iron, carotene, thiamine, riboflavin, nicotinic acid, and vitamin C. In traditional Chinese medicine, winter melon, considered sweet and cooling, goes to the Lung, Stomach, and Bladder channels to clear Heat, transform phlegm, quench thirst, and promote urination.

Wood Ear

See "black wood ear" and "white wood ear."

RECIPES

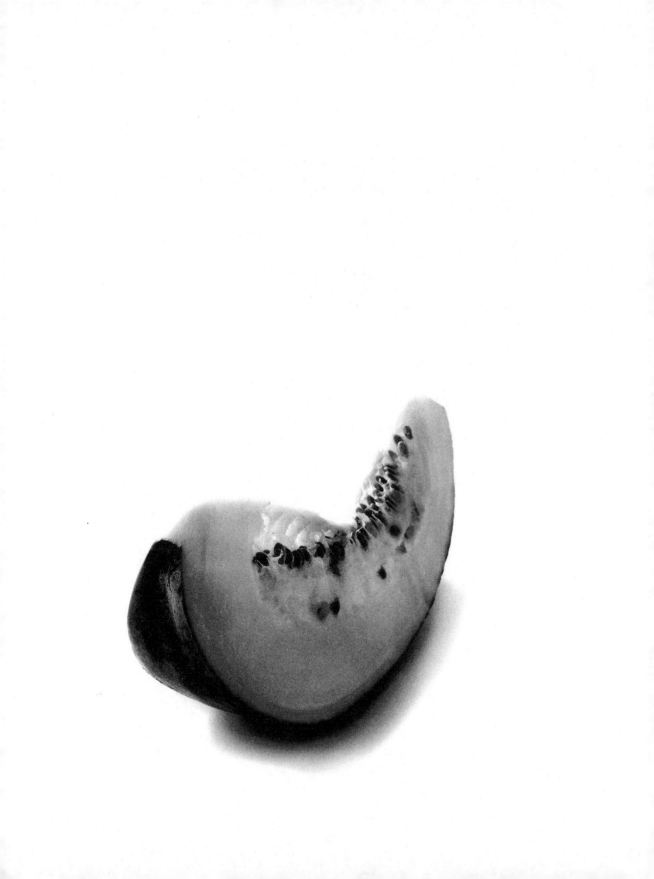

SUMPTUOUS SOUPS

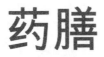

Food is medicine.

—EAST ASIAN PROVERB

VITALITY FISH SOUP

MAKES 3 TO 4 SERVINGS

This nourishing and energizing fish soup can be served alongside rice, vegetables, and/or side dishes. The fresher the fish, the better. If you prefer a light-colored broth to go with the white fish, season with salt instead of soy sauce.

INGREDIENTS

1 (1- to 2-inch) piece fresh ginger, slivered into $\frac{1}{16}$-inch slices

2 cloves garlic, minced

¼ cup (30 grams) goji berries (*gou qi zi*)

2 tablespoons rice wine or white wine

5 cups water

1 pound white fish, for example flounder, sole, or roughy, boned and cut into 1- to 2-inch chunks

½ pound bok choy, chopped into ½-inch pieces

2 green onions, ends trimmed, white part cut into ¼-inch rounds, green part cut into ½-inch pieces

2 teaspoons soy sauce or ½ teaspoon salt, or to taste

1 teaspoon dark sesame oil

Condiments: Rice vinegar, minced garlic, and/or chili oil

DIRECTIONS

1. Combine the ginger, garlic, goji berries, wine, and water in a large pot. Bring to a boil, then lower the heat and simmer, covered with the lid slightly ajar, for 15 minutes.

2. Add the fish, bok choy, and white part of the green onions to the soup, stir, and simmer for another 10 minutes.

3. Add the soy sauce, dark sesame oil, and green slices of the green onions. You can remove the ginger slices if you prefer or simply be prepared to eat around them.

4. Serve immediately, with condiments if desired.

A Comment on Condiments

Many traditional Chinese dishes, including many soups, are served with condiments, commonly soy sauce, minced ginger, vinegar, and various types of chili oil. Whereas some people prefer to savor the dish without these distractions, many take advantage of the extra flavors these toppings provide. The beauty of serving condiments on the side is that all the diners can have their meal just how they like it.

THEMES AND VARIATIONS

Sea bass or other kinds of fish can be substituted for the white fish. Chinese cabbage or spinach can be substituted for the bok choy (cook Chinese cabbage like bok choy, but since spinach cooks quickly, add it right before serving).

ESPECIALLY GOOD FOR

Anyone who wants to increase vitality, including older people, those recovering from an illness, and people who want to replenish their reproductive system (including women going through menopause).

FOR THOSE FAMILIAR WITH
TRADITIONAL CHINESE MEDICINE

This dish strengthens the Kidneys to counteract fatigue and insomnia, supplements the Lungs to help with weakness, shortness of breath, dry cough, and dry skin, and nourishes the Liver to help with dry eyes and poor vision.

Legend Has It

A stranger was walking in the mountains one day and came across a pretty young woman walking with a feeble old man.

"Why are you with this old man?" the stranger asked.

"Oh, him?" the woman replied. "This is my grandson. We look like this because I eat goji berries and he does not."

BUDDHIST TOFU SOUP

MAKES 4 TO 6 SERVINGS

This is a popular and easy dish that you may find on the menu in Chinese restaurants. Although the recipe calls for shiitakes, feel free to use whatever kind of mushroom you prefer. Use the freshest tofu you can find.

INGREDIENTS

8 to 10 (1 cup, or 1½ ounces) dried shiitake or other mushrooms

1 to 2 cups water

1 (12- to 14-ounce) package firm tofu, cut into ½-inch cubes

1 cup fresh bamboo shoot, cut into ½-inch cubes

4 cloves garlic, peeled and minced

1 (1-inch) piece fresh ginger, peeled and minced

6 cups vegetable broth (For recipes, see "Mixed and Sundry.")

1 cup chopped (½-inch slices) Chinese cabbage or bok choy

1 tablespoon dark sesame oil

1 tablespoon soy sauce, or to taste

2 tablespoons oyster sauce (optional) (Note: Mushroom-based vegetarian "oyster" sauces are available at Asian groceries.)

THEMES AND VARIATIONS

You can use fresh shiitakes instead of dried, substituting an additional cup of vegetable stock for the mushroom water. Asparagus can also be substituted for the bamboo shoot.

DIRECTIONS

1. Soak the shiitakes in the warm water for about 20 minutes. Reserve the water for later use. Remove and discard the mushroom stems, if desired. Chop the mushrooms into 1-inch pieces.
2. Combine the mushrooms, reserved mushroom water, tofu, bamboo shoot, garlic, ginger, and broth in a saucepan, bring to a boil, then lower the heat and simmer for about 10 minutes.
3. Add the Chinese cabbage to the soup. Cook for another 5 minutes.
4. Add the sesame oil, soy sauce, and oyster sauce (if using), then serve.

ESPECIALLY GOOD FOR

Anyone concerned about hypertension, high blood sugar, high cholesterol, weight control, or cancer prevention.

FOR THOSE FAMILIAR WITH
TRADITIONAL CHINESE MEDICINE

This dish strengthens the Spleen qi, harmonizes the Middle Burner, and drains Dampness.

Legend Has It

In Asia, bamboo is a symbol of longevity (it always has green shoots) and of strength and grace (its flexibility allows it to bend rather than break). One folktale tells of a sick woman who craved a healing soup made with bamboo shoots. Unfortunately, it was winter and her son could not find any. He was so sorry that he cried until his tears warmed the ground and bamboo shoots sprouted up, and he took the bamboo shoots home, to his mother's contentment.

BASIC MISO SOUP

MAKES 3 TO 4 SERVINGS

Miso soup—a staple in the Japanese diet—is based on miso paste, a healthy fermented paste made from soy. Because miso contains probiotics, the miso paste is traditionally added at the end of the preparation process and not boiled. Miso soup is often served for breakfast with rice, fish, and pickles, although this soup can also be found accompanying other meals. The Japanese view miso as a health food and use it as a home remedy for digestive problems, cancer, low libido, and tobacco poisoning. If you need to rewarm the soup later, try to avoid boiling it, as boiling will destroy the healthy microorganisms in the miso.

INGREDIENTS

1 tablespoon dried precut wakame seaweed

2½ cups *dashi* soup stock or water (For quick and easy *dashi* recipes, see "Mixed and Sundry.")

½ block (about 7 ounces) soft or firm tofu, cut into ½-inch cubes

3 to 4 tablespoons white miso paste, or 1½ to 2 tablespoons red miso paste, or to taste

1 medium-size green onion, chopped into ¼-inch pieces, roots and tough tips discarded

DIRECTIONS

1. Soak the wakame in water for 2 to 3 minutes. It will expand a lot, so don't be misled by its compact size in its dried form.
2. Place the *dashi* soup stock in a pot and bring to a boil.
3. Add the wakame and tofu to the pot, then simmer over low heat, covered with the lid slightly ajar, for about 5 minutes. Turn off the heat.
4. Remove 4 tablespoons of the stock from the pot and, in a bowl, mix it with the miso paste, making sure that all the lumps are stirred out. Gradually pour the miso mixture back into the pot and stir.
5. Garnish with the green onion.

THEMES AND VARIATIONS

Endless, including bean sprouts, burdock root, daikon, carrots, seafood, eggs . . . Don't feel limited by the variations we've included here!

ESPECIALLY GOOD FOR

Anyone who has a cold, is feeling under the weather, has an upset stomach, is recovering from illness, or is concerned about preventing cancer.

FOR THOSE FAMILIAR WITH
TRADITIONAL CHINESE MEDICINE

This dish harmonizes the *ying qi* and *wei qi*, releases the Exterior, and warms the Middle Burner.

PLEASING PUMPKIN-MISO SOUP

MAKES 2 SERVINGS

This creamy (without the cream) vegetable blend will leave your taste buds with pleasant memories.

INGREDIENTS

10 to 12 ounces pumpkin or winter squash, such as Japanese kabocha (about 2 cups when cubed)

1 (4-inch-square) piece kombu seaweed

1 (6-inch) piece of the white stem of a leek, sliced into ½-inch pieces

3 cups water

1 (1- to 2-inch) square (1 to 2 ounces) soft or firm tofu, cut into ½-inch cubes

2 tablespoons sweet white miso (*saikyo*)

A pinch of ground cinnamon

A pinch of ground nutmeg

THEMES AND VARIATIONS

If you are in the mood for a more savory version of this soup, omit the cinnamon and nutmeg, and garnish with chopped green onions.

DIRECTIONS

1. Seed, peel, and chop the pumpkin into 1-inch cubes. (An efficient way to chop a pumpkin is to cut it into wedges, cut off the skin if desired, then cut the wedges into cubes. A large, sharp cleaver can be a useful tool here since the raw vegetable can be tough. Another handy trick is to put the pumpkin in the microwave for 5 minutes to soften it before cutting and peeling.) The seeds can be reserved for roasting.

2. Combine the pumpkin, kombu, leek, and water in a pot. Bring to a boil, then lower the heat to low and simmer for about 20 minutes.

3. Add the tofu to the pot, and then simmer for another 5 to 10 minutes.

4. Remove the kombu. Using a hand blender, whir the soup until smooth. If you don't have a hand blender, pour the remaining contents of the pot into a blender or food processor and whir until it becomes a smooth puree.

5. Transfer the soup to a large bowl, and stir in the miso. (It can be helpful to put the miso in a small bowl first, adding the a few tablespoons of the puree and mashing them together to get out the lumps before adding the mixture into the larger bowl and stirring well.)

6. Add the cinnamon and nutmeg in about equal amounts, to taste, before serving.

ESPECIALLY GOOD FOR

Anyone who is concerned about diabetes, poor digestion, cold hands and feet, goiter, joint swelling, or weight control.

FOR THOSE FAMILIAR WITH
TRADITIONAL CHINESE MEDICINE

This dish is good for those with Spleen deficiency, or for people who need to reduce phlegm nodules, promote urination, or reduce edema.

GINGERY PUMPKIN SOUP

MAKES 2 SERVINGS

Here is a steaming soup, with the benefits of pumpkin and spices, for your fall table. Ongoing scientific research suggests that a chemical compound in Asian pumpkins improves insulin levels and lowers blood sugar. This dovetails with the Chinese tradition, in which pumpkin is also considered especially beneficial for people with the symptoms of diabetes.

INGREDIENTS

10 to 12 ounces pumpkin or winter squash (about 2 cups when cubed)

6 whole cloves

2½ cups vegetable or chicken stock (For recipes, see "Mixed and Sundry.")

2 tablespoons vegetable oil, such as canola or olive oil

1 small onion, diced

2 to 3 cloves garlic, peeled and minced

1 (1- to 2-inch) piece fresh ginger, peeled and minced

½ cup unflavored soy milk

A pinch of salt

A pinch of pepper

¼ cup fresh cilantro leaves, stems removed and discarded

DIRECTIONS

1. Seed, peel, and chop the pumpkin into 1-inch cubes. (An efficient way to chop a pumpkin is to cut it into wedges, cut off the skin if desired, then cut the wedges into cubes. A large, sharp cleaver can be a useful tool here as the raw vegetable can be tough. Another handy trick is to place the pumpkin in a microwave for 5 minutes to soften it before cutting and peeling.)

2. Combine the pumpkin, cloves, and stock in a pot. Bring to a boil, then lower the heat to low and simmer for about 20 minutes.

3. Add the onion, garlic, and ginger. Cook until the onions are translucent and soft (about 5 minutes).

4. When the pumpkin is done, remove the cloves from the broth (they will float on top of the liquid).

5. Combine the pumpkin mixture, the onion mixture, and the soy milk, using a hand blender to whir it into a smooth puree. If you don't have a hand blender, use a blender or food processor, working in batches if necessary. Add salt and pepper to taste.

6. Sprinkle the green cilantro leaves on top of the soup for a flavorful and colorful garnish.

THEMES AND VARIATIONS

You can add different vegetables to this soup, such as yam, celery, or carrot cut into 1-inch pieces; simmer them along with the pumpkin. Other types of milk may be substituted for soy milk, if you prefer. Canned pumpkin can work in a pinch if you don't have fresh pumpkin available.

ESPECIALLY GOOD FOR

Eating in the fall and winter, warming cold hands and feet. Also, pumpkin dishes are particularly helpful for people concerned about diabetes, beautifying the skin, constipation, or the prevention of prostate cancer, atherosclerosis, or gastric ulcers.

FOR THOSE FAMILIAR WITH
TRADITIONAL CHINESE MEDICINE

This dish is good for those with Spleen deficiency or for moistening the Lungs and Large Intestine.

CURRY FAVOR PUMPKIN SOUP

MAKES 2 SERVINGS

This simple soup goes down real smooth, offering the flavors and health benefits of both pumpkin and curry.

INGREDIENTS

10 to 12 ounces pumpkin or winter squash, such as Japanese kabocha (about 2 cups when cubed)

2½ cups chicken or vegetable stock (For stock recipes, see "Mixed and Sundry.")

2 tablespoons vegetable oil, such as canola or olive oil

1 small onion, diced

1 to 2 teaspoons curry powder

A pinch of salt

A pinch of pepper

Yuan Says

Although pumpkin and winter squash are good for diabetics, it's important not to overdo any one food for any health conditions. Remember your recommended foods are to add to—rather than replace—a balanced and varied diet.

DIRECTIONS

1. Chop the pumpkin pieces into 1-inch cubes, seeded and peeled. (Some pumpkins are quite tough, and are most easily handled by chopping the pumpkin into two, seeding it, then cutting it into wedges before peeling. A large, sharp cleaver can be helpful with this task; another handy trick is to put the pumpkin in the microwave for 5 minutes to soften it before cutting and peeling. The seeds can be reserved for roasting.)

2. Place the pumpkin cubes and stock in a pot. Bring to a boil, then lower the heat to low and simmer for about 20 minutes.

3. Heat the oil in a skillet over medium-high heat. Add the onion and curry powder. Cook until the onions are translucent and soft (about 5 minutes).

4. When both the onions and pumpkin are done, combine them in a blender or food processor. Whir into a smooth puree. You can also use a hand blender or immersion blender for this task.

5. Add salt and pepper to taste.

ESPECIALLY GOOD FOR

Anyone with diabetes, arthritis or other inflammatory condition, muscle stiffness and pain, a tendency to run cold, or fibromyalgia.

FOR THOSE FAMILIAR WITH
TRADITIONAL CHINESE MEDICINE

This dish addresses Spleen deficiency, Damp painful obstruction, and blockage of the channels.

DECONGESTING DAIKON SOUP

MAKES 4 SERVINGS

This tangy, full-bodied broth helps clear the Lungs to ease your breathing.

INGREDIENTS

1 small daikon radish, diced into ⅛-inch pieces (about 2 cups diced)

1 (1-inch) piece fresh ginger, peeled and grated or minced

1 tablespoon or 1 large piece (0.15 ounces, or 4 grams) dried tangerine peel (*chen pi*)

4 cups water

Salt

Condiments or garnishes: chopped green onions, chopped cilantro, lemon or lime juice, white pepper, and/or a few drops of sesame oil

DIRECTIONS

1. Combine the daikon, ginger, dried tangerine peel, and water in a pot. Bring to a boil, then lower the heat and simmer, covered, for about 30 minutes. The daikon will become soft.
2. Add salt to taste before serving.
3. Garnish or serve with condiments or garnishes, as desired.

ESPECIALLY GOOD FOR

Anyone suffering from a wet cough (eat a cup of this soup twice a day).

FOR THOSE FAMILIAR WITH TRADITIONAL CHINESE MEDICINE

This dish transforms phlegm in the Lungs and drains Dampness.

Words of Wisdom

When farmers put daikon on the market, doctors are out of business.

—CHINESE SAYING

Helpful Hints about Daikon

Related to the more familiar red radish you commonly see in the supermarket, daikon, which is usually white but sometimes tinged with green, comes in several varieties, the most common of which is 2 to 3 feet long and 2 to 3 inches wide. Others are shorter and squatter and can grow up to 50 pounds. (For more information on daikon, see "One Hundred Healthful Asian Ingredients.")

CLASSIC KOREAN SEAWEED SOUP

MAKES 4 SERVINGS

This Korean seaweed soup, known as myeok guk, *is a classic kitchen therapy dish served to postpartum mothers to help them recover after childbirth and to promote lactation. This soup is also served to those celebrating their birthday to commemorate their mother's pregnancy and labor—as well as to anyone who would enjoy a healthy soup to accompany a meal. This soup is often served with rice on the side; some people like to spoon rice into the soup while eating.*

INGREDIENTS

1 ounce (about ⅓ cup) dried seaweed, such as precut wakame

1 tablespoon sesame oil

2 cloves garlic, peeled and minced

3½ cups anchovy, bone, or vegetable stock (For recipes, see "Mixed and Sundry.")

1½ tablespoons soy sauce, or to taste

2 tablespoons brown sesame seeds (optional)

A pinch of pepper (optional)

DIRECTIONS

1. Soak the seaweed in water for 10 to 20 minutes, or until rehydrated. The seaweed will expand to more than three times its size. Drain and squeeze to remove excess water.

2. In a medium-size pot, heat the oil over medium heat, add the garlic, and cook until fragrant, about 30 seconds.

3. Add the seaweed and sauté for another 2 minutes.

4. Add the stock and soy sauce and raise the heat to high to bring the liquid to a boil.

5. Lower the heat, cover, and simmer for about 20 minutes or until the soup starts to appear milky. Cooking longer is okay, too, if you prefer more blended flavors.

6. If you are using sesame seeds and starting with the raw variety, place them in a dry skillet over medium-high heat and toast for about 5 minutes, until they become fragrant, golden, and begin to pop. Remove them immediately from the pan so they don't burn, and let them cool for at least 1 minute. Using a food processor or mortar and pestle, grind the seeds to release the flavors.

7. Sprinkle with sesame seeds and/or pepper, if desired.

THEMES AND VARIATIONS

Many versions of this recipe call for beef (use ¼ pound, cut into 2-inch strips, which can be browned with the garlic) or oysters (¼ pound, which also can be sautéed with the garlic). For vegetarians, mushrooms are a good substitute. Adding ground perilla seeds (3 tablespoons, when you add the broth) provides another delicious variation.

ESPECIALLY GOOD FOR

From the perspective of Korean culture, this soup is especially good for women who have given birth within the last month, and for anyone recovering from surgery. From the perspective of traditional Chinese medicine, the soup is especially good for anyone concerned with reducing soft masses (such as goiter, ovarian cysts, breast lumps, or lymph node swelling), lowering high blood pressure and high cholesterol, or preventing cancer.

FOR THOSE FAMILIAR WITH TRADITIONAL CHINESE MEDICINE

This dish helps soften hardness, clears Heat, drains Dampness, transforms phlegm, promotes urination, and reduces edema (swelling).

MUSHROOM MEDLEY–MISO SOUP

MAKES 4 TO 6 SERVINGS

A tasty variation of miso soup, with the added health benefits of mushrooms.

INGREDIENTS

3 medium-size (2 to 3 ounces) fresh shiitake mushrooms

2 bunches (2 to 3 ounces) fresh maitake mushrooms

8 medium-size (2 to 3 ounces) fresh oyster or other mushrooms

2 tablespoons dark sesame oil

¼ medium-size onion, diced

½ block (about 7 ounces) soft or firm tofu, cut into ½-inch cubes (optional)

1 medium-size green onion, ends trimmed, chopped into ¼-inch pieces

3½ cups *dashi* soup stock (For quick and easy *dashi* recipes, see "Mixed and Sundry.")

4 tablespoons white miso paste, or to taste

DIRECTIONS

1. Gently wash the mushrooms, and remove and discard any tough stems if desired. Slice the mushrooms into ½-inch pieces.

2. In a pot, heat the sesame oil. Add the onion and sauté over medium heat, stirring frequently, until translucent and golden, about 3 minutes.

3. Add the mushrooms, tofu (if using), and green onion, and sauté for another 2 minutes.

4. Add the soup stock to the pot and bring to a boil, then lower the heat and simmer for 2 minutes. Turn off the heat.

5. Remove 4 tablespoons of the stock from the pot and mix it with the miso paste in a bowl, making sure that all the lumps are stirred out.

6. Gradually pour the miso mixture back into the pot and stir before serving.

THEMES AND VARIATIONS

Mix and match the fresh mushrooms as desired. You can also substitute ½ ounce of each variety of dried mushroom. If you need to re-warm the soup later, try to avoid boiling it, as boiling will kill the healthy microorganisms in the miso.

ESPECIALLY GOOD FOR

People who want to increase their immunity, prevent cancer, or counteract problems such as lack of appetite, fatigue, and nausea.

FOR THOSE FAMILIAR WITH
TRADITIONAL CHINESE MEDICINE

This dish harmonizes digestion and addresses Spleen and Stomach qi deficiency.

WATERCRESS-MISO SOUP

MAKES 3 TO 4 SERVINGS

Miso soup provides a versatile base for whatever ingredients strike your fancy. Here, we suggest healthy and tasty greens, such as watercress.

INGREDIENTS

2 to 3 ounces fresh enoki, maitake, or other variety of mushroom

2½ cups *dashi* soup stock or water (For quick and easy *dashi* recipes, see "Mixed and Sundry.")

½ block (about 7 ounces) soft or firm tofu, cut into ½-inch cubes

3 to 4 tablespoons white miso paste, or 1½ to 2 tablespoons red miso paste, or to taste

½ bunch (¾ cup or 1¾ ounce) watercress

1 medium-size green onion, ends trimmed, chopped into ½-inch pieces

THEMES AND VARIATIONS

Other greens for this soup can include spinach, mizuna, or mustard greens. Dried mushrooms also work well; soak before using. If you need to re-warm the soup later, try to avoid boiling it, as boiling will kill the healthy microorganisms in the miso.

DIRECTIONS

1. Wash the mushrooms and chop off any roots or excess stems if desired.
2. Place the *dashi* soup stock in a pot and bring to a boil. Add the mushrooms and tofu to the pot, then simmer over low heat, covered with the lid slightly ajar, for about 5 minutes. Turn off the heat.
3. Remove 4 tablespoons of the stock from the pot and, in a bowl, mix it with the miso paste, making sure that all the lumps are stirred out.
4. Gradually pour the miso mixture back into the pot and stir.
5. Divide the watercress among the serving bowls. Spoon the soup over the watercress (this will cook the watercress). Garnish with the green onion.

ESPECIALLY GOOD FOR

Anyone who wants to increase immunity, reduce masses, control cholesterol, control weight, or counteract problems such as lack of appetite or fatigue.

FOR THOSE FAMILIAR WITH TRADITIONAL CHINESE MEDICINE

This dish moves the qi and Blood, drains Dampness, and strengthens the Spleen qi.

Helpful Hints about Miso

When shopping for miso, you will probably be faced with an array of choices. One of the most common distinctions is between white (*shiromiso*) and red (*akamiso*). The white miso is milder, often used in dressings; whereas the red variety offers a stronger flavor and is often used in stews. Don't be afraid to experiment to find out which kind of miso you like. But avoid any miso labeled "pasteurized," as it will not offer the same probiotic benefits as more unprocessed types. (For more information on miso, see "One Hundred Healthful Asian Ingredients.")

EASY EGGPLANT SOUP

MAKES 4 SERVINGS

This simple, delicious Japanese soup relies on some healthy staples. In Japan, eggplant (nasu) is a favorite vegetable to cook during the summer months.

INGREDIENTS

2 to 3 tablespoons dark sesame oil

3 small Japanese eggplants (about 12 ounces), ends removed, body cut widthwise into ¼- to ½-inch round slices

3½ cups kombu stock (see Quick Kombu *Dashi*, page 264, or *Dashi* of the Sea, page 265)

2 tablespoons white or red miso (the white variety is milder; the red, more flavorful), or to taste

2 tablespoons brown sesame seeds (unhulled)

DIRECTIONS

1. Heat the oil in a large skillet. Add the eggplant and cook over medium-high heat for about 5 minutes on each side, or until soft all the way through.

2. In a medium-size pot, warm the stock to just before boiling, then turn off the heat.

3. In a small bowl, mix a little stock with the miso and stir until well dissolved. Add the miso mixture into the rest of the stock and stir. Add the eggplant to the soup.

4. If your sesame seeds aren't already roasted, place them in a dry skillet and cook over medium-high heat, until the seeds are golden brown (about 5 minutes), shaking the pan frequently so they don't burn. When they are done, remove them from the skillet so they don't overcook, and let them cool for at least 1 minute.

5. Whir the sesame seeds lightly in a food processor or blender for about 15 seconds (or grind by hand, if you prefer, in a mortar and pestle; the Japanese traditionally use a ridged bowl called a *suribachi* to crush sesame seeds).

6. Transfer the soup to serving bowls, then garnish with the toasted sesame seeds.

> ### Yuan Says
> Eggplant is one of the few vegetables that has a purple color, which in traditional Chinese medicine is associated with moving the Blood.

THEMES AND VARIATIONS

You can use one regular eggplant from the supermarket if it's the only kind that's available, quartering its ¼- to ½-inch-thick slices so they are 2 to 3 inches across and fit into your soup bowls. Larger eggplants tend to be more bitter than the smaller Japanese variety, so soak the pieces in saltwater for 30 minutes or longer before cooking them, to help neutralize the bitterness.

ESPECIALLY GOOD FOR

Anyone who is concerned about high cholesterol or who wants to counteract pain and swelling or chronic musculoskeletal injuries.

FOR THOSE FAMILIAR WITH TRADITIONAL CHINESE MEDICINE

This dish clears Heat, cools and moves the Blood, moistens the Intestines, reduces swelling, and eases pain.

SAVORY SQUASH AND AZUKI BEAN SOUP

MAKES 4 TO 6 SERVINGS

This is a wholesome soup, a variation of which is popular in the macrobiotic kitchen, especially for those concerned about regulating blood sugar levels and reducing the craving for sweets.

INGREDIENTS

1 cup dried azuki beans

½ pound unpeeled kabocha, butternut squash, or other winter squash (about 2 cups, cubed)

1 to 2 teaspoons dark sesame oil

½ medium-size onion, diced

1 (1-inch) piece fresh ginger, peeled and grated

1 (4 by 6-inch) piece kombu seaweed

4 cups water, plus extra for soaking

4 tablespoons white miso paste (optional)

1 to 2 tablespoons soy sauce, or to taste

1 medium-size green onion, chopped into ¼-inch pieces, roots and tough tips discarded

Fast Facts about Azuki Beans

Azuki beans are especially popular in Japan, where they are the second-most-common legume after the soybean (*azuki* translates from the Japanese as "small bean"; soybean (*daizu*) translates as "large bean"). (For more information on azuki beans, see "One Hundred Healthful Asian Ingredients.")

DIRECTIONS

1. Soak the beans at room temperature in double their volume of water for at least 8 hours or overnight. Drain the beans.
2. Seed and chop the winter squash into 1-inch cubes. (If you find your squash is tough, as kabochas often are, an efficient way to chop it is to cut it into wedges, then cut the wedges into cubes. A large, sharp cleaver can be a useful tool. Another handy trick is to put the vegetable in a microwave for 5 minutes to soften it before cutting and peeling.)
3. Heat the sesame oil over medium-high heat in a medium-size saucepan. Add the onion and cook until golden brown, 3 to 5 minutes.
4. Place the beans, onion, ginger, kombu, and water in the pot and bring to a boil.
5. Lower the heat and simmer, covered with the lid slightly ajar, for 30 minutes. Remove the kombu.
6. Add the squash to the pot and simmer for another 45 to 60 minutes.
7. If you will be serving the soup immediately, mix together 1 tablespoon of warm water per tablespoon of miso paste (if using) in a small bowl, then stir the miso mixture into the soup. But hold off on adding the miso to any portions of soup that will be reheated and served later; adding that miso just before serving will preserve the miso's healthy probiotics.
8. Add soy sauce to taste. Sprinkle the green onion on the soup for a garnish.

ESPECIALLY GOOD FOR

Anyone who wants to increase energy levels, address chronic fatigue, reduce puffiness, or counteract diabetes.

FOR THOSE FAMILIAR WITH TRADITIONAL CHINESE MEDICINE

This dish strengthens the Spleen and Kidneys, helps to drain Dampness, and counteracts toxicity.

WHAT-TO-DO-FOR-A-HANGOVER SOUP

MAKES 2 TO 4 SERVINGS

This popular Chinese soup is traditionally served in the summer months (not just for hangovers), offering many layers of flavor despite the simplicity of its ingredients. There is no need to use the expensive, sheeted variety of nori seaweed used for sushi; instead, look for a variety used in soups, such as wakame.

INGREDIENTS

½ cup dried mung beans, rinsed

1 tablespoon (0.15 ounces, or 4 to 5 grams) precut wakame seaweed

4 cups water

2 teaspoons soy sauce or sodium-reduced soy sauce, or to taste

DIRECTIONS

1. Combine the mung beans, seaweed, and water in a medium-size pot of water. Bring to a boil, lower the heat, then simmer, covered, over low heat for 1 hour.
2. Add soy sauce to taste and serve as an appetizer or snack. (If you are trying to counteract fluid retention, go easy on the soy sauce and consider using the sodium-reduced variety.)

THEMES AND VARIATIONS

If you like miso soup, substitute 2 tablespoons of white miso paste or 1 tablespoon of red miso, or to taste, for the soy sauce. Before serving, remove 3 to 4 tablespoons of the stock from the pot and, in a separate bowl, mix it with the miso paste, making sure that all the lumps are stirred out before gradually stirring the miso mixture back into the soup. In Japan, miso not only has a reputation for increasing general health, but it is also used to counteract the effects of too much drinking, soothing the digestion and detoxifying the body.

ESPECIALLY GOOD FOR

Clearing the skin of, for example, acne or a rash; reducing fluid retention; or helping the body recover from a hangover or the buildup of toxins due to drinking, smoking, or taking many prescription drugs.

FOR THOSE FAMILIAR WITH TRADITIONAL CHINESE MEDICINE

This soup is cooling and good for treating Summer Heat, draining Damp Heat, and addressing toxic Heat.

Yuan Says

A patient recently came into my clinic, complaining of skin problems, especially acne. I examined his tongue—a key element of diagnostics in traditional Chinese medicine—and noticed that it had a thick coat on it, "Are you a heavy drinker?" I asked. He admitted he had had several drinks the night before. I prescribed this seaweed and mung bean soup to cleanse his system and relieve toxicity. He liked it and started eating it regularly—so regularly that when he came in to see me, I couldn't tell whether he had been drinking anymore from looking at his tongue; I had to start asking him, "Okay, be honest, have you been drinking lately?"

Words of Wisdom

With the first glass, a person drinks wine. With the second glass, the wine drinks the wine. With the third glass, the wine drinks the person.

—JAPANESE PROVERB

JAPANESE NEW YEAR'S SOUP

MAKES 4 SERVINGS

Here is one version of Japanese New Year's soup (ozōni), with shrimp, whose crooked back can represent old age and longevity. It is certainly tasty enough to have any time of year.

INGREDIENTS

4 medium-size (¾ ounce) dried shiitake mushrooms

1½ cups warm water

4 *mochi* rice cakes

3 cups *dashi* stock (For quick and easy *dashi* recipes, see "Mixed and Sundry.")

1 tablespoon sake

¼ pound shrimp, peeled and deveined

¼ pound spinach leaves, well washed, sliced into 3-inch pieces

2 tablespoons soy sauce, or to taste, or 4 tablespoons sweet white miso, or to taste

Mika Says

My Japanese grandmother liked to make her *ozōni* with chicken, mountain yam, fishcake, spinach, and tofu—and, of course, *mochi.* Family lore has it that on New Year's day you should eat one *mochi* for every year of your age—although this piece of advice is aimed at children, for practical reasons!

DIRECTIONS

1. Preheat the oven to 425°F and lightly oil a cookie sheet.
2. Soak the shiitake mushrooms in about 1½ cups of warm water for 20 minutes. Drain the mushrooms, reserving the water. Slice the mushrooms into ¼-inch slices, discarding the stems if desired.
3. Place the *mochi* on the prepared cookie sheet. Bake until they puff up, about 10 minutes. Check frequently to avoid burning the *mochi.* When they are done, remove them from the oven and set aside.
4. In the meantime, combine in a large saucepan the *dashi* stock, mushrooms, sake, and 1 cup of water from the mushroom soaking. Bring to a boil, then lower the heat to a simmer. Cook, covered, for about 5 minutes.
5. Add the shrimp to the soup pot and cook for 2 to 3 minutes. Stir the spinach leaves into the pot, and cook for about 30 seconds.
6. For a soy sauce–flavored soup, add soy sauce to taste. For a miso-flavored broth, remove 4 tablespoons of the stock from the pot and, in a separate bowl, mix it with the miso paste, making sure that all the lumps are stirred out, then gradually pour the miso mixture back into the pot and stir.
7. Place a piece of *mochi* in each serving bowl, then spoon the soup over the top before serving.

꧁ꕥ꧂

Helpful Hints about Mochi

Mochi, which is steamed rice pounded and formed into circles or rectangles ready for baking, is available at most Japanese and Asian food stores. When baked, *mochi*—associated with good luck and prosperity—transforms into a delightful combination of crispy and chewy textures.

THEMES AND VARIATIONS

There's no one way to make *ozōni*. In Japanese, the *o* is an honorific, the *zō* means "this and that," and the *ni* means "simmered," which leaves a lot of room for interpretation. Potential ingredients for *ozōni* include chicken, fish, fish cake, mountain yam, chestnut, burdock root, daikon, watercress, mizuna greens, mustard greens, Chinese cabbage, carrot, tofu, and scallions. In some variations of this recipe, the ingredients are cooked separately and combined right before serving.

Fresh shiitakes can be used instead of dried. Simply use an additional cup of *dashi* instead of the mushroom water.

ESPECIALLY GOOD FOR

Anyone who wants general nourishment or who is suffering from fatigue or from a long-term illness. Also, cancer patients recovering from chemo or radiation therapy.

FOR THOSE FAMILIAR WITH TRADITIONAL CHINESE MEDICINE

This dish strengthens qi, nourishes the Blood and yin, and generates fluids.

AUGMENTING ASPARAGUS SOUP

MAKES 4 TO 5 SERVINGS

This flavorful soup is popular in China. The dish is often made with ham, but we like it with seafood.

INGREDIENTS

1 heaping tablespoon (10 grams) dried lily bulb (*bai he*)

5 cups chicken or vegetable broth

½ cup rice wine or white wine

½ cup enoki mushrooms

1 heaping tablespoon (10 grams) goji berries (*gou qi zi*)

1 (1-inch) piece fresh ginger, peeled and minced

4 to 5 cloves garlic, peeled and minced

1 small bunch (¾ pound) asparagus, cut into 1-inch pieces, hard bottom ends of stalk discarded

½ pound crabmeat and/or shelled shrimp

¼ teaspoon salt, or to taste (optional)

1 tablespoon soy sauce, or to taste

¼ cup chopped fresh cilantro (optional)

Helpful Hints about Lily Bulb

Lily bulb, a starchy root vegetable that looks somewhat like milky-white flower petals when dried, offers a delicate flavor and has been used in herbal preparations for centuries. (For more information on lily bulb, see "One Hundred Healthful Asian Ingredients.")

DIRECTIONS

1. Soak the lily bulb in warm water for 30 minutes. Drain.
2. In a medium-size pot, bring the broth and wine to a boil, then add the lily bulb, enoki mushrooms, goji berries, ginger, and garlic.
3. Bring the soup back to a boil, then lower the heat and simmer, covered with the lid slightly ajar, for about 25 minutes.
4. Add the asparagus stalks and crabmeat and/or shrimp, and cook for about 1 minute. Then add the asparagus tips and cook another 4 to 5 minutes, until the asparagus is tender.
5. Add salt, if desired, and/or soy sauce to taste (the ideal amounts will depend on the type of stock you used), and garnish with the cilantro (if using) before serving.

THEMES AND VARIATION

If you can't find enoki mushrooms, substitute shiitake or oyster mushrooms.

ESPECIALLY GOOD FOR

Serving in the fall, when the fall crop of asparagus is ripe. Anyone with a dry cough or other respiratory conditions, insomnia, irritability, palpitations, menopausal discomfort, or concerns about preventing cancer.

FOR THOSE FAMILIAR WITH
TRADITIONAL CHINESE MEDICINE

This dish is good to moisten the Lungs, clear Heat, counteract coughs (including but not limited to dry coughs), quiet the Heart, and calm the spirit.

STEADYING SPINACH EGG DROP SOUP

MAKES 4 SERVINGS

This is a healthy treat for spinach-lovers. You can make a large batch of this soup and keep it in the refrigerator for a few days, ready to reheat and serve with dinner.

INGREDIENTS

2 tablespoons (15 grams) dried lily bulb (*bai he*)

5 cups water, plus extra for soaking

2 tablespoons powdered kudzu, arrowroot, cornstarch, or other thickener

1 medium-size bunch (about ¾ pound) spinach, well washed and chopped into 1-inch pieces

1 medium-size egg

Juice of ½ large lemon, or to taste

2 tablespoons soy sauce, or to taste

1 teaspoon dark sesame oil

1 teaspoon honey, or to taste (optional)

2 medium-size green onions, chopped into ¼-inch pieces, roots and tough tips discarded

ESPECIALLY GOOD FOR

Individuals with a dry cough or asthma brought on by hot weather, women going through menopause, anyone feeling irritable, or individuals suffering from muscle aches.

DIRECTIONS

1. Soak the lily bulb in warm water for about 30 minutes. Drain.
2. Combine the lily bulb and 5 cups of water in a medium-size pot and bring to a boil. Lower the heat and simmer, covered with the lid slightly ajar, for about 30 minutes, or until the lily bulb is soft.
3. Mix the kudzu in a small bowl with a little cold water so it dissolves and won't clump, and add the mixture to the soup. Stir.
4. Add the spinach, stir, and cook until the spinach is done (less than 1 minute). Turn off the heat.
5. In a separate bowl, beat the egg. Stirring rapidly, pour the egg into the soup in a slow, steady stream, pouring from a height of 8 to 10 inches (for a prettier result, pour the egg through the tines of a fork).
6. Add the lemon juice, soy sauce, sesame oil, and honey (if using), stir, and garnish with the green onions.

FOR THOSE FAMILIAR WITH TRADITIONAL CHINESE MEDICINE

Spinach is considered sweet and cold, with properties that can regulate qi, moisten the Intestines, and invigorate the Blood. Lily bulb is considered slightly cold, sweet, and slightly bitter, with properties that moisten the Lungs, clear Heat, and calm the spirit.

A Taste of History

Spinach came to China during the Tang dynasty (618 to 907 CE), along the great Silk Road, the trade routes connecting China to India, Persia, and beyond. One of the first vegetables brought into China, spinach was initially called the "Persian vegetable" because of its origin, then the "red-root vegetable" due to its appearance. Spinach grew well in its new home, and could be cultivated in all seasons in areas south of the Yangtze River. Eggplant, cilantro, green onions, cucumbers, and carrots are other plant foods that arrived in China during this time.

SIMPLE WINTER MELON SOUP

MAKES 2 TO 3 SERVINGS

Winter melon soup is a popular Chinese dish, often served in banquets or in Cantonese restaurants. For fancy banquets, the soup is cooked in the winter melon itself, and designs are carved into the melon to heighten the elegant effect. This is a simple recipe for winter melon soup that's easy to cook at home—no banquets required.

INGREDIENTS

6 (5 ounces fresh; 1 ounce dried) fresh or dried shiitake mushrooms
1 (1-pound) wedge winter melon
3 cups chicken, bone, or vegetable stock (For recipes, see "Mixed and Sundry.")
1 (½-inch) piece fresh ginger, slivered into ¹⁄₁₆-inch slices
¼ pound shrimp, shelled and deveined
Salt, soy sauce, or sodium-reduced soy sauce (optional)
1 to 2 teaspoons dark sesame oil
1 medium-size green onion, chopped into ½-inch pieces, roots and tough ends discarded

Helpful Hints about Winter Melon

Winter melon—actually a kind of large squash tasting somewhat like zucchini but resembling a watermelon in size—is available fresh, in slices or whole, or canned. In Asian markets, winter melon can be sold as *dong gua* (Chinese), *tōgan* (Japanese), or *donggwa* or *donga* (Korean). (For more information on winter melon, see "One Hundred Healthful Asian Ingredients.")

DIRECTIONS

1. If you are using dried mushrooms, soak them in ½ cup of warm water for 20 minutes, or until soft. If you are using fresh mushrooms, simply rinse. Cut off and discard the stem if desired, then slice the mushrooms into ¼-inch pieces.
2. Peel the melon wedge (this will be easier if you peel the skin thickly, as the melon closer to the skin is tougher). Scrape off and discard the stringy inner fibers and seeds. Cut the melon into ½-inch slices, then cut the slices widthwise into 1-inch pieces.
3. Place the stock, melon, ginger, and mushrooms into a saucepan and bring to a boil. Lower the heat and simmer, covered with the lid slightly ajar, for about 15 minutes, or until the melon becomes slightly transparent and soft.
4. Add the shrimp and cook for about 5 more minutes.
5. Add salt or soy sauce to the soup to taste, if desired (if you have edema or high blood pressure, you'll want to go easy on the salt or use a low-sodium variety soy sauce; also note that the broth's saltiness before salting can vary according to the stock you used).
6. Remove the ginger pieces, if desired (or just eat around them).
7. Sprinkle sesame oil and green onions on top and serve.

Yuan Says

Although winter melon is harvested in the summer, this vegetable is called "winter melon" because the outside of the melon grows covered with white powder, resembling a winter frost. The vegetable also stores well, so it can be eaten in the winter months.

Winter melon soup helped impress on me that food can be medicine. After my family had moved to a poor neighborhood during the Cultural Revolution in China, we had an old man as a neighbor. He would eat his meals outside with his family, as most people did, and we would often hear him coughing and complaining about shortness of breath. But every month when he would get his check from the government, he would spend it on meat or fish and other ingredients to make a winter melon soup. When the meal was ready, I would watch him savor the soup with great delight. In the morning, the old man would tell his family how great he felt and how wonderful it was that he had slept through the night without having to wake up to relieve himself.

THEMES AND VARIATIONS

Vegetarians can omit the shrimp or substitute sliced tofu. For those who prefer the more traditional ham instead of shrimp, use about 1 ounce of ham, sliced, and add it to the bowls just before serving.

ESPECIALLY GOOD FOR

Anyone who wants to reduce swelling and puffiness, for example, from premenstrual syndrome or menopause; who wants to lose weight; who is experiencing prostate problems; or who has high blood pressure. To enhance the therapeutic effects of winter melon, leave the peel on and place the seeds in a bag made of cheesecloth or other porous material, simmer with the soup, and remove before serving.

FOR THOSE FAMILIAR WITH TRADITIONAL CHINESE MEDICINE

This dish clears Heat, expels Dampness, and promotes urination.

RENEWING RIB AND WINTER MELON SOUP

MAKES 4 SERVINGS

This is a wholesome soup with the benefits of winter melon. Here, the cooling effects of winter melon are balanced with the warming meat.

INGREDIENTS

¼ cup (30 grams) coix (Job's tears, *yi yi ren* in Chinese, or *hato mugi* in Japanese)

1 tablespoon vegetable oil, such as canola or olive oil

1 small onion, chopped into ½-inch pieces

3 cloves garlic, peeled and minced

1 to 2 pounds lamb, beef, or pork ribs

12 to 14 cups water

2 pounds winter melon (about 4 cups after cut up)

1 tablespoon (10 grams) apricot kernels (*xing ren*)

2 medium-size carrots, peeled and cut into ½-inch slices

1 to 2 sheets fresh, fresh-frozen, or dried tofu skin (*yuba*), cut into 1-inch strips (use kitchen shears)

Salt, soy sauce, or sodium-reduced soy sauce

2 green onions, chopped into ½-inch pieces, roots and tough tips removed

Condiments: soy sauce, vinegar, minced garlic, and/or chili oil

DIRECTIONS

1. Place the coix in water to soak.
2. Heat the oil in a skillet, add the onions and garlic, and cook over medium heat until the onions become translucent, about 3 minutes.
3. Place the ribs and 6 cups of water in a pot. Bring the water to a boil, then pour off the first batch of water. (This step will help make the final broth clearer; if you prefer to skim the soup instead, that's fine as well. In this case, there's no need to add water in the next step.)
4. Pour in 6 to 8 cups of fresh water, keeping the ribs in the pot. Bring the water to a boil again, add the onions and garlic, then lower the heat and simmer, covered with the lid slightly ajar, for about 1½ hours. (If you are substituting chicken pieces for ribs, this time period can be reduced to 30 minutes.)
5. In the meantime, peel the melon wedge (this will be easier if you peel the skin thickly, as the melon closer to the skin is tougher). Scrape off and discard the stringy inner fibers and seeds. Cut the melon into ½-inch slices, then cut the slices widthwise into 1-inch pieces.
6. Crush the apricot seeds with a rolling pin or glass jar (they should crush easily).
7. When the soup has done its first round of simmering as called for in step 4, add the winter melon, carrots, tofu skin, coix (drain first), and apricot kernel pieces, then simmer for another 30 minutes, or until the winter melon is soft.
8. Add salt or soy sauce to taste (Note: If you have edema or high blood pressure, you'll want to go easy on the salt/soy sauce; you may want to opt for a low-sodium variety of soy sauce, often sold as "lite").
9. Sprinkle the green onions on the soup. Serve with condiments, so each diner can add finishing touches to their own taste.

Helpful Hints about Tofu Skin

Tofu skin (a.k.a. tofu sheets, dried bean curd, soy milk skin, bean skim, *yuba* in Japanese, or *dou fu pi* in Chinese) is a product made from tofu. Popular in Chinese and Japanese cuisine (you may have had some at restaurants without realizing what it was), tofu skin is available in Asian markets (try the frozen foods section). This yellow-brown delicacy is usually made by heating soy milk in a shallow container, then harvesting and drying the "cream" that comes to the top. Tofu skin is also used to wrap dim sum dishes, bunched into sticks (called dried bean curd stick or *fu zhu*, literally, "tofu bamboo"), and shaped into meat substitutes.

THEMES AND VARIATIONS

You can substitute chicken pieces, for example, drumsticks or thighs, for the ribs, if you prefer; in this case, reduce the total cooking time to about 1 hour. You can also substitute pearl barley for the coix, if necessary.

ESPECIALLY GOOD FOR

Anyone who wants to reduce swelling and puffiness, for example, from premenstrual syndrome or menopause; address irritable bowel syndrome; prevent prostate cancer or address other prostate problems; strengthen bones; benefit the skin; or counter the effects of aging. Caution: Don't overdo the apricot kernels, as large doses can be toxic.

FOR THOSE FAMILIAR WITH
TRADITIONAL CHINESE MEDICINE

This soup supplements the qi, nourishes the Blood, and drains Dampness.

Legend Has It

Tofu skin is viewed as one of the most nutritious foods in the East. According to legend, the first Chinese emperor, Qui Shi Haung, was responsible for its popularity. When he began to feel the effects of age, he commanded his advisers to find an elixir to lengthen his life. After many false starts, the advisers hit on tofu skin, which became the emperor's favorite health food.

CLASSIC CHINESE GINSENG-CHICKEN SOUP

MAKES 6 TO 8 SERVINGS

This slightly bitter-tasting soup is a popular Chinese health food. You may choose to consume the ginseng pieces or eat around them while still benefiting from the broth.

INGREDIENTS

½ to ¾ ounce (15 to 20 grams) dried ginseng (*ren shen*), preferably sliced, or whole

2 to 3 pounds chicken pieces (purchased as drumsticks, thighs, etc., or chopped from ½ chicken)

8 (10 grams) Chinese red dates (*hong zao*), seeded

8 cups water, plus extra for soaking

2 tablespoons (15 grams) goji berries (*gou qi zi*)

½ teaspoon salt, or to taste

2 tablespoons soy sauce, or to taste (optional, or serve on the side)

2 green onions, green parts only, tough ends discarded, chopped into ½-inch pieces (save the white parts for some other use) (optional)

Condiments: rice vinegar, minced garlic, and/or hot chili oil (optional)

DIRECTIONS

1. If you are starting with sliced dried ginseng, soak the pieces for 1 hour at room temperature, then drain. If you are starting with a whole piece of dried ginseng, soak it in water at room temperature for at least 12 hours or overnight to soften, drain, and then slice.

2. In a large soup pot, combine the ginseng, chicken, Chinese red dates, and water and bring to a boil. Skim off any excess oil or fat.

3. Lower the heat and simmer, covered with the lid slightly ajar, for 40 minutes.

4. Add the goji berries and continue to simmer for another 15 minutes.

5. Add salt and/or soy sauce to taste, if desired.

6. Sprinkle the green parts of the green onion on the soup as a garnish. Serve with condiments if desired.

Fast Facts about Ginseng

The botanical name for Asian and American ginseng, *Panax*, means "all-heal" in Greek. Carl Linnaeus, the father of modern taxonomy, used the word for this genus due to its wide use in Chinese herbal medicine. (For more information on ginseng, see "One Hundred Healthful Asian Ingredients.")

THEMES AND VARIATIONS

Some people like to include Chinese yam (*shan yao*) or *he shou wu* in their ginseng soup.

This same basic recipe can be used with the Chinese herb cordyceps (Chinese caterpillar fungus, *dong chong xia cao* in Chinese), a mushroom relative, instead of ginseng to make a different variety of antiaging soup; in this case, use about ten pieces (¹⁄₁₀ ounce or 3 grams) of cordyceps. The soup can also be made with American ginseng (*xi yang shen*), which also contains some of the same chemical components as Asian ginseng, but it is considered cooling and more nourishing of the yin.

ESPECIALLY GOOD FOR

Anyone concerned with increasing vitality, immunity, endurance, and strength; recovering from an illness or childbirth; or counteracting chronic cough, wheezing, dizziness, or blurred vision.

FOR THOSE FAMILIAR WITH TRADITIONAL CHINESE MEDICINE

This soup supplements qi and nourishes the Blood and yin.

HEALTHFUL HERBAL CHICKEN SOUP

MAKES 6 TO 8 SERVINGS

The red dates and goji berries contribute a sweet taste to this healthful herbal chicken soup.

INGREDIENTS

2 to 3 pounds chicken pieces (purchased as drumsticks, thighs, etc., or chopped from ½ chicken)

8 cups water

A pinch of salt

1 (1-inch) piece fresh ginger, slivered into 1/16-inch slices

3 cloves garlic, peeled and minced

6 to 8 medium-size pieces (20 grams) dried Chinese yam (*shan yao* or *huai shan*)

6 medium-size pieces (about 20 grams) astragalus (*huang qi*)

1 rounded tablespoon (10 grams) goji berries (*gou qi zi*)

6 to 8 (10 grams) Chinese red dates (*hong zao*), seeded

2 tablespoons rice wine

2 green onions, chopped into ½-inch pieces, roots and tough tips discarded

3 tablespoons soy sauce, or to taste

DIRECTIONS

1. In a large soup pot, combine the chicken, water, and salt and bring to a boil. Skim off any excess oil or fat.
2. Tie the ginger, garlic, Chinese yam, and astragalus together in a piece of cheesecloth (just place the herbs in the center and tie the ends). This will make it easy to remove the herbs later.
3. Add the cheesecloth bag of herbs and the goji berries, Chinese red dates, and wine to the pot. Bring it back to a boil, then lower the heat and simmer, covered with the lid slightly ajar, for 45 to 60 minutes. Skim off any excess oil or fat.
4. When the soup is done, remove and discard the bag of herbs.
5. Add soy sauce to taste and garnish with the green onions.

A Word from the Ancients

Long-term consumption of Chinese yam sharpens the hearing, brightens the eyes, makes the body light, frees one from hunger, and prolongs life.

—*Divine Farmer's Materia Medica* (*Shen Nong Ben Cao*)

THEMES AND VARIATIONS

If you can find fresh Chinese yam and decide to use it instead of the dried variety, cut it into 1-inch pieces and add it to the soup with the goji berries and red dates (rather than placing it in the bag with the ginger and astragalus). Dried Chinese yam can also be placed directly in the soup and eaten (soak it first and cut it into bite-size pieces).

If you prefer, you can use either astragalus or Chinese yam instead of both.

ESPECIALLY GOOD FOR

Anyone concerned with increasing vitality, building immunity, controlling blood sugar levels, dizziness, insomnia, or diarrhea, strengthening bones, or maintaining good eyesight.

FOR THOSE FAMILIAR WITH
TRADITIONAL CHINESE MEDICINE

This soup supplements qi and nourishes the Blood.

Helpful Hints about Chinese Yam

Chinese yam (not to be confused with the sweet potato often sold as a "yam" in Western supermarkets) is the starchy root of a plant native to China, Japan, Korea, and Taiwan. Look for dried, sliced Chinese yam in packages containing chalky white pieces about 1 inch wide and 3 to 4 inches long. Fresh Chinese yam is also available; in Japanese markets look for *nagaimo* or *yamaimo*. (For more information on Chinese yam, see "One Hundred Healthful Asian Ingredients.")

STATE-OF-RETURN CHICKEN SOUP

MAKES 6 TO 8 SERVINGS

The key ingredients in this classic therapeutic dish are dang gui *(a.k.a. angelica sinensis root) and astragalus; if you are missing one of the other herbs, don't hesitate to cook the soup anyway.*

INGREDIENTS

2 to 3 pounds chicken pieces (purchased as drumsticks, thighs, etc., or chopped from ½ chicken)

8 cups water

A pinch of salt

1 (1-inch) piece fresh ginger, slivered into ¹⁄₁₆-inch slices

⅓ ounce (10 grams) *dang gui*

6 medium-size pieces (20 grams) astragalus (*huang qi*)

1 rounded tablespoon (10 grams) goji berries (*gou qi zi*)

6 to 8 (10 grams) Chinese red dates (*hong zao*), seeded

4 to 5 cloves garlic, peeled and minced

2 tablespoons rice wine

2 medium-size carrots, cut into ½-inch slices

2 medium-size celery stalks, cut into ½-inch slices

3 tablespoons soy sauce, or to taste

2 green onions, chopped into ½-inch pieces, roots and tough tips discarded

What's in a Name?

Dang gui—a major herb in traditional Chinese medicine—translates literally from the Chinese as "state of return," indicating its role in restoring regular menses.

DIRECTIONS

1. In a large soup pot, combine the chicken, water, and salt and bring to a boil. Skim off any excess oil or fat.
2. Tie the ginger, *dang gui*, and astragalus together in a piece of cheesecloth (just place the herbs in the center and tie the ends). This will make it easy to remove the herbs later.
3. Add the cheesecloth bag of herbs, goji berries, Chinese red dates, garlic, and wine to the pot. Bring back to a boil, then lower the heat and simmer, covered with the lid slightly ajar, for about 45 minutes. Skim off any excess oil or fat.
4. Add the carrots and celery to the soup and cook for another 10 minutes.
5. When the soup is done, remove the bag of herbs.
6. Add the soy sauce to taste and garnish with the green onions.

THEMES AND VARIATIONS

Root vegetables, such as turnips and potatoes, can round out this dish for heartier fare. If you think you'll prefer the taste of this dish with less *dang gui*, try using 3 to 5 grams.

ESPECIALLY GOOD FOR

Anyone feeling weak or getting over an illness; also, women recovering from childbirth or a heavy menstrual period, experiencing irregular bleeding, or who are having problems conceiving due to an irregular menstrual period. If you are pregnant, you may want to skip the *dang gui*.

FOR THOSE FAMILIAR WITH
TRADITIONAL CHINESE MEDICINE

This soup builds the Blood, supplements the qi, and regulates the *chong* and *ren* meridians.

CHANGE-OF-PACE CHICKEN, MUSHROOM, AND LOTUS SEED SOUP

MAKES 6 TO 8 SERVINGS

This is a lovely variation of an old healing favorite, chicken soup.

INGREDIENTS

6 (1 ounce dried; ⅓ pound fresh) dried or fresh shiitake mushrooms

25 (a little less than 1 ounce, or 25 grams) dried lotus seeds (*lian zi*)

2 to 3 pounds chicken pieces (purchased as drumsticks, thighs, etc., or chopped from ½ chicken)

8 cups water, plus extra for boiling

A pinch of salt

1 (1-inch) piece fresh ginger, slivered into ¹⁄₁₆-inch slices

2 tablespoons mirin or dry sherry

½ pound bok choy, cut into ½-inch slices

3 tablespoons soy sauce, or to taste

2 green onions, chopped into ½-inch pieces, roots and tough tips discarded

Helpful Hints about Lotus Seeds

These off-white, oval seeds are widely available in Asian groceries dried (sometimes called "lotus nuts" in this form) or canned. (For more information on lotus seeds, see "One Hundred Healthful Asian Ingredients.")

DIRECTIONS

1. If you are starting with dried mushrooms, wash and soak them in about a cup of warm water until the mushrooms are soft, about 30 minutes. If you are starting with fresh mushrooms, simply rinse. Remove and discard the stems if desired, then cut the mushrooms into ½-inch slices.

2. Boil about a cup of water, and place the lotus seeds in the boiling water for about a minute to blanch. Remove the lotus seeds from the water.

3. In a large soup pot, place the chicken, water, and salt together and bring to a boil. Skim off any excess oil or fat.

4. Add the ginger, mirin, lotus seeds, and mushrooms, and bring back to a boil.

5. Lower the heat to a simmer, and cook, covered with the lid slightly ajar, for about 30 minutes, or until the lotus seeds are soft. Skim off any excess oil or fat if desired.

6. Add the bok choy, then simmer for 10 minutes more. Remove the ginger pieces, if desired (or eat around them).

7. Add the soy sauce and green onions before serving.

ESPECIALLY GOOD FOR

Anyone who wants to counteract insomnia, digestive problems, poor appetite, premenstrual syndrome, depression, chronic diarrhea, irritable bowel syndrome, weak bones, or a weakened immune system.

FOR THOSE FAMILIAR WITH TRADITIONAL CHINESE MEDICINE

In this dish, the lotus seeds and mushrooms act to strengthen the Spleen and Kidney, nourish the Heart, and calm the spirit.

LOTUS ROOT–CHICKEN SOUP

MAKES 3 TO 4 SERVINGS

Soup is a popular way to prepare lotus root, a mild vegetable with an attractive lacy interior. When cooked briefly, the texture of lotus root is crisp and crunchy. When cooked for longer periods, lotus root becomes soft and almost powdery.

INGREDIENTS

2 to 3 whole pieces (14 ounces, or 400 grams) lotus root (*ou* in Chinese, *renkon* in Japanese)

6 cups water

2 pounds chicken pieces (purchased as drumsticks, thighs, etc., or chopped from ½ chicken)

4 pieces (½ ounce, or 15 grams) dried Chinese yam (*shan yao* or *huai shan*)

6 Chinese red dates (*hong zao*), seeded

2 tablespoons (15 grams) goji berries (*gou qi zi*)

1 small carrot, cut into ½-inch slices

A pinch of salt

2 bundles (4 ounces) dried cellophane (mung bean preferred) noodles

2 green onions, chopped into ½-inch pieces, roots and tough ends discarded

2½ tablespoons soy sauce, or to taste

2 teaspoons sesame oil

Condiments: soy sauce, chopped garlic, and/or chili oil (optional)

DIRECTIONS

1. Peel the lotus root, remove and discard the knobby ends, and slice the root thinly widthwise, placing each slice immediately into the water so the lotus root does not discolor.

2. Combine the lotus root, chicken, Chinese yam, Chinese red dates, goji berries, carrot, and salt into a large pot and bring to a boil. Lower the heat and simmer, covered with the lid slightly ajar, for about 40 minutes. Skim off any excess oil or fat if desired.

3. Add the cellophane noodles and green onions to the soup and simmer for another 5 minutes.

4. Add the soy sauce, and sprinkle the sesame oil onto the soup before serving with condiments.

Yuan Says

In many ways, soup is an ideal way to nurse your body back to health. The nutrition from food and herbs can be absorbed easily from a warm soup to help supplement the body. In China, people visiting friends and relatives in the hospital often bring homemade soup to show they care, the way people in the West bring flowers.

THEMES AND VARIATIONS

Don't be shy if you are inspired to add greens, such as spinach, to this soup.

ESPECIALLY GOOD FOR

Anyone concerned with increasing vitality, reducing fatigue and dizziness, building immunity, maintaining good eyesight, controlling weight, reducing high cholesterol, counteracting diabetes, strengthening bones, or reducing menopausal discomfort.

FOR THOSE FAMILIAR WITH
TRADITIONAL CHINESE MEDICINE

This soup strengthens the Spleen, supplements qi, and nourishes the Blood.

Helpful Hints about Lotus Root

When shopping for fresh lotus roots, which resemble 6- to 8-inch-long oblong gourds, look for specimens with a lighter beige peel, which indicates a fresher vegetable than the darker brown pieces. You may also encounter the peeled white flesh of the lotus root vacuum packed (whole or sliced) or canned. (For more information on lotus root, see "One Hundred Healthful Asian Ingredients.")

FLU SEASON SOUP

MAKES 4 SERVINGS

This may look like a Western soup, but it contains many ingredients used in the Chinese tradition to enhance the immune system and strengthen the body.

INGREDIENTS

¾ cup (about 90 grams) pearl barley or coix (Job's tears, *yi yi ren* in Chinese, or *hato mugi* in Japanese)

3½ cups water

1 tablespoon vegetable oil, such as canola or olive oil

½ medium-size onion, cut into ½-inch pieces

2 cloves garlic, peeled and minced

2 to 3 medium-size stalks celery, cut into ½-inch slices

1 cup cooked azuki beans, kidney beans, or black beans (*hei dou*), or a 15-ounce can, drained

2 teaspoons dried thyme

1 cup chicken or vegetable broth (for example, Immunity-Boosting Chicken Stock, page 270)

1 leek, well washed, cut into ¼-inch slices, roots and the tough tips discarded

½ cup fresh or frozen green peas

Black or white pepper

Salt

A handful of arugula, roughly chopped into 1- to 2-inch pieces (about ¼ cup chopped)

DIRECTIONS

1. Combine the barley and water in a large pot, bring to a boil, then lower the heat and cook, uncovered, at a gentle simmer for about 30 minutes.

2. Heat the cooking oil in a large pan over medium heat, then add the onion and garlic. Cook, stirring, until golden brown.

3. Add the celery, beans, thyme, and broth to the pan. Cook, covered, for 15 minutes. Gently stir the beans against the side of the pan to break them open. (If at any point during this or later steps, the mixture becomes too thick or the ingredients threaten to stick to the bottom of the pan, add water.)

4. Add the bean mixture to the pot of barley, along with the leeks and peas, and season with pepper.

5. Simmer for another 15 minutes or so, until the barley is soft.

6. Add salt to taste (the amount will vary, depending on the amount of salt in your stock).

7. Sprinkle the arugula on top of the dish as a garnish.

Yuan Says

In China, cooking is considered a key step in bringing out the healthful properties of foods and herbs. Long, slow cooking is considered especially good for younger and older people, and those with chronic disease, helping them to absorb key nutrients from the food.

Fast Facts about Arugula

You might associate arugula, a pungent green of the mustard family, with Italian or French cuisine, but it is also used around the world (including in Asia, where in China it is known as *zi ma cai*, and in Australia, where it is known as "rocket leaf.") In ancient Rome, the herb was believed to be an aphrodisiac. In China, arugula is considered less of a medicine than a food, with neutral to cooling properties and the ability to stimulate the appetite.

THEMES AND VARIATIONS

If you are starting with dried beans, measure out ⅓ cup, then soak them for at least 8 hours, or overnight. Drain and place them in a pot with about 1 cup of water. Cover the pot, boil, and then lower the heat to a simmer. Azuki beans will cook in about 45 minutes. Kidney beans will require about 1½ hours.

ESPECIALLY GOOD FOR

Making during the flu season; serving to anyone with a cold or the flu, who wants to maintain general good health, or who is concerned about the effects of aging (such as hair loss, gray hair, and poor memory).

FOR THOSE FAMILIAR WITH
TRADITIONAL CHINESE MEDICINE

Because this soup has many wholesome and diverse ingredients, it helps restore balance to the body, strengthening *wei qi*, stabilizing the exterior, and supporting the body's normal qi and Kidney qi.

Barley Cooking Tips

If you are using barley, either the pearl or pot varieties can work well in this recipe. Pearl barley will cook in 35 to 60 minutes; pot barley is less refined (although still removed from a tight hull surrounding the grain to be edible) and may take up to 1½ hours to cook (15 to 20 minutes less if soaked several hours beforehand).

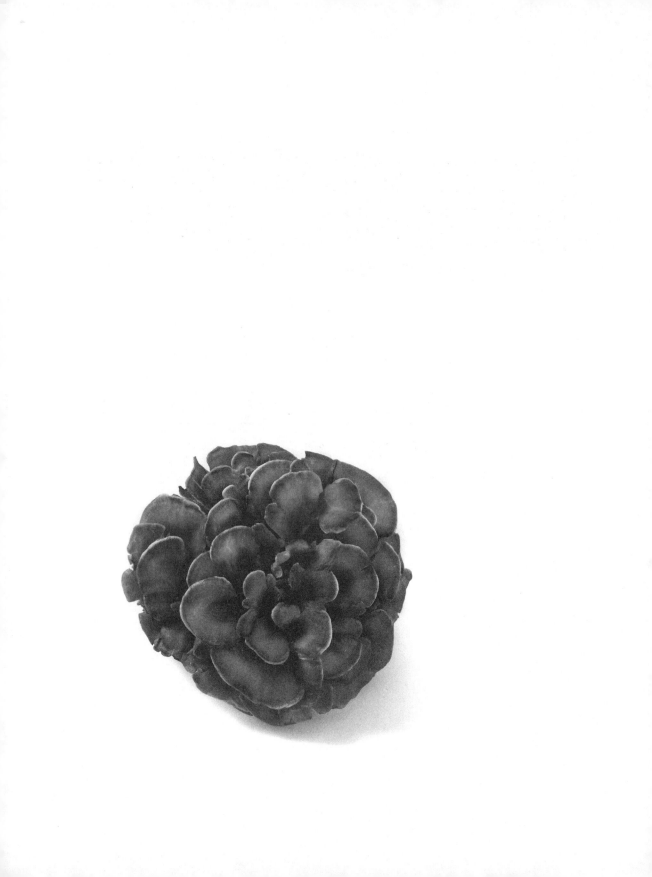

SAVORY SIDE DISHES, OR VEGETARIANS' DELIGHT

上工治未病

*Anyone who takes medicine
and neglects diet wastes
the skills of the physician.*
—CHINESE PROVERB

POTENT PAN-FRIED PUMPKIN

MAKES 2 SERVINGS

This seasonal dish is popular in China in the fall, and once you taste its superb flavors you'll know why.

INGREDIENTS

15 to 18 ounces pumpkin, such as
    a small Hokkaido or kabocha
    (about 3 cups when cubed)
¼ cup walnuts
1 tablespoon (10 grams) apricot
    kernels (*xing ren*)
2 tablespoons vegetable oil, such
    as canola or olive oil
¼ cup raisins
½ cup water
Salt
Ground cinnamon (optional)

DIRECTIONS

1. Seed and chop the pumpkin into 1-inch cubes, leaving the peel on. (An efficient way to chop a pumpkin is to cut it into wedges, then cut the wedges into cubes. A large, sharp cleaver can be a useful tool since the raw vegetable can be tough. Another handy trick is to put the pumpkin in the microwave for 5 minutes to soften it before cutting and peeling.)

2. Crush the walnuts and apricot kernels into small pieces (using a rolling pin or glass jar will work; putting a piece of waxed paper between the nuts and kernels and the rolling pin will keep the pieces from jumping all over).

3. Heat the oil in a medium-size lidded skillet, then brown the pumpkin over medium-high heat, stirring frequently.

4. Add the walnuts, apricot kernels, and raisins, with just enough water to keep the mixture moist.

5. Cover and cook over low heat until soft, about 20 minutes, checking occasionally to make sure the mixture isn't drying out (if it is, add a touch more water).

6. Add salt to taste; sprinkle with cinnamon, if desired; and serve as part of a meal or as a snack.

Fast Facts about Raisins

The Northwestern region of China, especially Xinjiang Province, which borders on Kazakhstan, Russia, and Mongolia, is known as "the home of fruit and melons" and is particularly famous for its raisins, which have had songs and poems dedicated to them. In Xinjiang, which has been cultivating grapes for at least two thousand years, raisins are dried in the shade, rather than the sun, using the force of the hot desert air. This preparation method produces raisins that retain a green color and fruity flavor absent in most other raisins. Look for Xinjiang raisins if you happen to be in an Asian grocery store.

In the Chinese tradition, raisins are thought to strengthen the Liver and Kidneys and to supplement qi and Blood, whereas fresh grapes primarily act to create body fluids. In the West, raisins and grapes (as well as wine—especially red wine), peanuts, cranberries, and blueberries have been identified as sources of resveratrol, which has been associated with anticancer, antiaging, and anti-inflammatory effects. (For more information on grapes and raisins, see "One Hundred Healthful Asian Ingredients.")

THEMES AND VARIATIONS

The Hokkaido pumpkin works well in this dish because it is firm and not too moist, but other kinds of pumpkin can be substituted. In addition, mixed nuts can be used instead of apricot kernels. If you like seafood, you can soak 1 to 2 tablespoons of dried shrimp in rice wine or water for about 30 minutes, or until soft, then chop them into small pieces before tossing with the pumpkin before serving.

ESPECIALLY GOOD FOR

Diabetics, who may crave a sweet taste, and anyone who wants to increase endurance. Studies in China have shown that while pumpkin offers a sweet flavor, it actually moderates blood sugar.

FOR THOSE FAMILIAR WITH TRADITIONAL CHINESE MEDICINE

This yin dish strengthens the Spleen, and helps manage appetite.

TERRIFIC TOFU AND MUSHROOMS

MAKES 4 SERVINGS

This flavorful presentation of tofu and mushrooms, two vegetarian staples, goes well with brown rice in this vegan dish.

INGREDIENTS

8 dried shiitake mushrooms
2 tablespoons sesame oil
1 (1-inch) piece fresh ginger, peeled and minced
2 cloves garlic, peeled and minced
2 green onions, cut into ¼-inch pieces, roots and tough tips discarded
1 (12- to 14-ounce) package firm tofu, cut into ½- to 1-inch cubes
2 tablespoons cold water
1 tablespoon powdered kudzu, arrowroot, cornstarch, or other thickener
1 tablespoon soy sauce, or to taste
1 teaspoon lemon juice, or to taste (optional)

DIRECTIONS

1. Soak the shiitake mushrooms in 1½ to 2 cups of water for 20 minutes, or until soft. Drain, reserving the liquid for later use. Cut off and discard the stem, if desired, and slice the remainder into ¼-inch pieces.
2. Heat the oil in a wok or skillet over medium-high heat. Add the ginger and garlic and cook for 30 to 60 seconds, until fragrant.
3. Add the shiitakes, green onions, and tofu.
4. Add 1 cup of the mushroom liquid, cover, and cook over medium-high heat for 5 to 7 minutes, turning the tofu once, until the tofu is cooked through.
5. In a small bowl, stir together the water and the kudzu until no lumps remain. Add the kudzu mixture and soy sauce to the tofu mixture and stir. Cook for another minute.
6. Flavor with lemon juice to taste, and serve with rice.

THEMES AND VARIATIONS

Other types of mushrooms, fresh or dried, can be substituted for the dried shiitakes. If you are using fresh mushrooms, use *dashi* or vegetable stock instead of mushroom water.

ESPECIALLY GOOD FOR

Anyone with fatigue, menopausal symptoms, diabetes, hypertension, or concerns about warding off cancer.

FOR THOSE FAMILIAR WITH
TRADITIONAL CHINESE MEDICINE

This dish strengthens qi and addresses yin deficiency.

COOL-AS-A-CUCUMBER SALAD

MAKES 2 SERVINGS

You might want to double up this recipe because this delicious salad can disappear fast! Try serving it with a soup or rice dish.

INGREDIENTS

1 medium-size cucumber, peeled
Salt
1 clove garlic, crushed and then minced
¼ cup white vinegar
2 tablespoons dark sesame oil

Good Inside and Out

Looking for a way to relieve sore, puffy eyes? Yuan recommends resting with cool cucumber slices on closed eyelids for 10 minutes. Another remedy for soothing red itchy eyes is cool, damp tea bags. Try it—you might be surprised how good it feels.

DIRECTIONS

1. Using a blunt instrument; such as the handle of a knife, pound the cucumber's surface to soften it slightly and increase its ability to absorb the salt and dressing. Cut the cucumber in half lengthwise. Scoop out the seeds with a spoon, if desired. Then cut the cucumber widthwise into thin slices or slivers.
2. Sprinkle and toss with salt, to taste.
3. Combine the cucumber, garlic, vinegar, and sesame oil in a bowl and mix well. Serve.

THEMES AND VARIATIONS

The Koreans make a similar refreshing chilled soup for the summer months, combining cucumbers, garlic, salt, and a spoonful of vinegar with water or chicken broth, and then garnishing the soup with green onions and/or toasted sesame seeds.

ESPECIALLY GOOD FOR

Eating in hot weather; serving to anyone who tends to run hot or who is displaying a poor appetite.

FOR THOSE FAMILIAR WITH
TRADITIONAL CHINESE MEDICINE

This dish helps to counteract Summer Heat.

OPEN SESAME EGGPLANT

MAKES 2 OR 3 SERVINGS

If you've ever been perplexed about how to serve eggplant, here's a great answer featuring garlic and sesame seeds.

INGREDIENTS

3 to 4 tablespoons dark sesame oil
3 cloves garlic, minced
1 medium-size eggplant (about
    1 pound), cut into 1-inch cubes
1 cup water
1 tablespoon rice wine
1½ tablespoons soy sauce
1 tablespoon sesame seeds

Good Inside and Out

As well as acting as a delicious ingredient for recipes, eggplant can be used externally as a home remedy for skin irritations. For a rash, grind a baked eggplant into powder, mix with sesame oil, then apply to the affected area. To soothe bee stings or centipede bites, cut open a fresh eggplant and rub directly onto the affected area. For pain and swelling of unknown causes, crush a fresh eggplant, mix with vinegar, and apply to the affected region.

DIRECTIONS

1. Heat the oil in a pan, then add the garlic, then the eggplant. Cook until the eggplant is golden brown on all sides. (You might want to brown the eggplant in two batches to distribute the oil more evenly, as the eggplant has a tendency to absorb it.)
2. Add the water to the pan. Bring to a boil, then lower the heat. Cover and cook for about 10 minutes, until soft.
3. Remove the lid, then add the rice wine and soy sauce. Cook, uncovered, for another 3 to 5 minutes.
4. In the meantime, toast the sesame seeds in a dry skillet over medium heat until golden brown, stirring or shaking frequently, about 5 minutes. When they are done, remove the seeds from the hot skillet so they don't overcook.
5. Transfer the eggplant mixture to a serving dish and sprinkle with the toasted sesame seeds. Serve warm.

THEMES AND VARIATIONS

If you prefer, you can boil or steam your eggplant for about 20 minutes, until soft, then add soy sauce, sesame oil, and toasted sesame seeds to taste.

ESPECIALLY GOOD FOR

Anyone who is concerned about high cholesterol or who wants to counteract pain or swelling.

FOR THOSE FAMILIAR WITH
TRADITIONAL CHINESE MEDICINE

This dish clears Heat, moves and cools the Blood, moistens the Intestines, reduces swelling, and eases pain.

SPECIAL SPICY SPINACH

MAKES 2 SERVINGS

No bland I-don't-want-to-eat-my-spinach here. Although this dish is vegetarian, seafood lovers can use dried shrimp or scallops as a garnish for an additional flavor.

INGREDIENTS

2 cups water
1 bunch spinach (about ¾ pound), washed well, then chopped into 2- to 3-inch pieces
1 teaspoon wasabi paste, or to taste
1 tablespoon soy sauce
2 tablespoons rice vinegar
1 tablespoon dark sesame oil

Helpful Hints about Wasabi

You can buy wasabi, a sinus-clearing hot relative of mustard, as a paste or a powder. Because of its popularity as a garnish for sushi, wasabi can sometimes be found in health food stores and regular supermarkets, in addition to Asian food stores. (For more information on wasabi, see "One Hundred Healthful Asian Ingredients.")

DIRECTIONS

1. Bring the water to a boil and add the spinach. Bring the water back to a boil, then drain well, squeezing out the excess water. Place the spinach in a serving bowl.
2. Prepare the sauce by combining the wasabi paste, soy sauce, vinegar, and sesame oil in a small bowl. Stir well.
3. Serve with sauce on the side, so everyone can determine how much zing to add, or toss the sauce with the spinach.

THEMES AND VARIATIONS

Soak about 1 teaspoon of dried shrimp or scallops in water for 30 to 45 minutes, until soft, then dice and toss with the spinach. Other flavorings to consider instead of wasabi include fresh ginger juice, which you can make by grating a piece of fresh ginger, then squeezing it (in your hands, with a garlic press, or through a piece of cheesecloth).

ESPECIALLY GOOD FOR

Eating in the summer, or serving to anyone who has a poor appetite or who is weak after a long illness or chemotherapy.

FOR THOSE FAMILIAR WITH TRADITIONAL CHINESE MEDICINE

This dish harmonizes the Middle Burner, promotes the movement of qi, and drains Dampness.

Mika Says

I love spinach, but for years I hesitated to buy it because I didn't want to face the task of removing the dirt from its gritty leaves, which never seemed to get quite clean enough. After experimenting with different methods, though, I've found that soaking and swishing the leaves in a large bowl of cold water is an efficient and effective method for removing the dirt. Drain and repeat the process until the leaves are clean. I now happily seek out spinach in the vegetable aisle.

CLEANSING SEAWEED SCRAMBLED EGGS

MAKES 2 SERVINGS

This simple, delicious recipe combines the popular kitchen therapy ingredients of seaweed and coix with an old standby—scrambled eggs. In Asia, coix has a reputation for beautifying the complexion. Seaweed, which is rich in minerals such as iodine, calcium, iron, zinc, copper, selenium, molybdenum, fluoride, and manganese, is known for helping to detoxify the body.

INGREDIENTS

2 tablespoons (30 grams) coix (Job's tears, *yi yi ren* in Chinese, or *hato mugi* in Japanese)

1 tablespoon dried precut wakame seaweed

3 eggs

1 tablespoon vegetable oil, such as canola or olive oil

A pinch of salt

A pinch of pepper

DIRECTIONS

1. Soak the coix in warm water for about 30 minutes, then drain.
2. Boil 2 cups of water, then add the coix and seaweed. Lower the heat and simmer, partially covered, for about half an hour, until the ingredients are soft. Drain and set aside.
3. Crack the eggs into a bowl and stir. Heat the oil in a pan, then add the eggs. Cook, stirring, until not quite done (they should still be moist).
4. Add the seaweed and coix and cook for 1 to 2 more minutes.
5. Add salt and pepper to taste, then serve.

Warren Says

One of the criticisms of the Western diet (along with all its other ills) has been its reliance on a small number of grains—especially corn, soy (mostly in a highly processed form), and wheat. Coix provides an opportunity to diversify your consumption of grains to include another nutritious and ancient species. Other grains you might want to try incorporating into your diet are millet, barley, quinoa, amaranth, and buckwheat.

Fast Facts about Eggs

Eggs are popular in Asian cuisine—not only chicken eggs, but also eggs of other birds, such as ducks. Eggs symbolize fertility and rebirth, as well as good luck, happiness, and tranquility (because they have no sharp edges); in China, eggs are a traditional gift when a child is born, colored red for good luck. In terms of cooking, eggs are found in many dishes—soups, scrambled, or served on rice, smoked, marinated in tea, steamed, or made into thin egg pancakes. In terms of traditional Chinese medicine, chicken eggs, considered neutral in temperature and sweet in flavor, are thought to supplement the qi, nourish Blood and yin, and moisten the body. The white moistens the Lungs and clears Heat in conditions such as reddened eyes and dry cough, whereas the yolk enriches the yin and Blood to counteract such problems as exhaustion, weakness, fatigue, and nervousness.

THEMES AND VARIATIONS

Shiitake mushrooms are a nice addition. Soak for 20 minutes if you are using dried shiitakes; if you are using fresh shiitakes, simply rinse. Slice the shiitakes into ¼-inch slices, then add to the pot of simmering seaweed and coix about 5 minutes before you drain them.

ESPECIALLY GOOD FOR

Anyone who wants to help cleanse his or her system of swelling or masses (such as goiter, ovarian cysts, breast lumps, or lymph node swelling), or who may suffer from hypothyroidism or goiter.

FOR THOSE FAMILIAR WITH TRADITIONAL CHINESE MEDICINE

This dish helps counteract stagnation and drain Dampness.

SIMPLE SEAWEED SALAD

MAKES 4 SERVINGS

This is a quick and tasty salad that is terrific as an appetizer or side dish.

INGREDIENTS

1 cup (about ¾ ounce) dried seaweed, such as *hiyashi* wakame
(which rehydrates into bright
green slivers) or *fueru* wakame
(a darker green, leafy variety;
look for the kind that is already
cut into pieces)

1 to 2 cloves garlic, minced

3 tablespoons rice vinegar

3 tablespoons soy sauce

2 tablespoons dark sesame oil

1 tablespoon unhulled sesame
seeds

DIRECTIONS

1. Cover the seaweed with cold water for 10 to 15 minutes, drain and press out the water, then cover with boiling water for 5 minutes.
2. Combine the garlic, rice vinegar, soy sauce, and sesame oil in a bowl.
3. Toast the sesame seeds in a dry skillet over medium heat until golden brown, stirring or shaking frequently, about 5 minutes. Set the sesame seeds aside to let cool in a dish or on a plate.
4. Drain the hot water from the seaweed, and squeeze out any excess water.
5. Combine the liquid ingredients and the seaweed, then toss well until the seaweed is evenly coated.
6. Sprinkle with the toasted sesame seeds as a garnish.

ESPECIALLY GOOD FOR

Anyone with a skin rash, acne, high cholesterol, masses (such as ovarian cysts, breast lumps, or fibroids), or cancer, or who wants to clear the body of toxins.

FOR THOSE FAMILIAR WITH
TRADITIONAL CHINESE MEDICINE

This dish helps counteract stagnation, clear Heat and toxic Heat, and drain Dampness.

What's in a Name?

Seaweed is eaten in coastal communities around the world, but it is so popular in Japan that much of the seaweed sold in the West is known by its Japanese name, including such varieties as nori (the delicate sheets used to wrap sushi), arame (pencil-size strips used for soups, stews, salads, and stir-fries), kombu (usually sold in sheets or strips and used as one of the three main ingredients to make the Japanese traditional soup stock *dashi*), hijiki (thin, dark threads used for soup, salad, and stir-fries), and wakame (leafy strips used in this recipe and others for salads, soups, and stir-fries). (For more information on seaweed, see "One Hundred Healthful Asian Ingredients.")

Yuan Says

I recommend seaweed to my patients all the time. Often in the West, people are told only what foods they should not be eating—don't eat sugar, don't eat beef, don't eat saturated fat—rather than what foods they should be eating. I think this is a mistake both in terms of health and quality of life. A broad spectrum of natural foods—including a variety of sea and land vegetables, grains, and fruits—is beneficial. So, try eating seaweed! It's good for you and you might find you'll want to enjoy it regularly.

THREE-COLOR NOODLE-SEAWEED SALAD

MAKES 4 TO 6 SERVINGS

This salad—one of our favorites—combines the crunch of carrots, the smoothness of seaweed, and the body of noodles in a tasty sauce.

INGREDIENTS

1 cup (about ¾ ounce) dried sea-weed, such as shredded *fueru* wakame

2 bundles cellophane (mung bean) noodles (about 4 ounces)

4 cloves garlic, minced

¼ to ⅓ cup rice vinegar

¼ cup soy sauce

3 tablespoons dark sesame oil

2 tablespoons sesame seeds

1 medium-size carrot, cut into matchstick-shape pieces, peeled if desired

2 medium-size green onions, cut into ½-inch lengths, roots and tips discarded

DIRECTIONS

1. Cover the seaweed and mung bean noodles with cold water (5 to 7 cups) for 15 minutes, drain, and press the remaining water out.

2. In the meantime, boil about 5 cups of water.

3. Once the seaweed and noodles have been drained of the cold water, cover them again with the boiling water, and let sit for 10 minutes.

4. In the meantime, combine the garlic, rice vinegar, soy sauce, and sesame oil in a bowl.

5. If they aren't already roasted, toast the sesame seeds in a skillet over medium heat until golden brown, stirring or shaking frequently, about 5 minutes. Set the sesame seeds aside to let cool in a dish or on a plate.

6. Drain the hot water from the seaweed and noodles, and squeeze out any excess water.

7. Combine the liquid ingredients and the seaweed, noodles, carrots, and green onions, then toss well.

8. Sprinkle the toasted sesame seeds over the top as a garnish.

ESPECIALLY GOOD FOR

Anyone with a skin rash, acne, high cholesterol, high blood pressure, soft masses (such as ovarian cysts, breast lumps, lymph node swelling, or fibroids), or cancer.

FOR THOSE FAMILIAR WITH
TRADITIONAL CHINESE MEDICINE

This dish helps counteract stagnation and drain Dampness, as well as clearing Heat.

FRESH LOTUS ROOT SALAD

MAKES 4 TO 6 SERVINGS

Lotus root is a surprisingly versatile vegetable, great in salads, soups, and juices. For salads, look for young roots as indicated by a light tan peel (older specimens will have a dark brown rind) and avoid those preserved in brine in vacuum-sealed bags.

INGREDIENTS

1 pound fresh lotus root (*ou* in Chinese, *renkon* in Japanese), peeled, ends trimmed
1½ tablespoons soy sauce
3 tablespoons rice vinegar
1 teaspoon honey or other natural sweetener (optional)
1 tablespoon dark sesame oil
2 tablespoons fresh cilantro leaves

THEMES AND VARIATIONS

Lotus root salad is sometimes made with raw sliced lotus root. In this case, it is considered especially good for cooling the Blood and for easing mild nosebleeds.

DIRECTIONS

1. Using a sharp knife, cut the lotus root widthwise into ⅛-inch thick slices. As you cut them, drop them into a bowl of cold water to prevent discoloration.
2. Bring 3 to 4 cups of water to a boil.
3. Drain the lotus root, place it back in the bowl, then pour the boiling water on top. Let the lotus root sit in the hot water for 5 minutes, then drain, rinse under cold water, and pat dry.
4. In a small bowl, mix together the soy sauce, vinegar, honey (if using), and sesame oil. Stir well. Heat the mixture briefly if the sweetener needs help dissolving.
5. Arrange the lotus root slices in an attractive pattern, and pour the dressing over the top. Let marinate for at least 30 minutes.
6. Garnish with cilantro before serving.

ESPECIALLY GOOD FOR

Eating on a hot summer day; serving to anyone who tends to run hot or who needs help with his or her digestion.

FOR THOSE FAMILIAR WITH
TRADITIONAL CHINESE MEDICINE

Fresh lotus root addresses Dryness from Heat and harmonizes the Spleen and Stomach.

SESAME–LOTUS ROOT STIR-FRY

MAKES 2 SERVINGS

This attractive and tasty dish shows off the lacy patterns of the lotus root, accented by the green garnish.

INGREDIENTS

2 tablespoons vinegar
1 section (⅓ to ½ pound) lotus root (*ou* in Chinese, *renkon* in Japanese)
1 tablespoon brown sesame seeds
1 tablespoon dark sesame oil
1 (1-inch) piece fresh ginger, peeled and minced
2 cloves garlic, peeled and minced
2 green onions, chopped into ¼-inch pieces, roots and tough tips discarded
1 tablespoon soy sauce

THEMES AND VARIATIONS

Feel free to add other vegetables—such as onions, snow peas, or shiitake mushrooms—to the stir-fry as well.

Mika Says

You might be surprised how popular mild and crunchy lotus root can be with kids. My kids love this dish, and keep asking whether we have lotus root so we can make some more.

DIRECTIONS

1. Place enough water in a bowl to cover the lotus root and add the vinegar.
2. Peel the lotus root, remove and discard the knobby ends, and slice the root thinly across the width, placing each slice in the vinegar mixture immediately so the lotus root does not discolor.
3. If your sesame seeds aren't already roasted, toast the sesame seeds in a dry skillet over medium heat until golden brown, stirring or shaking frequently, about 5 minutes. Turn off the heat, pour the sesame seeds into a bowl so they don't overcook, and set aside.
4. Heat the sesame oil in a frying pan or wok.
5. Add the ginger and garlic and cook until fragrant (10 seconds to a minute).
6. Drain the lotus root slices, then add them to the wok and cook, stirring frequently and making sure both sides get browned, over medium-high heat until the lotus root slices begin to look translucent, about 3 minutes.
7. Add the white part of the green onion, and cook for another 2 minutes or until the lotus root is done.
8. Add the soy sauce, sesame seeds, and remainder of the green onion and stir well. Serve.

ESPECIALLY GOOD FOR

Anyone suffering from fatigue, dizziness, menopause, diabetes, or the effects of childbirth; individuals who want to slow the graying of hair or hair loss.

FOR THOSE FAMILIAR WITH
TRADITIONAL CHINESE MEDICINE

This dish nourishes the Blood, and strengthens the Spleen and Kidney qi.

DOWN-TO-EARTH BURDOCK ROOT AND CARROT STIR-FRY

MAKES 4 SERVINGS

The crunchy, earthy taste of the burdock root is punctuated by the sweeter carrot. In Japan, this dish is often served with shichimi togarashi *(Japanese seven-spice blend) or crushed red pepper flakes.*

INGREDIENTS

- 1 medium-size burdock root (*niu bang gen* in Chinese, *gobō* in Japanese), chopped (about ½ pound, or 2 cups chopped)
- 1 tablespoon vegetable oil
- 1 tablespoon dark sesame oil
- 2 medium-size carrots (about ¼ pound), cut into matchstick-shape pieces
- 1 tablespoon soy sauce
- 2 tablespoons mirin or dry sherry
- 1 to 2 tablespoons brown sesame seeds, preferably roasted

DIRECTIONS

1. Scrub the burdock root (scrape with the back of a knife if necessary, but avoid peeling) and cut it into matchstick-shape pieces. Place the pieces directly into cold water so they don't discolor.
2. Heat the vegetable and sesame oils in a skillet or wok over medium-high heat. Drain the burdock root, and add it to the pan. Cook, stirring frequently, for about 2 minutes.
3. Add the carrots, and cook, continuing to stir frequently, for about another 5 minutes, or until the vegetables are almost done.
4. Add the soy sauce, mirin, and sesame seeds, and stir well, cooking for another 2 minutes.

Words of Wisdom

For every new food you eat, you gain seven days of life.
—JAPANESE SAYING

Helpful Hints about Burdock Root

When shopping for fresh burdock in an Asian food store, choose firm and crisp roots. They are often hard to miss among the other vegetables because these long, brown roots are often more than three feet long. For those with a garden, burdock root also grows easily from seed in many parts of North America, and can be harvested its first year after two to four months of growth, or in the spring of its second year. If you choose to grow your own, be prepared to exercise your muscles, digging deep to harvest the long root! (For more information on burdock root, see "One Hundred Healthful Asian Ingredients.")

THEMES AND VARIATIONS

If you find julienning the vegetables too exacting, the burdock root and carrots are sometimes cut into shavings, somewhat as you'd make when sharpening a pencil by hand. A more common variation of this recipe includes sugar, but we find that mirin adds enough sweetness to the dish for a balanced taste.

Adding lotus root is another possibility for this stir-fry.

ESPECIALLY GOOD FOR

Anyone who wants to counteract inflammation, infections, or water retention, or prevent atherosclerosis.

FOR THOSE FAMILIAR WITH
TRADITIONAL CHINESE MEDICINE

This dish helps clear toxic Heat and eliminate Dampness.

UMEBOSHI-SESAME ASPARAGUS

MAKES 2 TO 3 SERVINGS

This is a tasty way to enjoy asparagus, with an accent from umeboshi *(pickled red plum), which is popular in Japan as a condiment and a home remedy for digestive problems, infections, hangovers, and colds.*

INGREDIENTS

1 *umeboshi* pickled plum, seeded and chopped finely, or 1 tablespoon *umeboshi* paste

1 clove garlic, peeled and minced

2 tablespoons tahini or other sesame paste

1 teaspoon dark sesame oil

4 teaspoons lemon juice

2 to 4 tablespoons water

¼ teaspoon salt

1 medium-size bunch asparagus (about 1 pound)

Warren Says

As your mother probably told you, eat your vegetables to stay healthy—and she was right! We recommend buying organic produce, not only to avoid consuming harmful pesticides, but also because organic produce is often more nutrient-rich and better tasting than its commercially farmed counterpart, and organic farming is better for the environment. Or try your hand at growing your own vegetables!

DIRECTIONS

1. Combine the *umeboshi*, garlic, tahini, sesame oil, and lemon juice in a small bowl and stir well.
2. Add the water to the mixture 1 tablespoon at a time, stirring, until you have the desired consistency for the dressing.
3. Cut the asparagus into 2-inch pieces, discarding the woody ends of the stalks. Divide the cut asparagus pieces into stalks and tips.
4. Bring 2 to 3 cups of water to a boil (enough to cover the asparagus), then add the salt and asparagus stalks. After about 1 minute, add the asparagus tips. Simmer for about 2 minutes, or until the asparagus stalks are tender.
5. Drain the asparagus and rinse with cold water to preserve the color and stop the cooking.
6. Spoon the dressing over the asparagus, toss, and serve.

THEMES AND VARIATIONS

Another way to serve asparagus is with Creamy Umeboshi Dressing (see page 278).

ESPECIALLY GOOD FOR

Eating during dry weather; serving to individuals who want to regain energy, counteract a dry throat, mouth, or eyes, or soothe throat discomfort.

FOR THOSE FAMILIAR WITH
TRADITIONAL CHINESE MEDICINE

This dish supplements the Lung yin, clears Liver heat, nourishes the Blood and body fluids, and harmonizes the Stomach.

BLACK SESAME ASPARAGUS

MAKES 4 SERVINGS

This healthy vegetable dish is delicious no matter what culture you're from. Sugar is often ground with the sesame seeds in dishes of this sort, but we find that the mirin adds enough sweetness to balance the other flavors.

INGREDIENTS

1 medium-size bunch asparagus (about 1 pound)
A pinch of salt
3 tablespoons black sesame seeds
2 tablespoons mirin or dry sherry
1 tablespoon soy sauce
1 teaspoon lemon juice (optional)

According to Tradition

The Japanese have a special mortar and pestle called a *suribachi* (literally "grinding bowl") to hand grind sesame seeds and other foods and medicines. The inside of the glazed bowl consists of small grooves, and the pestle is made of wood so as not to wear down the ridges. *Suribachi* are available to purchase from Japanese stores and online vendors. (Although food processors don't have the same charm, they can achieve similar results.)

DIRECTIONS

1. Cut the asparagus into 2-inch pieces, discarding the woody ends of the stalk. Divide the cut asparagus pieces into stalks and tips.
2. In a medium-size pot, bring 2 to 3 cups of water to a boil (enough to cover the asparagus), then add the salt and asparagus stalks. After about 1 minute, add the asparagus tips. Lower the heat and simmer for about 2 minutes, or until the asparagus stalks are tender.
3. Drain the asparagus and rinse with cold water to preserve their color and stop the cooking.
4. Toast the sesame seeds in a dry skillet over medium heat, stirring or shaking frequently, about 5 minutes. When they are done, immediately pour them out of the skillet so they don't overcook, and let them cool for at least 1 minute.
5. Place the seeds in a food processor and whir until powdery (or grind by hand in a mortar and pestle).
6. Stir the sesame powder, mirin, soy sauce, and lemon juice (if using) together, then drizzle the mixture over the asparagus before serving.

ESPECIALLY GOOD FOR

Anyone who seeks longevity and facial beauty, who is concerned about preventing cancer, or who wants to counteract hair loss, gray hair, or frequent urination.

FOR THOSE FAMILIAR WITH
TRADITIONAL CHINESE MEDICINE

Here, the black sesame seeds build yin and Blood and moisten the Intestines to counteract constipation, while the asparagus clears Heat and moistens the Lungs.

KOREAN-STYLE BEAN SPROUTS

MAKES 4 TO 6 SERVINGS

Bean sprouts, both mung bean sprouts and soybean sprouts, are a popular vegetable in Asia, grown for thousands of years and especially valued in the winter when other vegetables are scarce. Bean sprouts are a good source of vitamins A, C, and E, as well as protein.

INGREDIENTS

2 teaspoons brown sesame seeds

¾ pound (6 cups) mung bean sprouts (commonly sold as "bean sprouts"), rinsed and drained

1 tablespoon soy sauce

2 tablespoons rice or cider vinegar

2 tablespoons sesame oil

2 cloves garlic, peeled and minced

A pinch of salt

Black or red pepper (optional; omit if you want to maximize the bean sprouts' cooling effects)

THEMES AND VARIATIONS

Bean sprouts are also delicious stir-fried over high heat for about 1 minute.

DIRECTIONS

1. If your sesame seeds aren't already roasted, toast them in a dry skillet over medium heat until golden brown, stirring or shaking frequently, about 5 minutes. Pour them out of the hot skillet into a bowl so they don't overcook. Set aside.

2. Place about 6 cups of water in a medium-size pot (enough to cover the sprouts later), then bring the water to a boil. Turn off the heat and add the sprouts to the pot. Let them sit for 2 to 3 minutes. Drain.

3. In a bowl, make the dressing by mixing together the soy sauce, vinegar, sesame oil, garlic, salt, and pepper (if using).

4. Combine the mung bean sprouts and the sauce, and toss well.

5. Garnish the dish with the sesame seeds. Serve at room temperature or chilled.

ESPECIALLY GOOD FOR

Eating in the summer; serving to individuals who want to slow the aging process or address skin conditions such as acne, boils, and canker sores.

FOR THOSE FAMILIAR WITH
TRADITIONAL CHINESE MEDICINE

Mung bean sprouts clear Heat and increase yang energy.

SOYBEAN SPROUT AND WOOD EAR SALAD

MAKES 2 TO 3 SERVINGS

A healthy, natural vegetarian dish popular in China.

INGREDIENTS

A handful (⅓ ounce, or 10 grams) dried black wood ear (*hei mu er*)

1 small red bell pepper (optional)

2 cups (4 to 5 ounces) fresh soybean sprouts, rinsed

2 tablespoons rice vinegar

2 tablespoons sesame oil

2 to 3 cloves garlic, peeled and minced

1 teaspoon soy sauce

¼ teaspoon honey (optional)

1 to 2 green onions, chopped into ¼-inch pieces, roots and tough ends discarded

Salt

Yuan Says

In many Chinese and Japanese recipes that use soy sauce and/or vinegar, you'll find sugar as an ingredient, although usually only a small amount. The idea is to balance the flavors so the dish doesn't taste too harsh. You can apply the same principle with honey or other natural sweeteners, which were used in the past when sugar was not was not widely available. Today, products labeled "seasoned vinegar" usually include a sweetener, so there is no need to add it separately.

DIRECTIONS

1. Soak the wood ear for 30 minutes in warm water, where it will expand to two to five times its original size. Rinse the wood ear, remove and discard the fibrous base, and cut into ¼-inch strips. Place the wood ear and about 2 cups of water in a pot. Bring to a boil, then lower the heat and simmer for about 3 minutes. Remove the wood ear with a slotted spoon and place the pieces in a large bowl.

2. Seed the red pepper (if using), removing and discarding the stem, and cut it into ¼ by 2-inch pieces. You can leave these raw or cook them in the hot water for about 2 minutes, removing with a slotted spoon. Place the red pepper pieces in the bowl with the wood ear.

3. Place the soybean sprouts in the pot of water and bring to a boil. Lower the heat to a simmer and cook for about 3 minutes, until softened but not soggy. Drain and place the soybean sprouts in the bowl with the wood ear and red pepper.

4. In a small bowl, mix the vinegar, sesame oil, garlic, soy sauce, and honey (if using) together. Warm the mixture if the honey needs help dissolving.

5. In a large bowl, combine the wood ear, soybean sprouts, garlic, red pepper, and green onions. Toss the ingredients with the sauce, and add salt to taste.

6. Ideally, let the dish sit for 30 minutes to let the flavors blend before serving as an appetizer or side dish.

ESPECIALLY GOOD FOR

Anyone with atherosclerosis, high cholesterol, anemia, poor memory, or who wants to build immunity or lose weight. Caution: People with hemorrhagic diseases or pregnant women should avoid eating large quantities of wood ear.

FOR THOSE FAMILIAR WITH TRADITIONAL CHINESE MEDICINE

This dish clears Heat, drains Dampness, nourishes the yin, and moistens the Lungs.

JAPANESE-STYLE GREENS

MAKES 4 SERVINGS

Variations on this delicious and healthy recipe for greens can be found throughout East Asia.

INGREDIENTS

1 large bunch leafy greens, such as spinach or chard, tough stems discarded

A pinch of salt

2 teaspoons dark sesame oil

1 tablespoon rice vinegar

1½ tablespoons soy sauce

1 tablespoon brown sesame seeds

Mika Says

My Japanese grandmother's recipes included greens we don't usually think of eating today, such as green pepper leaves. To me, this is a reminder that in times past people ate what was available from the land and sea. While this posed its own challenges (often including getting enough to eat), the situation also pushed people to eat what we now aspire to in a healthy diet, including fresh seasonal vegetables and a variety of different foods.

DIRECTIONS

1. Fill a large pot with about ½ inch of water and bring to a boil. Add the greens and salt and cook, stirring constantly, until tender. Spinach will take only a couple minutes; other greens may take longer, up to 7 minutes.

2. When the greens are done, drain them and place in cold water to stop the cooking and set the color. Press into a ball to squeeze out the extra water, and slice into ½-inch pieces.

3. In a small bowl, mix together the sesame oil, vinegar, and soy sauce.

4. If your sesame seeds aren't already roasted, toast them in a dry skillet over medium heat until golden brown, stirring or shaking frequently, about 5 minutes. When they are done, remove them from the hot skillet so they don't overcook.

5. Toss the greens with the dressing, and then garnish with the sesame seeds.

ESPECIALLY GOOD FOR

Spinach is especially good for anyone suffering from high blood pressure, headache and dizziness, or the effects of too much alcohol.

FOR THOSE FAMILIAR WITH
TRADITIONAL CHINESE MEDICINE

Spinach, which is sweet and cool, clears Heat, stops bleeding, generates body fluids, and nourishes the Blood. Other greens may have different properties.

SEAWEED–SWEET POTATO SIMMER

MAKES 4 TO 6 SERVINGS

This healthy and tasty combination of land and sea vegetables is simmered Japanese style. We like this dish with spicy Togarashi Topping (see page 282).

INGREDIENTS

⅓ cup dried hijiki seaweed

1½ cups water

2½ tablespoons soy sauce, or to taste

2 tablespoons mirin or dry sherry

2 tablespoons dark sesame oil

1 medium-size sweet potato, (about 1 pound), cut into matchstick-shape pieces

2 tablespoons brown sesame seeds

THEMES AND VARIATIONS

Burdock and carrot can be used instead of sweet potato.

ESPECIALLY GOOD FOR

Anyone who wants to strengthen the body or who is concerned about reducing masses or nodules.

Legend Has It

According to Japanese folklore, hijiki seaweed lends health and beauty to those who consume small amounts regularly, and is responsible for the thick, black, lustrous hair of the Japanese people.

DIRECTIONS

1. Cut or break the hijiki into 1-inch pieces if necessary and place the seaweed into the water to soak for about 20 minutes. Drain the hijiki, reserving the water it was soaked in.

2. Measure 1 cup of the water from soaking the hijiki (which will be most of it), and mix this liquid with the soy sauce and mirin.

3. In a wok or sauté pan, heat the oil over medium-high heat. Add the sweet potatoes and cook, stirring frequently, for 2 to 3 minutes.

4. Add the hijiki to the pan and pour the liquid mixture on top. Stir. Lower the heat, cover, and simmer for about 3 minutes.

5. Uncover and cook for another 5 to 10 minutes, until most of the liquid has been absorbed.

6. Meanwhile, if your sesame seeds aren't already roasted, toast the sesame seeds in a dry skillet over medium heat until golden brown, stirring or shaking frequently, about 5 minutes. When they are done, remove them from the hot pan so they don't burn.

7. Place the vegetables in individual bowls, and sprinkle with sesame seeds before serving.

FOR THOSE FAMILIAR WITH TRADITIONAL CHINESE MEDICINE

Sweet potato supplements the Spleen and Stomach, while seaweed softens areas of hardness.

GINGER–SNOW PEA RICE

MAKES 3 TO 4 SERVINGS

This makes a delicious side dish or a snack, especially for someone recovering from stomach distress.

INGREDIENTS

1 cup uncooked short-grain white rice

1 teaspoon dark sesame oil

1 (1-inch) piece fresh ginger, peeled and grated

2 cups water

½ teaspoon salt, or to taste

¼ pound snow peas (about 1½ cups), strings removed, chopped into ½-inch pieces

---

Words of Wisdom

Let little seem like much, as long as it is fresh, natural, and beautiful.

— JAPANESE PROVERB

DIRECTIONS

1. Rinse the rice (place in a bowl, add cold water, swirl the rice around with your fingers, then drain; repeat until the water runs clear).

2. Heat the sesame oil in a saucepan over medium-high heat. Add the ginger and cook for about 1 minute.

3. Add the rice, water, and salt and bring the mixture to a boil. Lower the heat, cover, and simmer over low heat until the water is mostly absorbed, 10 to 13 minutes.

4. Add the snow peas and cook, covered, for 2 minutes longer.

5. Let the rice sit, covered, for 5 to 10 minutes before serving.

THEMES AND VARIATIONS

This recipe works well using a rice cooker. Sauté the ginger in a pan and add it to the rice cooker before starting, and follow the manufacturer's instructions for the water-to-rice ratio.

ESPECIALLY GOOD FOR

Soothing the digestion, warding off some types of common cold, warming cold hands and feet.

FOR THOSE FAMILIAR WITH
TRADITIONAL CHINESE MEDICINE

Ginger warms the Middle Burner, treats exterior Wind-Cold syndrome, warms the Lungs, and helps eliminate toxicity. Snow peas supplement the qi and nourish Blood.

CHRYSANTHEMUM BROCCOLI

MAKES 4 SERVINGS

This dish presents broccoli with floral overtones and the contrasting texture of the firm, crunchy wood ear.

INGREDIENTS

¾ ounce (20 grams) dried white wood ear (*bai mu er* or *yin er* in Chinese, *hakumokuji* or *shiro kikurage* in Japanese)

3 to 4 tablespoons (10 grams) dried chrysanthemum flowers (*ju hua*)

1 (1-pound) bunch broccoli, cut into bite-size pieces, discarding the stem (or reserving it for a soup stock)

2 tablespoons soy sauce or light soy sauce

2 tablespoons lemon juice

2 tablespoons sesame oil

½ teaspoon honey, maple syrup, or other natural sweetener (optional)

DIRECTIONS

1. Soak the white wood ear and chrysanthemum flowers in warm water for 15 to 20 minutes, then drain. Wash the wood ear, cut off its tough fibrous base, and slice it into ¼-inch wide strips.

2. In a large pot, bring to a boil enough water to cover the ingredients. Add the white wood ear, chrysanthemum flowers, and broccoli, and cook, covered, for 4 to 6 minutes, until the broccoli is tender. Drain the water and let the vegetables cool. Remove the chrysanthemum flowers.

3. In a small bowl, mix together soy sauce, lemon juice, sesame oil, and honey (if using) to make a dressing. (Warm the mixture slightly to help the honey dissolve, if needed.)

4. In a serving bowl, toss the vegetables with the dressing. Serve at room temperature.

THEMES AND VARIATIONS

If you want to avoid picking out the chrysanthemum flowers, you can place them in a tea bag or piece of cheesecloth for easy removal.

If you are strictly avoiding salt, this dish is still tasty with a drizzle of dark sesame oil instead of the dressing made with soy sauce.

ESPECIALLY GOOD FOR

Anyone concerned about preventing cancer or recovering from chemotherapy or radiation therapy; individuals experiencing red eyes, dry skin, acne, headache, or high blood pressure.

FOR THOSE FAMILIAR WITH TRADITIONAL CHINESE MEDICINE

This dish clears Heat and toxic Heat, moistens body fluids, and supplements yin.

BOK CHOY WITH WOOD EAR AND SHIITAKES

MAKES 2 SERVINGS

This delicious stir-fry combines the benefits of mushrooms, wood ears, greens, and herbs. Serve with rice.

INGREDIENTS

½ cup (¾ ounce, or 20 grams) dried black wood ear (*hei mu er* in Chinese, *kikurage* in Japanese)

A pinch of salt

4 medium-size (¾ ounce, or 20 grams dried; ¼ pound fresh) dried or fresh shiitake mushrooms

2 tablespoons sesame oil

1 (½-inch) piece fresh ginger, peeled and minced

1 to 2 cloves garlic, peeled and minced

1 medium-size green onion, chopped into ½-inch pieces, roots and tough tips discarded

1 medium-size cluster bok choy, (about ½ pound), cut into 1 by 2-inch strips grouped by color (white and green parts)

1 teaspoon soy sauce, or to taste

1 tablespoon powdered kudzu, arrowroot, cornstarch, or other thickener

2 tablespoons cold water

DIRECTIONS

1. Place the dried wood ear in a bowl of warm water with the salt and soak for about 30 minutes, or until soft (it will expand to two to five times its original size). If you are using dried shiitake mushrooms, soak them with the wood ear; if you are using fresh shiitakes, simply rinse them.

2. Cut the wood ear and shiitakes into ¼-inch pieces, discarding the fibrous base from the wood ear and, if desired, the stem from the shiitake.

3. Heat the sesame oil in a wok or sauté pan over medium-high heat.

4. Add the ginger, garlic, and green onions, and stir-fry for a few seconds, until fragrant.

5. Add the white stalks of the bok choy and stir-fry for 1 minute, stirring frequently.

6. Add the wood ear, shiitake mushrooms, and leafy part of the bok choy and stir-fry for about 3 minutes, stirring frequently.

7. Cover, lower the heat, and simmer for another 3 minutes, or until the vegetables are done. Stir in the soy sauce.

8. Mix the kudzu with about 2 tablespoons of cold water and stir out the lumps, then add the mixture to the wok. Cook for a minute, stirring, to mix the flavors together and set the thickener, then serve warm.

Fast Facts about Shiitakes

A Chinese farmer Wu San Kuang (sometimes spelled "Wu San Kwang" or "Wu San Kwung") is credited for inventing shiitake mushroom cultivation about one thousand years ago by inoculating with mushroom spores the notches he cut into logs. Today, temples still stand in his honor. (For more information on shiitake mushrooms, see "One Hundred Healthful Asian Ingredients.")

THEMES AND VARIATIONS

This dish can be made with only shiitakes or only wood ear, rather than both. Adjust the amounts accordingly.

ESPECIALLY GOOD FOR

Anyone who wants to replenish energy and stamina, boost immunity, control cholesterol, or counteract constipation. Caution: People with hemorrhagic diseases or pregnant women should avoid eating large quantities of wood ear.

FOR THOSE FAMILIAR WITH TRADITIONAL CHINESE MEDICINE

This dish supplements the qi, nourishes the Blood and yin, clears Heat and toxicity, and lubricates the Intestines.

SESAME CELLOPHANE NOODLES WITH MUSHROOMS AND BOK CHOY

MAKES 4 TO 6 SERVINGS

A version of this healthful dish is popular in Korea, where it is called japchae *(literally "mixture of vegetables"). It is commonly believed that a stir-fry vegetable version of this dish was invented in the 1600s for the Korean king Gwanghaegun. The king was so pleased with the dish that he promoted the liege, Yi Chung, who created it. The cellophane noodles became a key ingredient in this dish in the twentieth century.*

INGREDIENTS

⅓ cup (½ ounce, or 15 grams) dried black wood ear (*hei mu er* in Chinese, *kikurage* in Japanese)

5 dried shiitake mushrooms (1 ounce)

3 (2-ounce) bundles cellophane noodles, mung bean preferred

4 tablespoons sesame oil

3 cloves garlic, peeled and minced

1 (1-inch) piece fresh ginger, peeled and minced

1 small onion, diced

1 large carrot, cut into matchstick-shape pieces

2 clusters baby bok choy, or ¾ pound regular bok choy or Chinese cabbage, cut into ¼-inch strips

2 tablespoons mirin or dry sherry

3 to 4 tablespoons soy sauce, or to taste

2 tablespoons sesame seeds

Pepper (optional)

DIRECTIONS

1. Soak the wood ear for 30 minutes in warm water, where it will expand to two to five times its original size. Rinse the wood ear, remove and discard the fibrous base, and cut into 1 by ¼-inch strips.

2. Soak the dried shiitakes in warm water for 20 minutes, or until soft. Drain, reserving the water for later use. Squeeze the excess liquid from the mushrooms and, if desired, discard the stems. Cut the mushrooms into ¼-inch slices

3. Soak the noodles in a bowl of hot water for about 15 minutes, or until soft. Drain and cut the noodles into 3-inch pieces with scissors or a knife.

4. In a large wok or sauté pan, heat 2 tablespoons of the sesame oil over medium-high heat. Add the garlic, ginger, and onions, and stir-fry for about 2 minutes.

5. Add the carrot, then the bok choy. Continue to stir-fry for about 5 minutes, until the vegetables are cooked.

6. Mix together a sauce from ½ cup of the water from soaking the mushrooms, mirin, soy sauce, and the remaining 2 tablespoons of sesame oil.

7. Add the noodles to the wok, then pour in the sauce. Stir. Continue cooking until the noodles have been heated and the liquid has been absorbed, 5 to 10 minutes.

8. In the meantime, toast the sesame seeds in a dry skillet over medium heat until golden brown, stirring or shaking frequently, about 5 minutes. When they are done, remove them immediately from the hot skillet so they don't burn.

9. Sprinkle the sesame seeds on top of the noodles and add pepper (if using) to taste.

THEMES AND VARIATIONS

You can use fresh shiitakes instead of dried, substituting *dashi* or vegetable stock for the mushroom water in step 6.

ESPECIALLY GOOD FOR

Anyone with diabetes, cancer, high cholesterol, or constipation. Caution: People with hemorrhagic diseases or pregnant women should avoid eating large quantities of wood ear.

FOR THOSE FAMILIAR WITH TRADITIONAL CHINESE MEDICINE

This dish clears Heat, moves Blood, and regulates the Middle Burner.

MUSHROOM BROWN RICE

MAKES 2 TO 3 SERVINGS

Mushrooms and brown rice—what more could you ask for? In Japan, mushroom rice, kinoko gohan, is a popular side dish that can feature a wonderful variety of different mushrooms, cultivated and wild.

INGREDIENTS

1 cup uncooked short-grain brown rice

2 cups cold water

2 (⅓ ounce dried, or 2 ounces fresh) dried or fresh shiitake mushrooms

1 piece kombu seaweed, about 4 by 8 inches (optional)

½ cup (2 ounces) fresh mushrooms (enoki, maitake, oyster, another variety, or a mixture), cleaned and sliced, stems discarded if desired

1 (½-inch) piece fresh ginger, peeled and grated or minced

1 tablespoon soy sauce

1 tablespoon sake

¼ teaspoon salt (optional)

DIRECTIONS

1. Rinse the brown rice (place in a bowl, add cold water, swirl the rice around with your fingers, then drain; repeat until the water runs clear), then place the rice in a pot with the 2 cups of fresh cold water. Let the rice soak for 1 hour.

2. If you are using dried shiitakes, in a separate bowl soak them in warm water with the kombu seaweed (if using, to give the mushrooms extra flavor), for about 20 minutes, or until the mushrooms are soft; then, discard the kombu (or reserve for another use) and drain the mushrooms. If you are using fresh shiitakes, simply rinse. Cut the shiitakes into ¼-inch slices, cutting off and discarding the stem, if desired.

3. Add the mushrooms, ginger, soy sauce, sake, and salt (if using) to the pot with the rice.

4. Cover, bring the mixture to a boil, then lower the heat to low and simmer for about 30 minutes, or until the water is absorbed and the rice is mostly cooked.

5. Turn off the heat and let the rice stand for another 10 minutes before serving.

THEMES AND VARIATIONS

This dish works well by combining all the ingredients in a rice cooker and following the manufacturer's guidelines for the rice-to-water ratio.

ESPECIALLY GOOD FOR

Anyone who wants to build immunity or ward off cancer, reduce high cholesterol or high blood pressure, or address a skin rash.

FOR THOSE FAMILIAR WITH TRADITIONAL CHINESE MEDICINE

This dish strengthens the qi, nourishes the Blood, strengthens the Spleen, drains Dampness, and benefits the skin.

A Story of Unintended Consequences

In one tale from China, a young woman married into a well-to-do family. When she moved in with the family and her husband, as was traditional, she hoped her situation would improve from her original poverty-stricken surroundings. Unfortunately, her mother-in-law took a strong dislike to the young woman. Not only was she expected to do the most difficult work in the household, she was left to consume brown rice instead of the beautiful refined white rice enjoyed by the others. Strangely enough, however, the rest of the family became ill with symptoms later associated with beriberi, caused by a lack of vitamin B_1. The young woman was the only one who remained strong and healthy, thanks to the brown rice in her diet. While today white rice is supplemented with B vitamins, brown rice still offers a strong nutritional profile, including fiber. In terms of traditional Chinese medicine, brown rice is seen as especially good for the Spleen and Kidneys, whereas white rice focuses on the Spleen and Stomach. (For more information on rice, see "One Hundred Healthful Asian Ingredients.")

TRIPLE-MUSHROOM MÉLANGE

MAKES 2 TO 3 SERVINGS

This dish is a mushroom lover's delight. In Asia, mushrooms are traditionally associated with longevity.

INGREDIENTS

½ cup (2 to 3 ounces) fresh enoki mushrooms

2 to 3 (2 to 3 ounces) large fresh shiitake mushrooms

½ cup (2 to 3 ounces) fresh king oyster mushrooms or other fresh mushrooms

2 tablespoons olive oil

2 cloves garlic, peeled and minced

1 cup vegetable broth

1 tablespoon powdered kudzu, arrowroot, cornstarch, or other thickener

2 tablespoons water

Salt

DIRECTIONS

1. Wash the mushrooms, remove and discard any tough stems, and slice into ½-inch pieces.
2. Heat the olive oil in a pan, then add the garlic. Sauté for about 30 seconds, until the garlic becomes fragrant.
3. Add the mushrooms and sauté for 2 minutes.
4. Add the vegetable broth, and cook, loosely covered, for another 8 minutes.
5. In a small bowl, mix the kudzu with the 2 tablespoons of water to remove any lumps, then add the mixture to the pan. Stir well, add salt to taste, then serve.

ESPECIALLY GOOD FOR

Anyone with high cholesterol, high blood pressure, or concerns about preventing cancer or increasing immunity.

FOR THOSE FAMILIAR WITH
TRADITIONAL CHINESE MEDICINE

Mushrooms are thought to benefit the five internal organs, strengthen the qi, nourish the Blood, help the digestive system, and calm the spirit.

Helpful Hints about Enoki Mushrooms

When shopping for enoki mushrooms, which can be recognized by their long, slender stems and tiny caps, look for specimens with firm, white, shiny caps, and avoid those with brownish stalks. Before cooking, rinse the mushrooms and cut off the roots at the base of the cluster. (For more information on mushrooms, see "One Hundred Healthful Asian Ingredients.")

MOVE-THE-QI DAIKON SALAD

MAKES 4 TO 6 SERVINGS

Variations of this easy, pungent salad are found across Asia. In Japan, daikon-carrot salad is a traditional New Year's dish.

INGREDIENTS

1 cup daikon (white radish) cut into matchstick-shape pieces

1 small carrot, cut into matchstick-shape pieces

3 tablespoons rice vinegar

¼ to ½ teaspoon honey or other natural sweetener (optional)

1 teaspoon sesame oil

Salt

Grated zest of 1 lemon or small orange

DIRECTIONS

1. Toss the daikon and carrot together in a serving bowl.
2. In a separate small bowl or pot, combine the vinegar with the honey (if using) and stir. (Briefly heat the vinegar to help the sweetener dissolve, if desired). If you opt not to use a sweetener, use the vinegar by itself.
3. Pour the sweetened vinegar and sesame oil on top of the vegetables and mix well. Season with salt to taste.
4. Let the mixture marinate for 20 to 30 minutes.
5. Garnish the salad with the grated citrus zest before serving.

THEMES AND VARIATIONS

One common option is to salt the julienned daikon and carrots, let them sit for 10 minutes, then rinse them before soaking in the vinegar; this will soften the vegetables and mellow the taste of the daikon, but may make the salad saltier.

For a more targeted therapeutic alternative for those trying to quit smoking or who are bothered by a phlegmy cough, try a simple daikon and dried tangerine peel salad. In this case, soak the dried tangerine peel for 15 minutes, drain, then add to the julienned daikon and toss with dressing. Anyone who is trying to kick the smoking habit can eat one small portion of the salad every day. Consider making a big batch and keeping it in the refrigerator for up to a week. You might find that cigarettes just don't taste as good as they used to.

ESPECIALLY GOOD FOR

Anyone with a tendency toward indigestion, who has a wet cough, or who is trying to quit smoking.

FOR THOSE FAMILIAR WITH TRADITIONAL CHINESE MEDICINE

This dish helps move qi, counteract food stagnation, and clear phlegm from the Lungs.

KOREAN FIVE-GRAIN RICE

MAKES 6 TO 8 SERVINGS

This dish, known as ogokbap *or* chapgokbap *in Korea, is traditionally eaten on the holiday known as Jeongwol Daeboreum, which celebrates the first full moon after the New Year. Traditionally served with a variety of fruits and nuts and considered somewhat of a national health food, the dish symbolizes a rich harvest in the year to come, as well as the five good things in life—longevity, wealth, good health, children, and a peaceful death. Consider serving* ogokbap *with Korean kimchi.*

INGREDIENTS

¼ cup dried black soybeans

¼ cup dried red beans

3½ cups water (plus extra for soaking)

¼ teaspoon salt

¼ cup (60 grams) pearl barley or coix (Job's tears, *yi yi ren* in Chinese, *hato mugi* in Japanese, *yulmu* in Korean)

1 cup uncooked short-grain white rice

¼ cup millet

¼ cup pine nuts

DIRECTIONS

1. Rinse the black and red beans, then place them in a large saucepan. Cover with water and bring to a boil. Boil over high heat for 1 minute. Remove from the heat, cover, and let it sit for 1 hour to soften.

2. Drain the beans, rinse them, drain again, and place 3½ cups of fresh water and the salt in the saucepan. Bring the beans to a boil, uncovered, then lower the heat, cover, and simmer for 45 minutes.

3. Stir the barley into the pot and cook the mixture, covered, for 10 minutes.

4. In the meantime, in a separate bowl, place the rice in water to soak.

5. After the barley has cooked for its 10 minutes, stir in the millet and cook, covered, for another 20 minutes.

6. Drain the rice, then add the rice to the pot and cook for about 25 minutes, covered, or until the mixture is tender. Add more water during this time if necessary (there should usually be ¼ to ½ inch of water over the rice; if you add more water, bring the water to a boil before lowering the heat to a simmer).

7. Place the pine nuts in a dry skillet over medium-high heat and toast until golden and fragrant, 3 to 5 minutes. Sprinkle the pine nuts over the rice as a garnish before serving.

THEMES AND VARIATIONS

The exact combination of grains in this dish varies from region to region, although the rice is a constant.

If you are a fan of brown rice (as we are), try this dish with short-grain brown rice. In this case, here are step-by step directions:

1. Rinse the black and red beans, then place them in a large saucepan. Cover with water and bring to a boil. Boil over high heat for 1 minute. Remove from the heat, cover, and let it sit for 1 hour to soften.

2. Drain the beans, rinse them, drain again, and place 3¾ cups of fresh water and the salt in the pot. Around this time, put the rice on to soak.

3. Bring the beans to a boil, then lower the heat and simmer, covered, for 45 minutes.

4. Stir the barley into the pot and cook the mixture, covered, for 10 minutes. After the barley has cooked for its 10 minutes, stir in the millet.

5. Drain the rice and stir it into the mixture. Cook, covered, for another 45 minutes, or until the mixture is tender. Check frequently toward the end to make sure it doesn't burn. (Add a few tablespoons of hot water if the rice looks as if it is drying out and might start crusting over the bottom of the pot; if you have inadvertently added too much water, cook with the lid off for several minutes, to let the moisture escape.)

6. Place the pine nuts in a dry skillet over medium-high heat and toast until golden and fragrant, 3 to 5 minutes. Sprinkle the pine nuts over the rice as a garnish before serving.

Warren Says

People watching their budget will appreciate the fact that beans are an extremely cost-effective (as well as delicious and nutritious) source of protein. In general, saving money is quite compatible with eating healthy food. The key to both is starting from whole, natural ingredients and cooking for yourself, rather than relying on prepared food.

ESPECIALLY GOOD FOR

Anyone who wants to build sustained energy, help memory, retard hair loss, or address insomnia.

FOR THOSE FAMILIAR WITH TRADITIONAL CHINESE MEDICINE

This dish strengthens the Spleen and addresses diarrhea and unwanted weight loss due to Spleen deficiency, as well as strengthening the Kidneys.

BLACK AND WHITE WOOD EAR TOFU

MAKES 4 SERVINGS

Don't be intimidated by the wood ear, which is sold dried in Asian grocery stores. It is a relatively neutral-tasting ingredient that adds color and a pleasant, firm texture, here set off by the smooth, creamy tofu.

INGREDIENTS

½ ounce (15 grams) dried black wood ear (*hei mu er* in Chinese, *kikurage* in Japanese)

½ ounce (15 grams) dried white wood ear (*bai mu er* or *yin er* in Chinese, *hakumokuji* or *shiro kikurage* in Japanese)

2 tablespoons olive oil

2 cloves garlic, peeled and minced

1 (15- to 19-ounce) package firm tofu, cut into 1-inch cubes

1¼ cups vegetable or chicken broth

¼ cup fresh cilantro leaves

Salt

Condiments: Black pepper, hot chili oil, or *togarashi* (For a recipe, see page 282.)

DIRECTIONS

1. Soak the black and white wood ear for 30 minutes in warm water, where it will expand to two to five times its original size. Rinse the wood ear, remove and discard the fibrous base, and cut into ¼-inch strips.

2. Heat the oil in a medium-size pan over medium heat, then add the garlic. Cook for about 30 seconds until fragrant.

3. Add the wood ear and cook, stirring occasionally, for 3 to 5 minutes.

4. Add the tofu, then the broth. Bring to a boil, then lower the heat and simmer, covered, for 5 minutes.

5. Add salt to taste (the amount will vary depending on the stock you use; people with high blood pressure will want to minimize salt use), garnish with cilantro, and serve with condiments.

ESPECIALLY GOOD FOR

Anyone with high cholesterol or high blood pressure, or individuals who want to prevent atherosclerosis.

FOR THOSE FAMILIAR WITH TRADITIONAL CHINESE MEDICINE

This dish addresses qi and Blood deficiency, as well as nourishing yin.

SPICY CUCUMBER AND WOOD EAR SALAD

MAKES 3 SERVINGS

This dish, which can be served as an appetizer or side dish, hails from Sichuan province, an area renowned for its excellent (and spicy) food.

INGREDIENTS

⅓ ounce (10 grams) dried black wood ear (*hei mu er* in Chinese, *kikurage* in Japanese)

1 (1 by 1⅓-inch) bunch (about 2 ounces) enoki mushrooms

1 cucumber

⅓ teaspoon salt, or to taste

2 teaspoons soy sauce, or to taste

1 tablespoon rice vinegar or lemon juice

⅓ teaspoon chili oil, or 3 small fresh hot peppers, or dried Sichuan or chili peppers to taste

⅓ teaspoon honey (optional)

2 tablespoons dark sesame oil

2 cloves garlic, peeled and minced

ESPECIALLY GOOD FOR

Anyone concerned about high cholesterol, diabetes, cancer, or menopause.

DIRECTIONS

1. Soak the wood ear for 30 minutes in warm water, where it will expand to two to five times its original size. Rinse the wood ear, remove and discard the fibrous base, and cut into ¼-inch strips. Cut off the root of the enoki mushrooms (about 1 inch from the bottom), separate the mushrooms, then wash and drain them.

2. In a small saucepan, bring 2 cups of water to a boil. Add the wood ear and cook over medium heat for 2 to 3 minutes, until they have softened. Remove with a slotted spoon.

3. Add the enoki mushrooms and cook for 3 to 4 minutes, until soft. Drain.

4. Peel the cucumber, cut it in half lengthwise, and scoop out the seeds. Slice the cucumber, widthwise, into thin pieces and sprinkle them with salt.

5. In a small bowl, mix together the ingredients for the sauce—soy sauce, rice vinegar, chili oil, honey (if using), sesame oil, and garlic. Heat the mixture briefly if the honey needs help dissolving.

6. Combine the wood ear, cucumbers, and enoki mushrooms in a bowl, then pour the sauce on top. Toss well.

FOR THOSE FAMILIAR WITH
TRADITIONAL CHINESE MEDICINE

This dish nourishes yin, generates fluids, and drains Dampness.

Legend Has It

One story tells of a student who was eager to graduate from his study of herbs. His teacher said, "Bring me an herb that is not medicinal and you can be done." At first the student felt quite fortunate, but after a few days he came back empty-handed and sadly told his teacher, "I'm afraid I will never be able to graduate." When the teacher asked why, he replied, "I have looked all over, at many trees and grasses, and although I cannot name all of them, I have not been able to find a single one that is not medicinal." The teacher laughed and said, "Good, now you are done with your studies."

MISO-TAHINI GREEN BEANS

MAKES 3 SERVINGS

This dish makes it easy to eat your vegetables. Although tahini is often associated with Middle Eastern cuisine, it is similar to traditional East Asian sesame paste and is more widely available in the West. For those who prefer a version made with the entire sesame seed rather than the hulled kernel, opt for the Asian variety (commonly available at Asian food stores) or tahini specifically labeled as made from whole seeds (available from natural food stores).

INGREDIENTS

2 tablespoons tahini or other
 sesame paste
1 tablespoon lemon juice
1 tablespoon white miso
1 clove garlic, peeled and minced
2 tablespoons water, or to taste
¾ pound green beans, cut into
 1½-inch pieces
A pinch of salt

DIRECTIONS

1. Mix the tahini, lemon juice, white miso, garlic, and water together in a small bowl and stir until the mixture becomes a smooth paste. This may take a few minutes

2. Bring a pot of water to a boil. Add the green beans and the salt. Cook, uncovered, over medium heat for about 5 minutes, or until done. Drain.

3. Spoon the dressing over the beans, toss well, and serve.

ESPECIALLY GOOD FOR

Promoting sustained energy and longevity, addressing conditions such as high cholesterol, high blood pressure, and puffy joints.

FOR THOSE FAMILIAR WITH TRADITIONAL CHINESE MEDICINE

Here, the green beans strengthen qi and nourish Blood; the sesame nourishes the Blood and generates body fluids; the miso and lemon harmonize the Middle Burner; and the garlic warms the Stomach, strengthens the Spleen, and moves the qi.

Warren Says

I once had a patient who said his idea of eating vegetables was the lettuce on a Big Mac. Unfortunately, his health reflected that attitude.

Yuan Says

In China, I used to enjoy shopping for vegetables according to the season. It was an art. When a vegetable such as beans first appeared in the markets, it was usually expensive because it was the first of the crop—but we hadn't seen it for a while, so we all looked forward to eating it. Then it became a kind of game: should we buy it today or wait until the price drops a little more? In the United States, the vegetables in the supermarket are the same all year round. It's nice that they are accessible, but unfortunately we become disconnected from the natural cycles of the seasons. And don't fruit and vegetables taste so much better when they are fresh and in season?

GARLIC GREEN BEANS

MAKES 2 TO 3 SERVINGS

In this dish, a garlicky sauce enlivens the more subtle flavor of the familiar green bean or more exotic Asian long bean (which commonly reaches 18 inches in length and can grow well past that).

INGREDIENTS

2 tablespoons rice vinegar

2 tablespoons soy sauce

2 teaspoons rice wine or dry sherry

¼ to ½ teaspoon chili oil or chili sauce

2 teaspoons dark sesame oil

2 tablespoons vegetable oil, such as canola or olive oil

3 to 4 medium-size garlic cloves, peeled and minced (about 4 teaspoons)

¾ pound green beans or long beans, washed, ends trimmed, and cut into 1- to 2-inch pieces

2 teaspoons powdered kudzu, arrowroot, cornstarch, or other thickener

1 tablespoon water

Fast Facts about Garlic

Garlic appears in ancient writings of the Chinese, Egyptians, Babylonians, and Indians as far back as five thousand years ago, and has been used medicinally in many cultures throughout its long history. Garlic's antibacterial activity is widely accepted, and it was used as an antiseptic by the Russian soldiers fighting on the front line during World War I. (For more information on garlic, see "One Hundred Healthful Asian Ingredients.")

DIRECTIONS

1. Stir together the rice vinegar, soy sauce, rice wine, chili oil, and sesame oil in a small bowl.
2. Heat the vegetable oil in a skillet or wok over medium heat, then add the garlic. Cook until fragrant (about 30 seconds).
3. Add the green beans and stir-fry for about 5 minutes, or until cooked.
4. Add to the pan the mixture of seasonings from step 1. Cook over low heat for about a minute to reduce the liquid.
5. In a separate small bowl, dissolve the kudzu in a tablespoon of cold water, stirring to get rid of the lumps.
6. Add the kudzu to the pan and stir. Serve!

ESPECIALLY GOOD FOR

Anyone who wants to help blood circulation, increase appetite, or relieve stress.

FOR THOSE FAMILIAR WITH TRADITIONAL CHINESE MEDICINE

The sauce reflects garlic's ability to warm the Stomach, strengthen the Spleen, promote the movement of qi, reduce stagnation, and counteract toxicity, while green beans supplement the qi and nourish the Blood.

BALANCING BITTER MELON EGGS

MAKES 1 TO 2 SERVINGS

Bitter melon is somewhat of an acquired taste, even in Asia. This vegetable is indeed quite bitter, but some people love it. Are you one of them? In this dish, the eggs and garlic round out the bitter flavor.

INGREDIENTS

1 medium-size (8-inch-long) bitter
   melon (*ku gua* in Chinese, *goya*
   in Japanese)
2 eggs
1 tablespoon soy sauce
A pinch of white pepper
2 tablespoons vegetable oil, such
   as canola or olive oil
2 cloves garlic, peeled and minced
Salt (optional)

DIRECTIONS

1. Cut the bitter melon in half lengthwise and scoop out the seeds with a spoon. Cut it in half lengthwise again, then slice into ¼-inch pieces across its width.

2. In a separate bowl, beat the eggs, adding the soy sauce and pepper.

3. Heat the oil in a skillet until hot, then add the garlic and bitter melon slices. Sauté for about 3 minutes, until the melon begins to soften.

4. Pour the eggs into the pan and let them set and slightly brown on one side (about 30 seconds), then flip them over to the other side to finish cooking (about a minute). Add salt to taste.

Words of Wisdom

Sour, sweet, bitter, pungent: all must be tasted.

—CHINESE PROVERB

Helpful Hints about Bitter Melon

Bitter melon, a vegetable that often looks like a bumpy cucumber, appears in East Asian, Southeast Asian, and Indian cuisine and can be found fresh in most Asian grocery stores. (For more information on bitter melon, see "One Hundred Healthful Asian Ingredients.")

THEMES AND VARIATIONS

Feel free to add other vegetables, such as onions and tomatoes, or herbs, such as goji berries. Some people simply sauté the bitter melon in some oil with garlic, and leave out the egg. If you want to mellow the bitter taste, you can boil it in water for a few minutes before sautéing.

ESPECIALLY GOOD FOR

Anyone with a skin rash, acne, heartburn, or concerns about diabetes, high blood sugar, or high cholesterol. Caution: Avoid eating bitter melon if you are trying to conceive.

FOR THOSE FAMILIAR WITH
TRADITIONAL CHINESE MEDICINE

This dish counteracts Heat and Damp Heat, and promotes urination to reduce edema (swelling).

Yuan Says

One of the touchstones of traditional Chinese medicine is the idea of balance among the five *zang fu*, or internal organs, and the five tastes of food (sour, bitter, sweet, spicy, and salty) for a healthy body. In our diet, we often miss this bitter flavor, linked to the Heart. Bitter melon can help fill in this gap.

PAN-FRIED BITTER MELON AND POTATOES

MAKES 4 SERVINGS

Although bitter melon is an acquired taste, some people swear by it. Here, the turmeric provides an interesting accent for both the bitter melon and potatoes.

INGREDIENTS

1 medium-size bitter melon (*ku gua* in Chinese, *goya* in Japanese)
2 tablespoons vegetable oil, such as canola or olive oil
2 teaspoons turmeric
2 cloves garlic, peeled and minced
1 medium-size onion, cut into ½-inch chunks
2 medium-size potatoes, cut into ½-inch chunks
Salt

DIRECTIONS

1. Cut the bitter melon in half lengthwise and scoop out the seeds with a spoon. Cut it in half lengthwise again, then slice into ½-inch pieces across its width.
2. Heat the oil in a large sauté pan, then add the turmeric, then the garlic, onions, potatoes, and bitter melon.
3. Cook, covered, over medium heat, stirring occasionally, for about 20 minutes, or until the potatoes are cooked through. Add salt to taste.

ESPECIALLY GOOD FOR

Anyone with a skin rash, acne, heartburn, or concerns about diabetes or high blood sugar. Caution: Avoid eating bitter melon if you are trying to conceive.

FOR THOSE FAMILIAR WITH
TRADITIONAL CHINESE MEDICINE

This dish counteracts Heat and Damp Heat, and promotes urination to reduce edema (swelling).

Yuan Says

Another way to consume bitter melon is by juicing it with other fruits and vegetables; this mellows the bitter flavor so it isn't dominant, while still providing benefits from the vegetable. In a juicer, try combining ¼ bitter melon (peeled and seeded), with ½ apple, 1 stalk of celery, ½ tomato, and ½ carrot. Or combine a piece of bitter melon with ½ carrot, ½ green bell pepper, ½ cup of pomegranate fruit, and 1 fig. Or juice part of a bitter melon with ½ cup of blueberries, ½ kiwi, 1 stalk of celery, and ½ carrot. In general, juicing a combination of fruits and vegetables is popular among my Chinese friends to promote health and fight off such conditions as high cholesterol, high blood pressure, diabetes, and cancer. You can make the juices in large batches and freeze them in convenient serving sizes.

LEEK AND WAKAME WITH MISO SAUCE

MAKES 2 TO 4 SERVINGS

This simple side dish blends flavors from the sea and the land. Although maple syrup is not a traditional sweetener in Asian cooking, it has become quite popular in Japan and is often called for in macrobiotic cooking.

INGREDIENTS

3 to 4 tablespoons (½ to ¾ ounce) dried pre-cut wakame seaweed

2 leeks, washed well and cut into ½-inch pieces

2 tablespoons white miso

½ teaspoon pure maple syrup or other natural sweetener (optional)

½ teaspoon wasabi paste

2 tablespoons rice vinegar

2 teaspoons unhulled brown sesame seeds

DIRECTIONS

1. Soak the wakame in water for about 5 minutes. It will expand greatly.
2. Boil about 2 cups of water (or however much is necessary to cover the leeks) in a medium-size saucepan. Place the leeks in the pot, cover, and cook for 3 to 4 minutes. Drain and let cool.
3. To make the dressing, in a separate bowl, combine the miso, maple syrup (if using), wasabi, and rice vinegar and stir until smooth.
4. Mix together the leeks and wakame, then toss with the dressing.
5. Toast the sesame seeds in a skillet over medium heat until golden brown, stirring or shaking frequently, about 5 minutes; remove them from the skillet when they are done so they don't burn.
6. Garnish the leeks and wakame with the toasted sesame seeds before serving.

ESPECIALLY GOOD FOR

Anyone with high cholesterol, high blood pressure, masses or soft swellings (such as goiter, ovarian cysts, breast lumps, or lymph node swelling), or a skin rash.

FOR THOSE FAMILIAR WITH
TRADITIONAL CHINESE MEDICINE

This dish transforms phlegm, drains Dampness, and aids digestion.

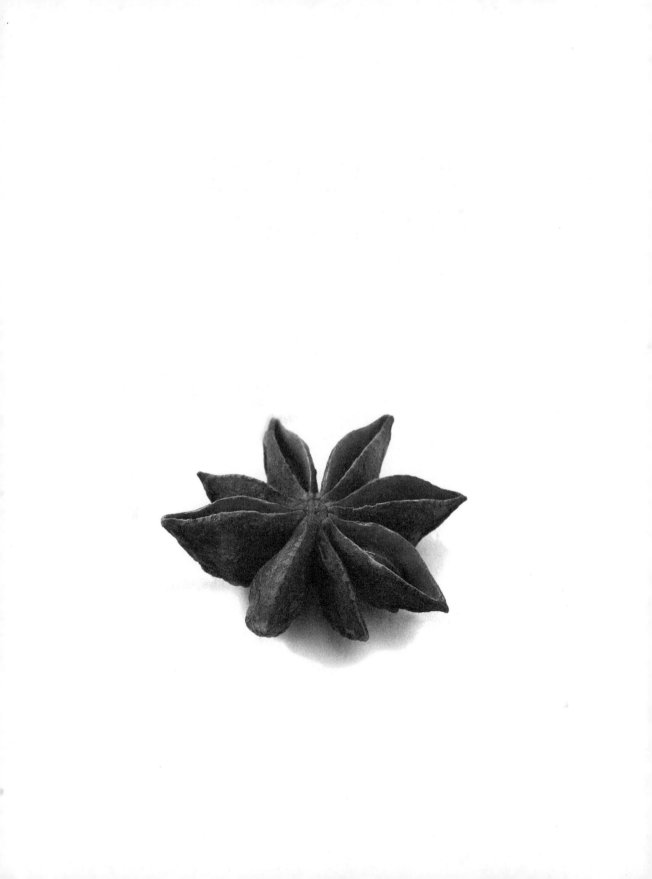

MARVELOUS MAIN DISHES

养生之道

Whatever the father of disease,

its mother is wrong food.

—CHINESE PROVERB

SOOTHING SHRIMP WITH ASPARAGUS AND GOJI BERRIES

MAKES 2 SERVINGS

The delicate flavors of this dish—one of our favorites—will comfort and nourish you.

INGREDIENTS

2 tablespoons goji berries
  (*gou qi zi*)
3 tablespoons rice wine
2 tablespoons sesame oil
1 (½-inch) piece fresh ginger,
  peeled and minced
2 cloves garlic, peeled and minced
¾ to 1 pound medium-size shrimp,
  shelled and deveined
1 pound asparagus, cut into 1-inch
  pieces, hard, white ends
  discarded
2 teaspoons powdered kudzu,
  arrowroot, cornstarch, or other
  thickener
1½ tablespoons water
1 tablespoon soy sauce, or to taste

Helpful Hints about Goji Berries

When shopping for goji berries—which are now widely available not only at Asian markets, but also at natural food stores and even some regular supermarkets—look for dried fruit that still looks plump, and avoid any produce that is bright orange-red, which might be an indication of artificial coloring. (For more information on goji berries, see "One Hundred Healthful Asian Ingredients.")

DIRECTIONS

1. Cover goji berries with the rice wine and marinate for 30 minutes or longer.
2. In a wok or skillet, heat 1 tablespoon of the sesame oil over medium-high heat.
3. Add the ginger and garlic and cook until fragrant, 30 to 60 seconds.
4. Add the shrimp and stir-fry for about 3 minutes, or until cooked through. Transfer the shrimp to a bowl and set aside.
5. While the pan is still hot, add another tablespoon of sesame oil to the pan, then add the asparagus stalks and stir-fry for about a minute. Then add the asparagus tips and stir-fry for another 3 minutes, or until the asparagus is cooked through.
6. Add the shrimp, goji berries, and 2 tablespoons of the wine the goji berries were soaked in.
7. Mix the kudzu in a small bowl with a little cold water to avoid clumping, then add it to the pan and stir well.
8. Add soy sauce to taste and serve with rice.

THEMES AND VARIATIONS
This dish is also terrific with scallops instead of shrimp.

ESPECIALLY GOOD FOR
Anyone experiencing fatigue, dizziness, menopause, night sweats, diabetes, blurred vision, or depression.

FOR THOSE FAMILIAR WITH TRADITIONAL CHINESE MEDICINE
This dish strengthens the Liver and Kidneys, clears Heat from yin deficiency, and strengthens muscles and tendons.

WASABI FISH COOKED IN SAKE

MAKES 2 SERVINGS

This dish, suitable for company, offsets the mild tastes of fish and sake with a hint of pungent wasabi, which is sometimes called Japanese horseradish.

INGREDIENTS

1 to 2 tablespoons dark sesame oil
1 (1-inch) piece fresh ginger, peeled and minced
2 cloves garlic, peeled and minced
2 to 3 fillets mahi mahi or other mild fish
1 teaspoon soy sauce
½ teaspoon wasabi paste
3 tablespoons sake

DIRECTIONS

1. Heat the sesame oil in a skillet over medium heat, and add the ginger and garlic. Cook until fragrant, 30 to 60 seconds.
2. Add the fish, and cook for 2 to 3 minutes (depending on the thickness of the fillets) on each side.
3. In the meantime, in a small bowl, mix together the soy sauce, wasabi, and sake.
4. When the fish has cooked, pour the liquid over the fish, turning to distribute the sauce.
5. Cook for about 1 minute, or until the fish is done and the liquid is reduced.

ESPECIALLY GOOD FOR

Anyone with cold hands and feet, premenstrual syndrome, or abdominal distention.

FOR THOSE FAMILIAR WITH
TRADITIONAL CHINESE MEDICINE

This dish supplements and regulates the qi, warms the yang, and relieves Cold stagnation.

Fast Facts about Sake

Sake, a type of rice wine, has a long history as a part of festivals, ceremonies, and social gatherings in Japan, where it is usually served warm in tiny porcelain cups. It also has an important role in traditional Japanese cooking. In Japan, sake symbolizes the miracle of nature, as well as abundance and wealth. The Koreans have a rice wine similar to sake, known as *jeongju*. The Chinese have the slightly less sweet Shaoxing wine (named after its region of origin), which is also served warm in small cups and is used extensively in cooking. *Jeongju*, Shaoxing wine, or vermouth can be substituted for sake in recipes.

SPRING SEAFOOD STEW

MAKES 2 TO 3 SERVINGS

If you like seafood, you'll love the subtle flavors of this dish. Use whatever combination of your favorite seafood you prefer.

INGREDIENTS

2 tablespoons vegetable oil, such olive or canola

1 pound assorted fish, shelled and deveined shrimp, sea scallops, and/or other seafood, fish deboned and cut into 1- to 2-inch cubes

1 (1-inch) piece fresh ginger, peeled and minced

3 medium-size green onions, chopped into ¼-inch pieces, grouped into green and white parts, roots and tough tips discarded

½ pound asparagus, cut into 1-inch pieces, tough, white stem discarded

1 cup white wine

A pinch of salt

1½ tablespoons powdered kudzu, arrowroot, cornstarch, or other thickener

3 tablespoons water

Lemon wedges or lemon juice (optional)

DIRECTIONS

1. Heat the oil in a pan, then sauté the seafood, ginger, and the white part of the green onions for 3 minutes, or until the seafood is browned.

2. Add the asparagus, wine, and salt. Cover, bring back to a boil, then simmer over low heat for about 3 more minutes, until the asparagus and seafood are cooked through.

3. Mix the kudzu in a small bowl with a little cold water to avoid clumping, then add it to the pot and stir well. Add to the pan, stir, and cook for another minute so the thickener sets.

4. Sprinkle the dish with the green portion of the green onion, add salt to taste, then serve with lemon wedges, if desired.

ESPECIALLY GOOD FOR

Eating when the weather is changing from cool to warmer; also, serving to anyone with a cough, sore throat, or discomfort in the area of the ribs.

FOR THOSE FAMILIAR WITH
TRADITIONAL CHINESE MEDICINE

This dish strengthens the qi, regulates Liver qi, moistens the Lungs, clears Heat, and calms the spirit.

Fast Facts about Seafood

In Chinese mythology, fish are a symbol of wealth and abundance, as well as a token of harmony, reproduction, and marital happiness. The ancient Chinese used small carvings of fish as good-luck charms, and pools filled with carp or goldfish to signify abundance and harmony. In Japan, the carp (and its ornamental variety, koi) is symbolic of perseverance in the face of adversity, an association that probably originated from a Chinese legend about carp that would swim against the current up the Yellow River to become dragons.

In traditional Chinese medicine, seafood is generally thought to strengthen the qi, while being easier to digest than meat. Different types of seafood have different additional properties:

- Fish tend to strengthen the Spleen and Stomach, eliminate Dampness, and regulate Blood to help with conditions such as low energy, edema, and excessive postpartum bleeding. Freshwater fish are usually neutral and sweet, whereas ocean fish are usually neutral to cold and salty like their natural environment.
- Shrimp, prawns, and lobster, which are considered warm and sweet, enrich the Blood and strengthen the qi and Kidney yang, addressing conditions such as weakness, impotence, and lower back pain.
- Crab, considered cold and salty, clears Heat, moves the Blood, and unblocks the channels, benefiting the joints and helping with arthritis.
- Scallops, which are cold and sweet, benefit the five internal organs and nourish Kidney yin, addressing conditions such as dizziness, hot flashes, dry mouth, weakness in the lower back and knees, nighttime urination, emotional upset, and insomnia.

Caution: Avoid seafood if you have seafood allergies or gout.

SILVER-WRAPPED FISH WITH TANGERINE PEEL

MAKES 2 SERVINGS

A light, healthy, traditional recipe with the ease and convenience of cooking with foil.

INGREDIENTS

- 1 large piece (0.15 ounces or 4 grams) dried tangerine peel (*chen pi*), or 1 tablespoon of shredded pieces
- 1 pound mild fish (such as mahi mahi, halibut, or haddock)
- 1 tablespoon powdered kudzu, arrowroot, cornstarch, or other thickener
- 2 to 3 tablespoons cold water
- ¼ teaspoon salt
- ¼ teaspoon pepper
- 2 tablespoons soy sauce
- 1 tablespoon vegetable oil, such as canola or olive oil
- 1 (1-inch) piece fresh ginger, peeled and grated or minced
- 1 medium-size green onion, chopped into ¼-inch pieces, roots and tough tips discarded

DIRECTIONS

1. Preheat the oven to 350°F.
2. Soak the dried tangerine peel in warm water until soft, about 15 minutes. Remove it from the water. If necessary, scrape off the white pith and cut the peel into small pieces. (Many herb shops sell tangerine peel already shredded and depithed, in which case you can skip this step.)
3. Place each piece of fish on a separate piece of aluminum foil.
4. In a small bowl, mix the kudzu with the cold water, then brush this mixture over the fish. Season the fish with salt, pepper, soy sauce, and vegetable oil.
5. Place the ginger, green onion, and dried tangerine peel on top.
6. Fold the aluminum foil around the fish and securely roll the edges together to make a sealed packet. (Use two pieces of foil if necessary to seal or cover any rips in the foil.)
7. Place the aluminum packets on a baking pan or cookie sheet and bake for about 15 minutes, or until cooked.
8. If you'd like, serve the foil packets individually so everyone can open up their own serving. While the foil will be cool, be careful not to burn your fingers when the steam rushes out!

Helpful Hints about Tangerine Peel

Whereas in Western cuisine orange or tangerine peel is used fresh and grated as a tangy ingredient, in Chinese cuisine, dried, aged tangerine peel is prized. Tangerine peel can be bought from Asian markets in small packages of dried strips, or you can dry your own from fresh peel in your own kitchen. (For more information on tangerine peel, see "One Hundred Healthful Asian Ingredients.")

THEMES AND VARIATIONS

If you prefer to steam the fish in a more traditional manner, cook it in a steamer or on a rack in a covered wok with water in the bottom.

ESPECIALLY GOOD FOR

Anyone who wants sustained energy or who would like to soothe coughs, relieve chest congestion, or ease mild abdominal pain and distention.

FOR THOSE FAMILIAR WITH
TRADITIONAL CHINESE MEDICINE

This dish strengthens the qi of the Spleen and Lungs.

Yuan Says

There's a saying in China that your parents give you your health for the first half of your life, but your health in the second half is what you've given yourself. Taking care of yourself with diet, exercise, and stress management will pay off in health, well-being, and good looks.

SALMON WITH WOOD EAR AND CELLOPHANE NOODLES

MAKES 3 TO 4 SERVINGS

This dish brings together a meaty fish that contrasts with the light and tangy cellophane noodles. We especially like this combination with wild salmon from the Pacific Northwest.

INGREDIENTS

½ cup (¾ ounce, or 20 grams) dried black wood ear (*hei mu er* in Chinese, *kikurage* in Japanese)

2½ cups vegetable or chicken stock (For stock recipes, see "Mixed and Sundry.")

1 tablespoon mirin or dry sherry

¼ teaspoon salt

A pinch of white or black pepper

2 bundles (4 ounces) dried cellophane (mung bean preferred) noodles

2 tablespoons vegetable oil, such as canola or olive oil

1 (1-inch) piece fresh ginger, peeled and minced

2 cloves garlic, peeled and minced

2 fresh boneless salmon fillets (about 1 pound), cut into 1-inch-wide strips

1 teaspoon sesame oil

1 teaspoon lemon juice, or to taste

1½ tablespoons soy sauce, or to taste

¼ cup fresh cilantro leaves

DIRECTIONS

1. Soak the black wood ear in warm water for 30 minutes (it will expand a lot). Drain, then cut the wood ear into ¼-inch strips, discarding the fibrous part around the base.

2. In a medium-size pot, combine the stock, wood ear, mirin, salt, and pepper. Cover, and bring the mixture to a boil. Turn off the heat.

3. Add the cellophane noodles to the pot and stir until the noodles are covered with the broth. Cover the pot and set aside.

4. Heat the vegetable oil in a skillet over medium-high heat, then add the ginger and garlic. Cook for 30 to 60 seconds, until fragrant.

5. Add the salmon slices to the skillet and cook for about 2 minutes without stirring. Gently turn the fish over to the other side, trying not to break the pieces, and cook another 2 minutes or until the fish is done to your taste.

6. Transfer the noodle mixture to a serving dish and add the sesame oil, lemon juice, and soy sauce to taste.

7. Place the salmon, ginger, and garlic on top of the noodles. Garnish with the cilantro before serving.

Helpful Hints about Cellophane Noodles

Although cellophane noodles can be made of sweet potatoes, potatoes, and cassava, we prefer the mung bean variety because it resists dissolving during cooking. You can find cellophane noodles, sold in bundles like small packages of yarn, in an Asian market or in the international section of a well-stocked supermarket. (For more information on cellophane noodles, see "One Hundred Healthful Asian Ingredients.")

ESPECIALLY GOOD FOR

Anyone with high blood pressure, high cholesterol, diabetes, prostatitis, menopausal symptoms, or the desire to improve his/her complexion.

FOR THOSE FAMILIAR WITH TRADITIONAL CHINESE MEDICINE

This dish strengthens the qi and nourishes and invigorates Blood.

FIVE-COLOR STIR-FRY WITH SCALLOPS AND GINKGO

MAKES 3 SERVINGS

This attractive and tasty offering provides a variety of flavors, textures, and colors. Five is considered a balanced number in Chinese medicine and philosophy, as expressed in the five elements (wood, fire, earth, metal, and water), five climates (wind, heat, dampness, dryness, and cold), five yin organs (Liver, Heart, Spleen, Lung, and Kidney), five flavors (sour, bitter, sweet, spicy, salty)—and five colors (green, red, yellow, white, and black).

INGREDIENTS

6 (1 ounce dried; 5 ounces fresh) dried or fresh shiitake or other mushrooms
2 tablespoons dark sesame oil
2 cloves garlic, peeled and minced
1 (1-inch) piece fresh ginger, peeled and minced
1 pound sea scallops
10 to 15 (2 ounces) snow peas, strings removed
1 small bell pepper, seeded and cut into ¼-inch slices
18 canned ginkgo nuts, drained
2 teaspoons powdered kudzu, arrowroot, cornstarch, or other thickener
1 tablespoon water
2 tablespoons vegetable or chicken stock (For recipes, see "Mixed and Sundry.")
1 tablespoon rice wine
Salt or soy sauce

DIRECTIONS

1. If you are using dried mushrooms, soak them in water for 20 minutes, or until soft. Remove the stems, if desired, and cut into 4-inch slices.

2. Heat the sesame oil in a wok or skillet. Add the garlic and ginger and cook until fragrant (30 to 60 seconds, depending on how hot your pan is).

3. Add the scallops, and stir-fry over medium-high heat for about 5 minutes, or until they turn white and opaque. Remove the scallops from the pan so they don't overcook, and set aside.

4. Add the mushrooms and cook, stirring, for about 1 minute. Add the snow peas, bell pepper, and ginkgo nuts, and stir-fry for 3 to 5 minutes.

5. In the meantime, in a small bowl, mix the kudzu with a little cold water to avoid clumping.

6. Add the stock and wine to the pan, and stir in the kudzu mixture. Return the scallops to the pan and stir again.

7. Add salt or soy sauce to taste, and serve with rice.

Yuan Says

In traditional Chinese medicine, one important concept is that you try to keep good energy in the body, while encouraging bad energy to exit. Ginkgo nuts focus on the first part of this equation, helping the body to hold in good energy rather than lose it to the outside.

Helpful Hints about Ginkgo

Ginkgo nuts—considered something of a delicacy in China and Japan, eaten roasted or used in soups, stir-fries, and desserts—can be purchased fresh, in their tan-colored shell, or canned. Caution: Ginkgo nuts can be slightly toxic in large quantities, so avoid overeating (more than 10 to 15 at a time, or eating frequently over the long term) and make sure to cook them. (For more information on ginkgo, see "One Hundred Healthful Asian Ingredients.")

THEMES AND VARIATIONS

You can substitute shrimp if scallops are not available.

If you are starting with fresh ginkgo nuts instead of canned, don't despair. First, remove the fruit around the seed if you need to (only necessary if you are collecting them from nature; they are sold in the shell without the fruit), then crack open the shells with a nutcracker (or gently with a hammer) and remove the ginkgo nuts. Place the ginkgo nuts in boiling water for about 40 minutes. The dark inner peel should begin to flake off in the water. Drain the ginkgo nuts, and remove the rest of the peel by rubbing it off; as long as the nuts are warm the skin should rub off easily. Finally, take a toothpick or skewer and push it through the nut from end to end, pushing out the bitter core. The ginkgo nuts are now ready for cooking in your stir-fry.

ESPECIALLY GOOD FOR

Providing a balanced diet that promotes longevity, since this dish contains the five colors representing all five elements. The ginkgo nuts can also act to ease asthma, wheezing, and frequent urination, and to help prevent senile dementia.

FOR THOSE FAMILIAR WITH TRADITIONAL CHINESE MEDICINE

This dish strengthens the Kidneys, builds qi and Blood, and preserves the Lung qi.

FISH DISH FOR VIGOR

MAKES 2 SERVINGS

This is a popular, tasty, and easy recipe using Chinese dates, one of our top ten herbs, and goji berries, another widely favored ingredient. This dish goes well served over brown rice.

INGREDIENTS

8 pieces (15 grams) dried Chinese red dates (*hong zao*), cut into ¼-inch cubes

2 tablespoons (15 grams) goji berries (*gou qi zi*)

1 pound mild fish, such as mahi mahi, haddock, or halibut, cut into 2-inch chunks

1 (½-inch) piece fresh ginger, peeled and minced

2 medium-size green onions, chopped into ¼-inch pieces, roots and tough tips discarded

¼ cup rice wine or white wine

A pinch of salt

1 tablespoon dark sesame oil

1 medium-size tomato, seeded and cut into 1-inch dice

1 cup vegetable stock (For stock recipes, see "Mixed and Sundry.")

1 bunch (about ¾ pound) spinach, well washed, cut into 2-inch pieces

2 tablespoons powdered kudzu, arrowroot, cornstarch, or other thickener

3 tablespoons water

1 tablespoon soy sauce, or to taste

Condiments: Soy sauce, minced garlic, vinegar, or chili oil

DIRECTIONS

1. Soak the Chinese red dates and goji berries for 20 to 30 minutes. Drain.
2. Combine the fish, ginger, green onions, wine, and salt in a non-reactive bowl (made of glass, stainless steel, or ceramic) and marinate for about 20 minutes, tossing occasionally.
3. Heat the sesame oil in a skillet over medium heat (not too high a heat for sesame oil), then pan-fry the tomato in the oil for about 2 minutes.
4. Place the stock in a large pot with the tomatoes, goji berries, and Chinese red dates, then cover and bring to a boil. Lower the heat and simmer for 5 minutes.
5. Add the fish and marinade to the pot. Cover and bring back to a boil, then lower the heat and simmer for 5 to 7 minutes, until the fish is done. Add the spinach to the pot, cover, and cook for another minute.
6. Mix the kudzu in a small bowl with a little cold water to avoid clumping, then add it to the pot and stir well. Add the soy sauce and salt to taste.
7. Serve this dish warm with condiments on the side as desired.

ESPECIALLY GOOD FOR

Eating as a summer meal on a hot day or serving to anyone who is weak, needs to replenish body fluids, or is recovering from chemotherapy or radiation.

FOR THOSE FAMILIAR WITH TRADITIONAL CHINESE MEDICINE

This dish strengthens qi and nourishes Blood.

Warren Says

Most Westerners are familiar with the use of cornstarch or flour as a thickener, but other starchy plants have traditionally filled this role in Asia. Try Eastern thickeners, such as powdered kudzu root, arrowroot, or water chestnut, to add variety to your diet.

SILVER-WRAPPED CHICKEN WITH GALANGAL AND GINGER

MAKES 4 SERVINGS

This delicious chicken dish blends a variety of delicious flavors and herbs, without special equipment or fussy preparation.

INGREDIENTS

3 tablespoons (0.42 ounces or 12 grams) dried tangerine peel (*chen pi*)

1 small roasting chicken, cut up, or 3 to 4 pounds of chicken pieces

½ teaspoon salt

½ teaspoon white pepper

1 (1- to 2-inch) piece fresh ginger, peeled and cut into ⅛-inch slices

1 (1- to 2-inch) piece fresh galangal (lesser galangal preferred), peeled and cut into ⅛-inch slices (1 to 2 tablespoons, sliced)

2 tablespoons mirin or dry sherry

2 to 3 tablespoons (20 grams) goji berries (*gou qi zi*)

DIRECTIONS

1. Preheat the oven to 425°F.
2. Soak the dried tangerine peel in warm water until soft, about 15 minutes. Remove from the water and scrape off the white pith and shred if necessary (some dried tangerine peel from the herb shop comes already shredded and depithed).
3. Place each piece of chicken on a piece of aluminum foil, and sprinkle the chicken with the salt, pepper, ginger, galangal, tangerine peel, mirin, and goji berries.
4. Fold the aluminum foil around each piece of chicken and roll the edges together to make a sealed packet.
5. Place the aluminum packets on a baking pan or cookie sheet and bake them for about 35 minutes, or until the chicken is cooked.
6. If you'd like, serve in the aluminum packet, so the diners can open their own portion. Although the foil will be cool, be careful not to burn your fingers when the steam rushes out!

THEMES AND VARIATIONS

You can substitute powdered galangal for the fresh variety. One tablespoon of fresh lesser galangal is roughly equal to ½ tablespoon (1½ teaspoons) of the powdered form.

ESPECIALLY GOOD FOR

Anyone who wants to increase strength or soothe some types of chronic epigastric or abdominal pain.

FOR THOSE FAMILIAR WITH TRADITIONAL CHINESE MEDICINE

This dish warms the Stomach, supplements qi, nourishes Blood, strengthens the Liver and Kidneys, and helps prevent eye problems that sometimes develop with age.

Helpful Hints about Galangal

Galangal—a member of the ginger family used as both as a spice and as a medicine—can be purchased as a whole root, sliced and frozen, or in powdered form. When buying fresh galangal, look for rock-hard rhizomes (you'll need a sharp knife to cut them) and store in the refrigerator wrapped in a paper towel. (For more information on galangal, see "One Hundred Healthful Asian Ingredients.")

LIFE-FORCE CHICKEN AND MUSHROOMS IN WINE

MAKES 4 SERVINGS

This is a delicious and hearty dish, especially tasty with a vegetable such as bok choy on the side. If you have any leftovers, you're in for a treat; like many stews, this one only gets better overnight.

INGREDIENTS

⅓ ounce (10 grams) dried black wood ear (*hei mu er* in Chinese, *kikurage* in Japanese)

8 (1½ ounces dried; ½ pound fresh) dried or fresh shiitake mushrooms

¼ cup soy sauce

2 tablespoons rice wine or medium-dry sherry

1 teaspoon dark sesame oil

1 (1-inch) piece fresh ginger, peeled and minced

1 to 2 cloves garlic, peeled and minced

3 green onions, chopped into ¼-inch pieces, roots and tough tips discarded

1 tablespoon powdered kudzu, arrowroot, cornstarch, or other thickener

1½ cups water, plus extra for soaking

1 small chicken, cut up, or 3 to 4 pounds of chicken pieces

DIRECTIONS

1. Soak the wood ear in warm water until soft, about 30 minutes (they will expand a lot). If you are using dried shiitake mushrooms, also soak them for 30 minutes, or until soft. (Simply rinse fresh shiitakes.)

2. Cut the wood ear into 1-inch pieces. Cut the tough stems off the shiitakes and discard, if desired, and cut the shiitakes into ¼-inch slices.

3. Create a marinade by mixing together the soy sauce, rice wine, sesame oil, ginger, garlic, and green onions. Mix the kudzu in a small bowl with about 2 tablespoons of water to keep it from clumping, then add to the marinade and stir until smooth.

4. Place the chicken pieces, wood ear, and shiitakes into the marinade, toss well to coat, then let sit at room temperature for about 30 minutes.

5. Pour 1½ cups of water into a heavy pot and add the chicken, wood ear, shiitakes, and marinade. Bring to a boil, then lower the heat and simmer for about 30 minutes, or until the chicken is cooked.

ESPECIALLY GOOD FOR

Anyone feeling weak or getting over an illness. Throughout Asia, dishes of this kind are also often given to new mothers to increase their strength after childbirth.

FOR THOSE FAMILIAR WITH
TRADITIONAL CHINESE MEDICINE

This dish builds the Blood, supplements the qi, and harmonizes the Middle Burner.

PERILLA-ROASTED DRUMSTICKS

MAKES 4 SERVINGS

This dish might remind you of teriyaki chicken, but with some additional fragrant overtones provided by perilla leaf, which is a member of the mint family.

INGREDIENTS

2 teaspoons vegetable oil
½ cup white wine
4 tablespoons soy sauce
A pinch of salt
1 (1-inch) piece fresh ginger, peeled and minced
4 cloves garlic, peeled and minced
8 chicken drumsticks (about 3 pounds)
8 fresh perilla leaves (*zi su ye* in Chinese, *shisoyo*, akajisō, aoba, aojiso, or ōba in Japanese)

DIRECTIONS

1. Preheat the oven to 350°F. Rub a roasting pan with the oil.
2. Mix the wine, soy sauce, salt, ginger, and garlic in a large bowl.
3. Wrap each drumstick with a perilla leaf and marinate the drumsticks in the liquid mixture for at least 30 minutes, turning the drumsticks over after 15 minutes so both sides have a chance to absorb the sauce.
4. Place the drumsticks on the oiled pan and bake for about 40 minutes, or until done.

ESPECIALLY GOOD FOR

Providing general nutrition, and serving to anyone who is concerned about managing blood sugar or has a tendency toward stomach cramps and nausea.

FOR THOSE FAMILIAR WITH
TRADITIONAL CHINESE MEDICINE

This dish harmonizes the Spleen and Stomach, supplements qi, and nourishes Blood.

Helpful Hints about Perilla Leaves

To buy fresh perilla leaves, look in the produce section of an Asian food store (in a Japanese food store, the leaves might be labeled ohba or ōba [the sushi bar variety of shiso]). Chinese herb stores can supply perilla leaves in a dried form. If you come across perilla in a can, note that it is probably seasoned with soy sauce, hot pepper, and other spices (delicious with rice, but not so good for cooking). (For more information on perilla leaves, see "One Hundred Healthful Asian Ingredients.")

FIVE-SPICE POWDER CHICKEN

MAKES 6 SERVINGS

There's nothing as easy and pleasing as roast chicken, and this version will fill your house with mouth-watering aromas.

INGREDIENTS

1 large piece (0.15 ounces or 4 grams) dried tangerine peel (*chen pi*), or 1 tablespoon of shredded pieces

2 cloves garlic, peeled and minced

1 (1-inch) piece fresh ginger, peeled and minced

Juice of ½ lemon

1 teaspoon Chinese five-spice powder (*wu xiang fen*) (For recipe, see "Mixed and Sundry")

¼ teaspoon Sichuan peppercorns or other kind of pepper

2 tablespoons vegetable oil

2 tablespoons dark sesame oil

½ teaspoon salt

2 tablespoons brown sesame seeds

1 (4- to 5-pound) roasting chicken, giblets removed

DIRECTIONS

1. Preheat the oven to 450°F.
2. Soak the dried tangerine peel in warm water until soft, about 15 minutes. Remove from the water. If necessary, scrape off the white pith and cut into small pieces. (Some herb shops sell tangerine peel already shredded and depithed, in which case you can skip this step.)
3. In a food processor, whir together the tangerine peel, garlic, ginger, lemon juice, five-spice powder, Sichuan peppercorns, vegetable oil, sesame oil, and salt until it is the consistency of a paste.
4. Stir the sesame seeds into the paste.
5. Wash the chicken, pat dry, and evenly coat the exterior and interior of the chicken with the tangerine peel paste.
6. Place the chicken on a rack in a baking pan and roast for 20 minutes.
7. Lower the heat to 375°F, and roast for another 50 minutes or so (ovens and chickens vary), until the leg bone rotates easily in its socket and the juices run clear rather than pink when you tip them out of the cavity of the bird.
8. Remove the chicken from the oven and let it rest for 5 minutes before carving.

THEMES AND VARIATIONS

If you don't have dried tangerine peel on hand, the dish still works well without it.

ESPECIALLY GOOD FOR

People with a tendency toward stomach distress (such as bloating, gas, or poor appetite), fatigue (perhaps due to chronic stress), and aches and pains or low pain tolerance.

FOR THOSE FAMILIAR WITH
TRADITIONAL CHINESE MEDICINE

This dish benefits the Liver and Spleen, addressing Liver qi stagnation with Spleen deficiency.

Fast Facts about Five-Spice Powder

Since Chinese five-spice powder (*wu xiang fen*) contains each of the five flavors—sour, bitter, sweet, pungent, and salty—some people believe that the ancients were trying to put together a mixture representing all five elements in making the blend. (For more information on five-spice powder, see "One Hundred Healthful Asian Ingredients.")

GINKGO CHICKEN IN FOIL

MAKES 5 TO 6 SERVINGS

This is a feast in a packet. Traditionally, bamboo leaves were used as a wrapper, but today foil is more convenient.

INGREDIENTS

12 (2¼ ounces dried; 7½ ounces fresh) dried or fresh shiitake or other mushrooms
½ chicken, cut up, or about 3 pounds of chicken pieces
¼ teaspoon salt
24 canned ginkgo nuts, drained
⅓ cup plus 1 tablespoon sake
½ to ¾ cup grated daikon radish
2 green onions, chopped into ¼-inch pieces, roots and tough tips discarded
⅓ cup soy sauce
2 tablespoons lemon juice
¼ teaspoon *togarashi* or chili powder, or to taste (optional)

Warren Says

The popular memory supplement made from ginkgo biloba leaf is actually a recent phenomenon, outside of the Chinese tradition. Traditionally, Chinese medical practitioners use the seed, rather than the leaf, of this ancient plant species.

DIRECTIONS

1. Preheat the oven to 425°F.
2. If you are using dried shiitake mushrooms, soak them in water for 20 minutes, or until soft. (If you are using fresh shiitakes, simply rinse.) Slice the mushrooms into ½-inch pieces, and remove and discard the tough stems.
3. Place each piece of chicken on a piece of aluminum foil.
4. Top the chicken with the mushrooms, and sprinkle with salt. Place the ginkgo nuts on top of the chicken, then sprinkle the chicken, mushrooms, and ginkgo nuts with 1 tablespoon of the sake.
5. Fold the corners of the foil together around the chicken and its toppings to make well-sealed packages (use two pieces of foil if necessary).
6. Place the aluminum packets on a baking pan or cookie sheet and bake for about 35 minutes, or until the chicken is cooked.
7. Meanwhile, make the dipping sauce. If you prefer to remove some of the alcohol from the sake, heat the remaining ⅓ cup of sake in a pot, remove the pot from the heat, and then set the sake on fire using a long match. Allow the sake to cool.
8. In a bowl, mix together the sake with the daikon, green onions, soy sauce, lemon juice, and *togarashi* (if using) to complete the sauce, which can be served on the side.
9. When the chicken is done, each diner can open his or her own foil-wrapped packet, and spoon the sauce on top as desired.

Yuan Says

One of the most impressive trees I have ever seen was a ginkgo tree in Qufu, Shandong Province, growing outside of a Confucian temple, where they are often planted. Because of the reverence given to this particular temple family, the Kong family, whose most famous member is Kong Fuzi (whom we know as Confucius), the temple—and the tree—had escaped harm from the many wars that had ravaged the Chinese countryside. The ginkgo tree was many hundreds of years old, with a huge trunk, towering over everything with its beautiful fan-shaped leaves. The longevity of the ginkgo tree was probably how the ginkgo nut first became associated with health-giving properties.

THEMES AND VARIATIONS

If you are starting with fresh ginkgo nuts instead of canned, all is not lost. First, remove the fruit around the seed if you need to, then crack the shells open with a nutcracker (or gently with a hammer) and remove the ginkgo nuts. Then place the ginkgo nuts in boiling water for about 10 minutes. The dark inner peel should begin to flake off in the water. Drain the ginkgo nuts, and remove the rest of the peel by rubbing it off; as long as the nuts are warm, the skin should rub off easily. Finally, take a toothpick or skewer and push it through the nut from end to end, pushing out the bitter core. The ginkgo nuts are now ready for cooking. Caution: Ginkgo nuts can be slightly toxic in large quantities, so avoid overeating (more than 10 to 15 at a time, or eating frequently over the long term) and make sure to cook them.

ESPECIALLY GOOD FOR

Anyone who wants to increase energy, improve memory, or address problems such as frequent urination, asthma, wheezing, or swelling of the ankles.

FOR THOSE FAMILIAR WITH TRADITIONAL CHINESE MEDICINE

This dish supplements the qi, nourishes the Blood, strengthens the Kidneys, and preserves the Lung qi.

CLASSIC KOREAN GINSENG-STUFFED POULTRY

MAKES 2 SERVINGS

This dish—known as samgyetang *in Korean—is one of the most famous and widespread kitchen therapy dishes of Korea. Served most often in the summer to replenish fluids lost to heat, this dish is also believed to ward off disease, help people adapt to stress, and prevent ailments such as the common cold. Some restaurants in Korea serve nothing but their own special version of this dish, whose specific recipe is kept a closely guarded secret. Traditionally, each person is served a small bird of his or her own in a steaming bowl of broth.*

INGREDIENTS

2 roots (18 to 20 grams) fresh or dried Asian ginseng (*ren shen*)

4 dried or fresh chestnuts, shelled and skinned (optional)

½ cup sticky rice (a.k.a. sweet rice or glutinous rice)

2 (1½-pound) Cornish Game hens or other spring chickens

Salt

4 to 6 cloves garlic, peeled

4 Chinese red dates (jujubes or *hong zao*), seeded

6 to 8 cups water

1 teaspoon dark sesame oil

Black pepper

DIRECTIONS

1. If you are starting with dried ginseng rather than fresh, wash and then soak it in warm water for at least 12 hours or overnight, until it becomes pliable, then cut it into 1/2-inch pieces. Similarly, if you are starting with dried chestnuts rather than fresh, soak them overnight.

2. Wash and then soak the sticky rice in cold water for 30 minutes or more, then drain.

3. Wash the poultry and sprinkle with salt, inside and out.

4. Stuff each bird with half of the rice, one ginseng root, 2 to 3 cloves of garlic, 2 Chinese red dates, and 2 chestnuts (if using). To keep the stuffing in, secure the flap of skin over the cavity (bamboo skewers or toothpicks can work well, or sew the flaps together with thread or string). Putting the Chinese red dates and chestnuts in the bird last can be helpful as they can act as a stopper to help keep the rice inside.

5. Place the birds in a pot where they will fit snugly, and add enough water to cover them. We like to use a separate pot for each bird, so you will need less water to cover each bird and the broth will thereby become richer.

6. Cover the pot(s) and bring the water to a boil. Lower the heat to a simmer, and cook for about 1½ hours, until the poultry is thoroughly stewed.

7. Five minutes before removing the soup from the heat, sprinkle the sesame oil on top of the poultry.

8. When the poultry is done, add salt and pepper to taste. Serve one bird for each person in a bowl with its broth.

THEMES AND VARIATIONS

Traditional recipes call for fresh ginseng, which can be difficult to find in the West, but you might be able to secure some from a Korean market from June through October. In this case, no soaking or chopping into pieces is necessary. Many Korean markets also sell packages containing all the dried ingredients you'll need to make *samgyetang*.

Some people also like to use ginkgo nuts, goji berries, pine nuts, walnuts, peanuts, sesame seeds, and/or pumpkin seeds in the stuffing, either whole or ground in a blender. Ginger is another possible ingredient. Some people like to put some of the stuffing ingredients directly in the broth as well as inside the chicken. A garnish of green onions and/or toasted sesame seeds can add a nice touch.

If you are starting with fresh chestnuts in the shell (in season from October through March), you will need to shell and skin them; to remove the shell and inner skin, use a sharp knife to cut an X in the side of the chestnuts. Boil for 7 to 8 minutes, then peel and skin them immediately (this will become more difficult as they cool down, so leave them in the hot water until you are ready.) The Koreans have a special tool for the often painstaking task of shelling chestnuts, which looks somewhat like a cross between needle-nose pliers and scissors, sometimes available in the kitchen section of a Korean market.

For extra nourishment, the Koreans sometimes use black chicken, or *ogolgye* (literally "black-boned chicken"), sometimes available from Asian butchers or well-stocked Asian supermarkets.

ESPECIALLY GOOD FOR

Anyone who is feeling run down, weak, or overwhelmed; individuals recovering from illness or feeling the effects of age; people who need extra reserves of endurance (ginseng has been used by serious athletes to enhance performance). Many practitioners advise those who are under forty and already vigorous to limit use of the herb, as its powerful effects could unbalance the body, resulting in headaches, flushed face, and insomnia (the traditional antidote for too much ginseng is mung bean soup).

FOR THOSE FAMILIAR WITH TRADITIONAL CHINESE MEDICINE

This dish strengthens the qi, particularly in the Lungs and Spleen, as well as the Stomach. It also nourishes the Blood, generates fluids, and quenches thirst.

SILVER-WRAPPED LAMB WITH SICHUAN PEPPERCORN AND STAR ANISE

MAKES 2 SERVINGS

This easy, delicious version of lamb is cooked in foil, which keeps the meat moist and allows several delightful and distinct flavors to blend together.

INGREDIENTS

1 medium-size piece (0.1 ounces or 2.5 grams) dried tangerine peel (*chen pi*), or 2 teaspoons of shredded pieces

1 to 1½ pounds lamb chops

1 (½-inch) piece fresh ginger, peeled and grated or minced

2 cloves garlic, peeled and minced

¼ teaspoon Sichuan peppercorns, ground, or to taste, or other ground pepper

1 to 2 teaspoons ground star anise, or 2 whole pieces of star anise, crushed

1 tablespoon soy sauce

THEMES AND VARIATIONS

If you don't have star anise on hand, anise (from an unrelated plant with some of the same chemical compounds) can be substituted. Although the two ingredients have a similar flavor, star anise is slightly more pungent and bitter.

Words of Wisdom

For longevity, eat until you are 70 percent full.

—CHINESE PROVERB

DIRECTIONS

1. Preheat the oven to 350°F.
2. Soak the dried tangerine peel in warm water until soft, about 15 minutes. Remove from the water and scrape off the white pith and shred if necessary (most dried tangerine peel from the herb shop comes already shredded and depithed). Dice.
3. Place each piece of lamb on a separate piece of aluminum foil. Place the tangerine peel, ginger, garlic, ground Sichuan peppercorns, star anise, and soy sauce on top, distributing these ingredients relatively evenly on the lamb pieces.
4. Fold the aluminum foil around the lamb and securely roll the edges together to make a sealed packet.
5. Place the packets on a baking pan or cookie sheet and bake for about 25 minutes, or until cooked.
6. If you'd like, serve the foil packets individually so all the diners can open up their own serving. While the foil will be cool, be careful not to burn your fingers when the steam rushes out!

ESPECIALLY GOOD FOR

Eating in the winter. Serving to people who run cold; anyone with cold hands and feet, cold abdominal pain, or cold joint pain; or women with premenstrual syndrome or who feel depleted from menstruation. (This dish is not so good for people who run warm.)

FOR THOSE FAMILIAR WITH TRADITIONAL CHINESE MEDICINE

This dish warms the Stomach, builds the Blood, strengthens Kidney yang, and eases pain and swelling.

CHAMPION CHICKEN WITH GOJI BERRIES

MAKES 4 SERVINGS

This fragrant dish will be a hit when you serve it, as the sweet goji berries and tangy ginger provide appetizing accents to the juicy chicken.

INGREDIENTS

2 tablespoons vegetable oil, such as canola or olive oil

2 cloves garlic, peeled and minced

1 (½- to 1-inch) piece fresh ginger, peeled and minced

1 roasting chicken, skinned and cut up, or 3 to 4 pounds of skinless legs and/or breasts

2 medium-size green onions, chopped into ½-inch pieces, roots and tough tips discarded

3 to 4 tablespoons rice wine or dry sherry

2 tablespoons soy sauce, or to taste

2 tablespoons (30 grams) goji berries (*gou qi zi*)

1½ cups water, or vegetable or chicken stock (For stock recipes, see "Mixed and Sundry.")

1 teaspoon dark sesame oil

DIRECTIONS

1. Heat the oil in a pan, then add the garlic and ginger and cook until the garlic is golden (about 5 minutes).
2. Place the chicken, garlic, ginger, green onions, wine, soy sauce, goji berries, and water in a pot.
3. Bring the mixture to a boil, then cover and lower the heat to a simmer. Cook for about 30 minutes, or until the chicken is cooked through.
4. Sprinkle the sesame oil on top as a finishing touch.
5. Serve in a bowl with some of the broth, or on top of rice with the broth as a gravy.

ESPECIALLY GOOD FOR

Anyone who wants to increase his or her strength, including women recovering from childbirth.

FOR THOSE FAMILIAR WITH TRADITIONAL CHINESE MEDICINE

This dish warms the Stomach, supplements the qi, nourishes the Blood, strengthens the Liver and Kidneys, and helps prevent eye problems that sometimes develop with age.

Legend Has It

A story set in the Tang Dynasty tells of a water well overgrown with goji berry vines, located near a Buddhist temple. Over the years, countless goji berries dropped into the well. The villagers who routinely drank from the well displayed remarkably good health and lived to a ripe old age.

FIVE-SPICE LAMB SKEWERS

MAKES 2 TO 3 SERVINGS

These skewers present a tasty and elegant treat, balancing different colors and flavors using a variety of ingredients.

INGREDIENTS

1½ tablespoons Chinese five-spice powder (*wu xiang fen*)

¼ teaspoon ground Sichuan or other pepper

1 pound lamb or other meat, cut into 1-inch cubes

1 to 2 yellow squash and/or zucchini, chopped into 1- to 2-inch pieces

1 red bell pepper, seeded and chopped into 1- to 2-inch pieces

1 small onion, chopped into 1- to 2-inch pieces

8 fresh shiitake mushrooms, stems discarded if desired

2 tablespoons olive oil

¼ teaspoon salt

DIRECTIONS

1. Preheat the grill.
2. In a large bowl, combine the five-spice powder and pepper, then stir in the lamb cubes. Mix well so the spices coat the lamb evenly.
3. Thread the skewers with lamb, squash, pepper, onion, and mushrooms.
4. Brush the vegetables with the oil, then sprinkle the skewers with salt.
5. Place the skewers on the grill and cook for 4 to 5 minutes. Turn over the skewers and cook for another 4 minutes or so before serving.

ESPECIALLY GOOD FOR

Eating in the winter, when the weather is cold. Serving to anyone feeling cold or who is experiencing fatigue, arthritic pain, menstrual pain, or cold sensations with premenstrual syndrome. Individuals who tend to run warm should avoid large quantities of this dish.

THEMES AND VARIATIONS

You can vary the vegetables you use on the skewers; for example, using cherry tomatoes.

A pan-fried version of Five-Spice Lamb is also delicious. In this case, cut the lamb into strips, mix it in a bowl with five-spice powder and pepper, then sauté the lamb in a pan with oil, garlic, and ginger for about 6 minutes. Serve the lamb over vegetables.

FOR THOSE FAMILIAR WITH TRADITIONAL CHINESE MEDICINE

This dish provides balance while strengthening Kidney yang, dispersing Cold, strengthening qi, and nourishing Blood.

WARMING FENNEL LAMB

MAKES 2 TO 3 SERVINGS

This hearty stir-fry uses lamb (the warmest of meats, according to traditional Chinese medicine), as well as the warming herbs ginger, green onion, cumin, chili, and fennel seeds. Serve with rice and vegetables.

INGREDIENTS

1 pound lamb, cut into ¾-inch cubes
1 tablespoon ground cumin
2 teaspoons rice wine
½ medium-size green onion, chopped into ¼-inch pieces, roots and tough tips discarded
2 tablespoons vegetable oil, such as canola or olive oil
1 (1-inch) piece fresh ginger, peeled and minced
Salt
1 teaspoon fennel seeds
Ground chili pepper (optional)

DIRECTIONS

1. Place the lamb in a large bowl. Sprinkle with the cumin, rice wine, and green onions as you stir the lamb. Mix well for a few minutes so that the lamb is evenly coated.
2. Heat the oil in a skillet or wok over medium-high heat. Add the ginger and cook for about 30 seconds, until fragrant. Add the lamb mixture and stir-fry for about 5 minutes, until nearly done.
3. One minute before removing the pan from the stove, add the fennel seeds and chili pepper (if using) and stir well. Serve.

ESPECIALLY GOOD FOR

Eating in the winter, when the weather is cold. Anyone feeling cold or experiencing fatigue.

FOR THOSE FAMILIAR WITH
TRADITIONAL CHINESE MEDICINE

This dish strengthens Kidney yang, disperses Cold, strengthens qi, and nourishes Blood.

STRENGTHENING STEW

MAKES 3 SERVINGS

This healthy stew basks in the influence of invigorating herbs. Dang gui *(angelica sinensis root) is sometimes called "female ginseng" due to its popularity as a woman's herb, but its benefits aren't limited to women.*

INGREDIENTS

4 tablespoons vegetable oil, such as canola or olive oil
1 small onion, chopped into ½-inch pieces
5 cloves garlic, peeled and minced
¾ pound grass-fed lamb (a shoulder or leg cut works well), cut into 1½-inch pieces
5 (5-inch) pieces (1 ounce, or 30 grams) astragalus root (*huang qi*)
¼ ounce (5 to 7 grams) *dang gui*
1 (1-inch) piece fresh ginger, peeled and slivered into ¹⁄₁₆-inch slices
4 cups water
⅛ teaspoon salt
¼ pound kale or other leafy greens, cut into 2-inch pieces
2 teaspoons soy sauce, or to taste
Chili oil (optional)

DIRECTIONS

1. Heat 2 tablespoons of the oil in a skillet, add the onions and garlic, and cook over medium-high heat until the onions become translucent (about 5 minutes). Transfer the onions and garlic to a large pot.

2. Pour another 2 tablespoons of oil in the skillet, and add the lamb. Cook over medium-high heat until browned on all sides, about 5 minutes. Place the lamb pieces in the pot with the onions and garlic.

3. Place the astragalus root, *dang gui*, and ginger slices in a piece of cheesecloth and tie the cloth loosely into a bag for easy removal later on (alternatively, you can pick out the pieces of root one by one before serving, or eat around them).

4. Place the cloth bag into the pot with the lamb, onions, and garlic. Add the water and salt. Bring the soup to a boil, then lower the heat and simmer for about 45 minutes.

5. Add the kale to the pot, and simmer for 15 to 20 minutes more (other types of greens can be added about 5 minutes before the cooking is done).

6. Remove the bag of astragalus root, *dang gui*, and ginger.

7. Add the soy sauce, and serve with chili oil, if you desire a spicy accent.

THEMES AND VARIATIONS

This dish can be made with chicken or Rock Cornish hen, for those who don't eat red meat. Interestingly, this dish is traditionally made with "black chicken" (*ogolgye*), which is rarely found in the West. Black chicken, whose nutrients are thought to be easily absorbed, is dark all the way through, including the meat and bones.

ESPECIALLY GOOD FOR

Anyone feeling weak or getting over an illness; also, women recovering from childbirth or a heavy menstrual period, facing irregular bleeding, or experiencing premenstrual syndrome. Caution: If you are pregnant, skip the *dang gui*.

FOR THOSE FAMILIAR WITH
TRADITIONAL CHINESE MEDICINE

This soup supplements the qi, builds the Blood, and disperses Cold. The combination of astragalus and *dang gui* is a classical Chinese herbal formula called *dang gui bu xue tang*.

Yuan Says

I had a patient who wanted to start a family with her husband, but who was worried she would not be able to become pregnant because she had always had irregular periods, sometimes twice a month, sometimes twice a year. I told her to eat this soup for a few days in a row once a month, whether she had her cycle or not. After a little while she moved away, and I thought we had lost touch. But about a year later, I opened the mail and she had sent me a picture of her beautiful new baby.

TEN-TREASURE DUMPLINGS

MAKES 8 TO 10 SERVINGS

Making dumplings can be a fun afternoon project, and who can resist the delicious results? You might want to make a big batch of these dumplings when you have time and keep them in the freezer so they'll be ready on a moment's notice.

INGREDIENTS

1 medium-size carrot, top trimmed
4 stalks celery
1 medium-size tomato
1 pound fresh mushrooms
2 medium-size green onions, ends trimmed
1 (1-inch) piece fresh ginger, peeled
3 cloves garlic, peeled
¼ pound ground turkey
¼ pound ground chicken
¼ pound ground lamb
¼ pound baby shrimp, or other shrimp cut into small pieces
1 medium-size egg
1 tablespoon sesame oil
½ teaspoon salt
¼ teaspoon pepper, or to taste
80 dumpling skins (available from Asian food stores and some supermarkets or, see Do-It-Yourself Dumpling Wrappers on page 276)
Dipping sauce, such as Delicious Dumpling Dipping Sauce, page 275

DIRECTIONS

1. Finely mince the carrot, celery, tomato, mushrooms, green onions, ginger, and garlic by hand or, more conveniently, by whirring one by one in a food processor. Place the minced ingredients in a large bowl.
2. Add the turkey, chicken, lamb, shrimp, egg, sesame oil, salt, and pepper to the bowl with the vegetables, then mix well to complete the dumpling stuffing.
3. Take one dumpling skin and wet its edges. Place a spoonful of the stuffing onto the center of the dumpling skin, squeeze out any air, then pinch the wrapper tightly along the edges, making a lumpy semicircle and sealing the stuffing inside. To ensure a tight seal, wet the outside edge of the dumpling wrapper again on one side and make five ⅛-inch pleats along the edges, pinching tightly. Don't overstuff, or the dough will tear. Repeat until you have used up the stuffing (which may take some time).
4. Boil a pot of water, then add the dumplings in batches. Boil until the dumplings float to the top. (If only a few float to the top, make sure the others aren't sticking to the bottom by stirring very gently.)
5. Add 1 cup of cold water, then bring to a boil again. One more time, add 1 cup of cold water then bring to a boil.
6. Remove the dumplings from the pot. Serve piping hot in a shallow dish with dipping sauce on the side.

Yuan Says

One of the wonderful things about the way I grew up is that we all sat down to eat as a large, extended family—grandparents, uncles, aunts, sisters, brothers. Because there were so many people, it was easy to serve a variety of dishes, from soups to vegetables, from fish to tofu, at every sitting. I have found that when living and eating as a small family of two to four people, it is much harder to have meals with such rich and healthy variety. Dishes such as dumplings, which contain many ingredients but can be served in individual portions, offer the benefits of eating a variety of foods without dozens of friends and relatives. One of the guiding principles of Chinese food therapy is eating a variety of foods, with different flavors—sour, bitter, sweet, spicy, and salty—different colors—red, yellow, green, white, purple, and black—and different natures—cold, cool, neutral, warm, and hot.

THEMES AND VARIATIONS

Don't feel bound by the types of meat listed here—the idea is variety, so feel free to substitute. The vegetables can also vary. Try squash instead of carrots, or throw in some enoki mushrooms. For a vegetarian recipe, see Vegetable Variety Pot Stickers (page 170).

If you want to freeze the dumplings for later use, lay them flat in a single layer on a baking sheet (not touching each other), then place them in the freezer for 20 to 30 minutes. You will then be able to combine the dumplings in a large zippered plastic bag and return them to the freezer without having them stick together. To rewarm frozen dumplings, place 2 tablespoons of oil in a nonstick pan. Place the dumplings in the pan, then add ⅔ cup of water. Heat, covered, over medium heat for about 8 minutes, until most of the water is gone, then uncover for a minute or so to boil off the remainder of the water.

ESPECIALLY GOOD FOR

Anyone who needs more diversity of nutrients, who has poor appetite or malnutrition, or who is recovering from chronic illness.

FOR THOSE FAMILIAR WITH TRADITIONAL CHINESE MEDICINE

This dish addresses qi and Blood deficiency.

VEGETABLE VARIETY POT STICKERS

MAKES 4 TO 6 SERVINGS

Here is a recipe for mouthwatering pan-fried vegetarian dumplings that we modestly declare better than anything you could buy in a store.

INGREDIENTS

1 bundle (2 ounces) dried cellophane (mung bean preferred) noodles

½ pound Chinese cabbage or bok choy

1 small carrot

3 stalks celery

1 small tomato

½ pound fresh shiitake or assorted mushrooms

1 green onion, ends trimmed

1 (½-inch) piece fresh ginger

1 tablespoon dark sesame oil

½ teaspoon salt

¼ teaspoon pepper, or to taste

1 medium-size egg

60 to 75 dumpling skins (available from an Asian grocery or some supermarkets, or see Do-It-Yourself Dumpling Wrappers on page 276)

4 tablespoons vegetable oil, such as canola or olive oil

½ cup water

Dipping sauce, such as Delicious Dumpling Dipping Sauce, page 275

DIRECTIONS

1. Soak the cellophane noodles in warm water for about 20 minutes. Drain and then chop into ½-inch pieces.
2. Mince the Chinese cabbage, carrot, celery, tomato, mushrooms, green onion, and ginger by hand or, more conveniently, by using a food processor, and place in a large bowl.
3. Add the chopped noodles, sesame oil, salt, and pepper and mix well.
4. In a wok or skillet, heat 2 tablespoons of vegetable oil over medium-high heat. Add the vegetable mixture, and stir-fry for 3 to 5 minutes, until fragrant and cooked.
5. Beat the egg in a small bowl, then stir it into the vegetable mixture. Turn off the heat.
6. Take one dumpling skin and wet its edges. Place one spoonful of the stuffing onto the center of the dumpling skin, squeeze out any air, then pinch the wrapper tightly along the edges, making a lumpy semi circle and sealing the stuffing inside. To ensure a tight seal, wet the semicircular edge of the dumpling wrapper again on one side and make five ⅛-inch pleats along the edges, pinching tightly. Repeat until the stuffing is used up (which may take some time).
7. In a skillet, heat 2 tablespoons of vegetable oil over medium-high heat, then place the dumplings in the pan, working in batches. Fry for 2 to 3 minutes, or until the bottoms of the dumplings are golden.
8. Add ½ cup water all at once (be careful of the splattering) and cover quickly. Cook for 5 to 7 minutes, until the water has mostly boiled off.
9. Uncover the skillet, lower the heat to medium-low, and cook for another 2 minutes.
10. Serve your dumplings warm, with the dipping sauce.

THEMES AND VARIATIONS

You can add tofu to the filling, but use a variety that has been smoked or deep-fried, so the excess water doesn't make the dumplings soggy. Asparagus is also tasty; pan-fry it for a minute longer than the other vegetables in the preparation stage. Chives are tasty, too. Save your green, leafy vegetables for another use, though, as they don't work well for the consistency of the filling.

If you prefer to boil your dumplings rather than pan-fry them, boil a pot of water, then add the dumplings. Cook until the dumplings float to the top. Add 1 cup of cold water, then bring the water to a boil again. One more time, add 1 cup of cold water, then bring to a boil. Remove the dumplings from the pot, drain well, and serve.

If you wish to freeze the dumplings for later use, after finishing step 6 (before frying) place them in a single layer on a baking sheet and put them in the freezer for 20 to 30 minutes; at that point, you can combine the dumplings in a large zippered plastic bag without having them stick together. To rewarm frozen dumplings, place 2 tablespoons of oil in a nonstick pan. Place the dumplings in the pan, then add $2/3$ cup of water. Heat, covered, over medium heat for about 8 minutes, until most of the water is gone, then uncover for a minute or so to boil off the remainder of the water.

ESPECIALLY GOOD FOR

Vegetarians or anyone who has high cholesterol or high blood pressure.

FOR THOSE FAMILIAR WITH TRADITIONAL CHINESE MEDICINE

This dish supplements qi and harmonizes the internal organs.

KUNG PAO CREATION

MAKES 2 SERVINGS

This is a staple from Yuan's kitchen and a popular dish in China's Sichuan Province.

INGREDIENTS

1 tablespoon powdered kudzu, arrowroot, cornstarch, or other thickener

2 tablespoons water

3 tablespoons soy sauce

1 tablespoon rice wine

¾ teaspoon sesame oil

¾ pound boneless chicken, pork, lamb, or other meat, or firm tofu, chopped into ½-inch pieces

3 tablespoons vegetable oil, such as canola or olive oil

4 cloves garlic, peeled and minced

1 (1-inch) piece fresh ginger, peeled and minced

3 to 7 whole dried hot chili peppers (depending on how spicy you like it), cut in half diagonally

⅓ cup roasted unsalted peanuts

3 to 4 green onions, chopped into ½-inch pieces, roots and tough tips discarded

DIRECTIONS

1. In a medium-size bowl, mix together the kudzu with about 2 tablespoons of water, until the lumps are gone. Add 1½ tablespoons of the soy sauce, 1½ teaspoons of the rice wine, and the sesame oil, and stir to make a marinade.

2. Place the meat in the marinade, mixing well. Let the mixture sit for 20 minutes.

3. In a small cup, mix together the remaining 1½ tablespoons of soy sauce and 1½ teaspoons of rice wine. Set aside.

4. Heat 2 tablespoons of vegetable oil in a wok or skillet over medium-high heat. Stir-fry the meat for about 5 minutes, until it is is about 80 percent cooked. Remove from the pan and set aside.

5. Add another tablespoon of vegetable oil, heat it, then add the garlic, ginger, and chili peppers, and stir-fry for 1 to 2 minutes. Return the meat to the pan, then stir-fry for another minute.

6. Add the unsalted peanuts, green onions, and the soy sauce mixture and stir.

7. Serve with rice and vegetables.

Yuan Says

A typical meal in China, even for a single family, consists of several dishes, a soup, and rice. If one dish emphasizes meat, others will feature vegetables. For larger festive gatherings, presenting eight or nine different dishes is common, not only to symbolize wealth and prosperity, but also to ensure that diners are offered a sufficient variety and balance of foods. A varied and balanced diet also decreases food cravings and hunger pangs, which can help with weight control.

Fast Facts about Meat and Poultry

According to traditional Chinese medicine, meat and poultry have therapeutic characteristics in common. They supplement qi, build Blood, and stimulate yang, making them ideal for counteracting fatigue and quickly replenishing energy following physical exertion, childbirth, or illness; they are invigorating for people who tend to be weak and lethargic. Meat and poultry also tend to be classified as warm to hot, making them good foods for eating in the cold seasons and for people who tend to run cold. Eat these foods only in moderation, however, as excess consumption can be harmful. With these commonalities in mind, specific meats and poultry offer different strengths:

- Chicken, which is the most neutral of these meats, is particularly good for weakness in the elderly and postpartum recovery. Turkey is similar to chicken.
- Beef, which is considered the strongest acting to replenish energy, is also particularly good for tendons and bones, as well as the Stomach, addressing lack of appetite.
- Lamb, which is considered especially warming, is particularly good at dispelling Cold, addressing such conditions as chills, aversion to cold, and cold extremities.
- Pork, which is the coolest of the meats listed here (although duck is cooler), moistens and nourishes the organs, addressing dry cough, dry skin, and thirst.

THEMES AND VARIATIONS

Try adding a beaten egg to the marinade for an interesting variation.

ESPECIALLY GOOD FOR

Supporting general nutrition; serving to anyone who runs cold, who has cold hands and feet, or who wants to stimulate the digestion after a long illness.

FOR THOSE FAMILIAR WITH TRADITIONAL CHINESE MEDICINE

This dish is warming, strengthens the qi, harmonizes the Spleen and Stomach, and nourishes the Blood. Individuals who tend to run warm should avoid large quantities of this dish.

A FLURRY OF CURRY

MAKES 4 SERVINGS

Curry is a mainstay throughout much of Asia. Here's a version we like, with coconut milk.

INGREDIENTS

2 to 3 tablespoons vegetable oil

3 cloves garlic, peeled and minced

1 (1-inch) piece fresh ginger, peeled and minced

1 medium-size leek, well washed and sliced into ¼-inch pieces, tough roots and tips discarded

1 small onion, cut into small dice

1 pound boneless and skinless chicken, other meat, or tofu, cut into 1-inch pieces

2 to 3 tablespoons curry powder

1 (13½-ounce) can coconut milk

2 tablespoons soy sauce

2 carrots, cut into ¼-inch slices

½ pound (1 small head) broccoli, cut into florets, stem discarded (or reserve for another use)

3 medium-size tomatoes, seeded and cut into ½-inch pieces

½ cup shelled fresh or frozen peas

DIRECTIONS

1. Heat the vegetable oil in a large wok or sauté pan over medium-high heat. Add the garlic and ginger and cook for 30 to 60 seconds, until fragrant.

2. Add the leek and onions and cook for 3 to 4 minutes. Transfer them from the pan to a small bowl and set aside.

3. Add more oil to the pan if necessary, then add the chicken. Stir-fry until browned on all sides. Return the onion mixture to the pan.

4. Add the curry powder and stir-fry in the pan for a minute to bring out the flavors.

5. Add the coconut milk, soy sauce, and carrots, bring to a boil, then lower the heat and simmer for 3 to 5 minutes.

6. Add the broccoli, tomato, and peas, and simmer for another 8 to 10 minutes, stirring occasionally.

7. Serve with rice.

Fast Facts about Curry

Curry, which originated in India, has spread throughout the Asia-Pacific region—and the world—in many wonderful variations. The Japanese are particularly enthusiastic about curry, and curry makes up one of the most popular dishes in that country; the Indonesians, Thais, and Malaysians also embrace this dish. In China, curry is eaten mostly in the southern and western regions. The trademark ingredient of a curry is a sauce made of curry powder or paste—actually a blend of spices, usually containing turmeric, coriander, cumin, and fenugreek, and sometimes also containing ingredients such as ginger, garlic, fennel seed, cinnamon, clove, mustard seed, cardamom, mace, nutmeg, and various types of pepper. Depending on the blend, its taste can range from mild to spicy. Many of the ingredients in curries, including turmeric, are considered warming and beneficial to health in the East Asian and South Asian traditions.

THEMES AND VARIATIONS

Vary the vegetables according to what is in season. Try zucchini, yellow squash, potatoes. . . .

ESPECIALLY GOOD FOR

Anyone with poor appetite, joint pain (such as in arthritis), or poor memory.

FOR THOSE FAMILIAR WITH TRADITIONAL CHINESE MEDICINE

This dish moves the qi and Blood, strengthens the Spleen qi, nourishes Blood, and relieves stagnation from Cold.

MAGNIFICENT MIZUTAKI

Everyone creates his or her own special sauce to taste for this Japanese hotpot (nabe). The Chinese also embrace hotpots, especially for winter meals. Typical ingredients include mushrooms, leafy greens, dumplings, tofu, bean sprouts, daikon, and thinly sliced meat or seafood.

INGREDIENTS

8 to 10 (1½ ounces dried; ½ pound fresh) dried or fresh shiitake mushrooms

16 cups water

2 (4 by 6-inch) pieces kombu seaweed

2 to 3 pounds boneless and skinless chicken, cut into 1½-inch pieces

1 tablespoon dried precut wakame seaweed (optional)

½ pound Chinese cabbage or bok choy, cut into ½-inch pieces

½ pound (½ package) firm tofu, cut into ½-inch cubes

3 bundles (6 ounces) dried cellophane (mung bean preferred) noodles

½ pound leafy greens, such as spinach, chrysanthemum greens, or mizuna

1 bunch (3.5 ounces, or 1½ cups) watercress (optional)

SAUCE

Juice of 3 to 4 lemons

Soy sauce

¼ cup grated daikon (optional)

Ground chili pepper or spicy *togarashi* topping (For a recipe, see page 282.) (optional)

DIRECTIONS

1. If you are using dried shiitakes, soak them in warm water for about 20 minutes or until soft, then drain. (If you are using fresh shiitakes, simply rinse.) Cut the mushrooms into ¼-inch slices, discarding the stems, if desired.

2. Place the water and kombu in a pot and begin heating it. Just before the water comes to a boil, remove the kombu.

3. Add the chicken pieces, mushrooms, and wakame. Bring to a boil, then lower the heat and simmer, uncovered, for 15 to 20 minutes.

4. Add the Chinese cabbage, tofu, and cellophane noodles to the pot and continue to simmer for another 5 minutes.

5. Add the leafy greens and watercress, and cook for 30 seconds.

6. Serve family style, with the pot in the center of the table. At the table, each diner should make a mixture of soy sauce, lemon juice, and daikon and/or hot pepper, if desired, in the bottom of his/her bowl. For those who need guidance, start with individual servings of about 2 teaspoons each of soy sauce, lemon juice, and daikon, then adjust to taste when you spoon the soup on top and mix. Yum!

THEMES AND VARIATIONS

Get creative! This dish can evolve every time you cook it. Broccoli is a wonderful addition. Green onions are lovely in the soup, too. And fish works instead of chicken. We also sometimes use chicken pieces on the bone, such as drumsticks and thighs, which imparts a rich flavor to the broth; in this case, cook for 35 minutes in step 3.

ESPECIALLY GOOD FOR

Eating in the winter during cold weather; supporting general nutrition and health; supplementing therapy for cancer; or addressing conditions such as goiter, fibroids, or other disorders involving masses.

Mika Says

This dish was a staple in our house when I was growing up and is still a staple now that I have a family of my own. It's perfect for a busy household, because you can make a big pot of delicious, healthy food with a small investment of time and eat it throughout the week. It also freezes well for later use.

FOR THOSE FAMILIAR WITH TRADITIONAL CHINESE MEDICINE

This dish helps build the qi and Blood, softens hardness, and transforms phlegm.

MOUTHWATERING MEAL IN A MINUTE

MAKES 2 SERVINGS

This simple, warm, and nutritious dish is a version of Japanese ochazuke, *a combination of rice and tea, with other ingredients on top. For a more traditional version, see Always-on-Call* Ochazuke, *page 201.*

INGREDIENTS

1 to 2 teaspoons brown sesame seeds

1½ cups water

1 rounded teaspoon green tea leaves, or 1 to 2 teabags

2 eggs

1 tablespoon dried precut wakame seaweed (optional)

⅓ cup shelled fresh or frozen peas

5 medium-size leaves spinach or other greens, well washed, stems discarded, chopped into 3-inch pieces

1½ cups cooked rice, preferably brown

1 to 1½ tablespoons soy sauce, or to taste

Togarashi (for a recipe, see page 282) or chili pepper (optional)

DIRECTIONS

1. If your sesame seeds aren't already roasted, toast the sesame seeds by putting them in a wide skillet over medium heat, shaking the pan occasionally. Continue frying until fragrant, 3 to 5 minutes. Remove the seeds from the hot skillet so they don't overcook, and set aside.

2. Boil about 1½ cups of water, turn off the heat, and add the tea. Let the tea steep for 3 to 5 minutes, or until the desired strength, then strain out the tea or remove the tea bag(s).

3. In a small saucepan, bring about 2 cups of water to a boil. Add the eggs, wakame (if using), and peas. Cook for about 3 minutes, until the white of the egg is cooked, but the yolk is still runny. Add the spinach and cook for 30 seconds, until the leaves are wilted. Turn off the heat.

4. Place the rice in serving bowls. With a slotted spoon, remove the poached eggs and other cooked items from the pot and arrange them on top of the rice.

5. Pour the tea over the rice and other ingredients. Add the soy sauce to taste.

6. Sprinkle the sesame seeds on top to garnish, and serve with *togarashi* or chili pepper on the side, if desired.

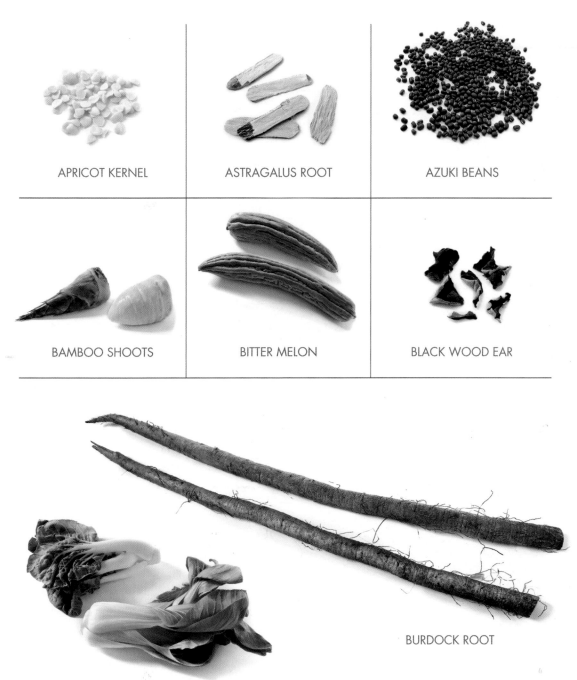

APRICOT KERNEL

ASTRAGALUS ROOT

AZUKI BEANS

BAMBOO SHOOTS

BITTER MELON

BLACK WOOD EAR

BURDOCK ROOT

BOK CHOY

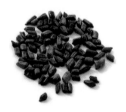

CASSIA SEEDS

CELLOPHANE NOODLES

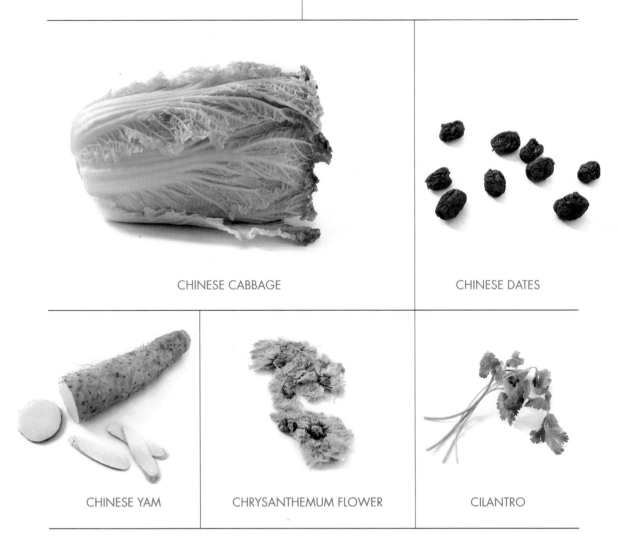

CHINESE CABBAGE

CHINESE DATES

CHINESE YAM

CHRYSANTHEMUM FLOWER

CILANTRO

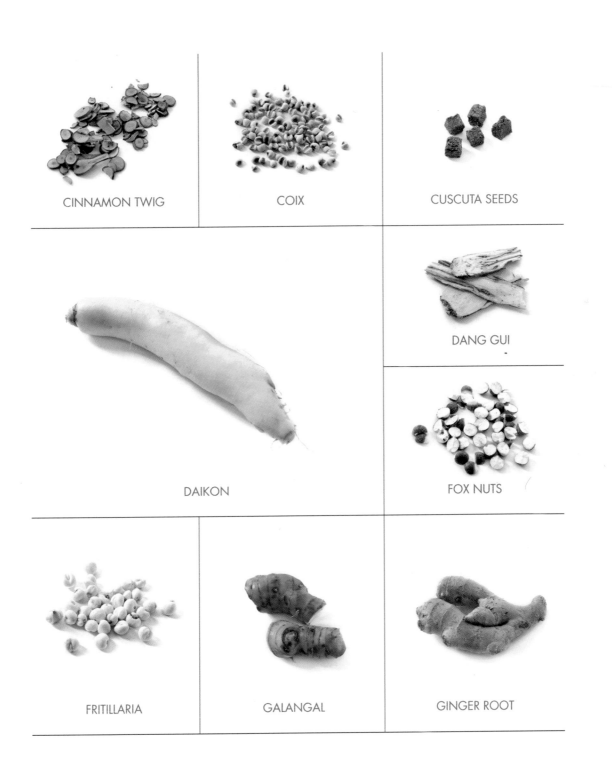

CINNAMON TWIG

COIX

CUSCUTA SEEDS

DANG GUI

DAIKON

FOX NUTS

FRITILLARIA

GALANGAL

GINGER ROOT

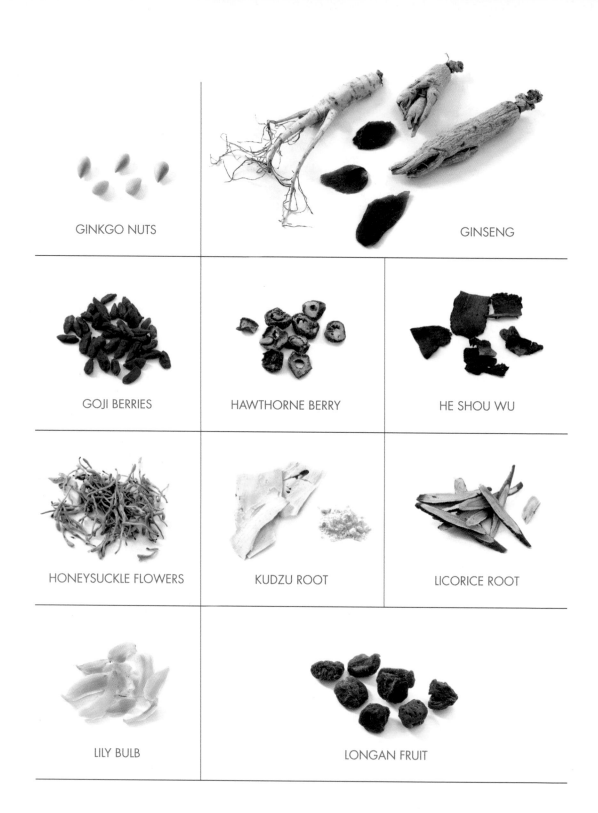

GINKGO NUTS

GINSENG

GOJI BERRIES

HAWTHORNE BERRY

HE SHOU WU

HONEYSUCKLE FLOWERS

KUDZU ROOT

LICORICE ROOT

LILY BULB

LONGAN FRUIT

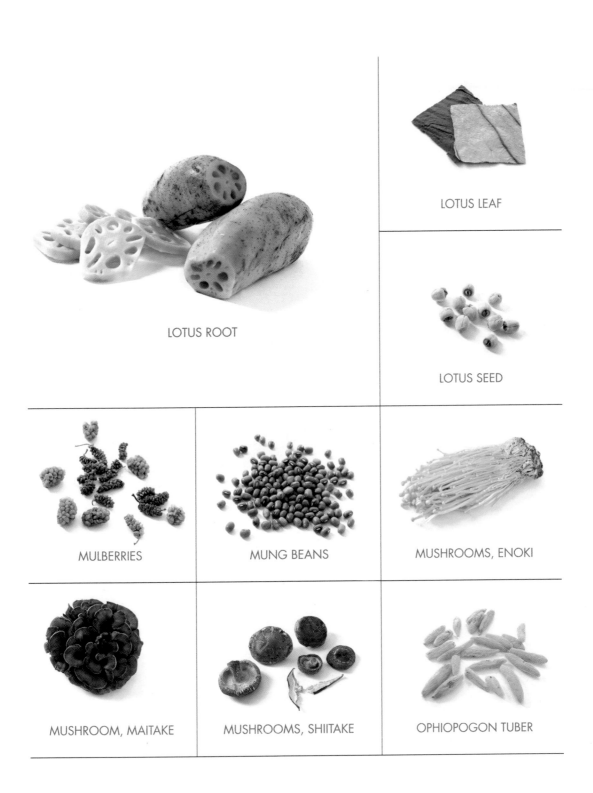

LOTUS LEAF

LOTUS ROOT

LOTUS SEED

MULBERRIES

MUNG BEANS

MUSHROOMS, ENOKI

MUSHROOM, MAITAKE

MUSHROOMS, SHIITAKE

OPHIOPOGON TUBER

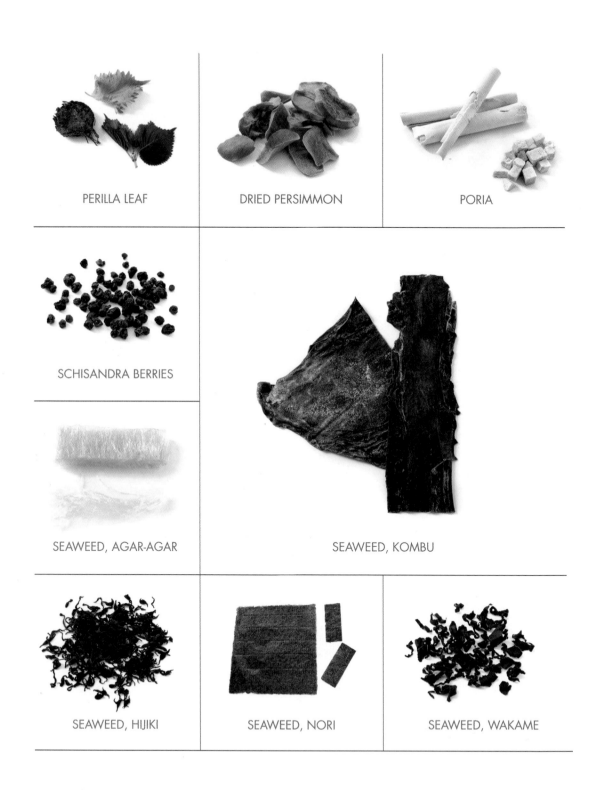

PERILLA LEAF

DRIED PERSIMMON

PORIA

SCHISANDRA BERRIES

SEAWEED, AGAR-AGAR

SEAWEED, KOMBU

SEAWEED, HIJIKI

SEAWEED, NORI

SEAWEED, WAKAME

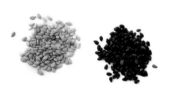

SESAME SEEDS

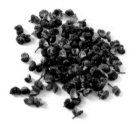

SICHUAN PEPPERCORN

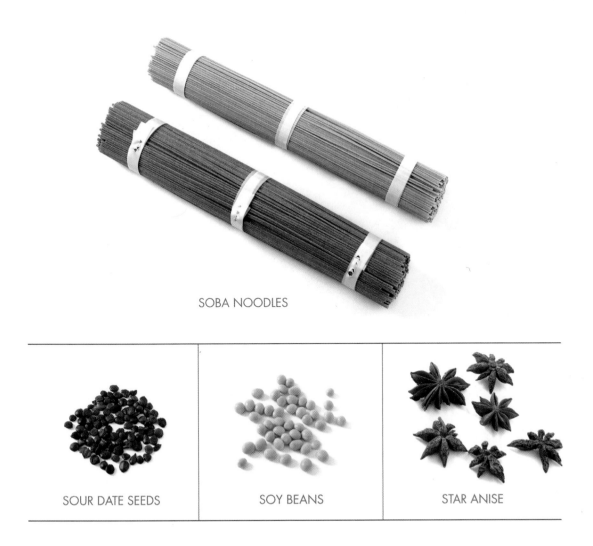

SOBA NOODLES

SOUR DATE SEEDS

SOY BEANS

STAR ANISE

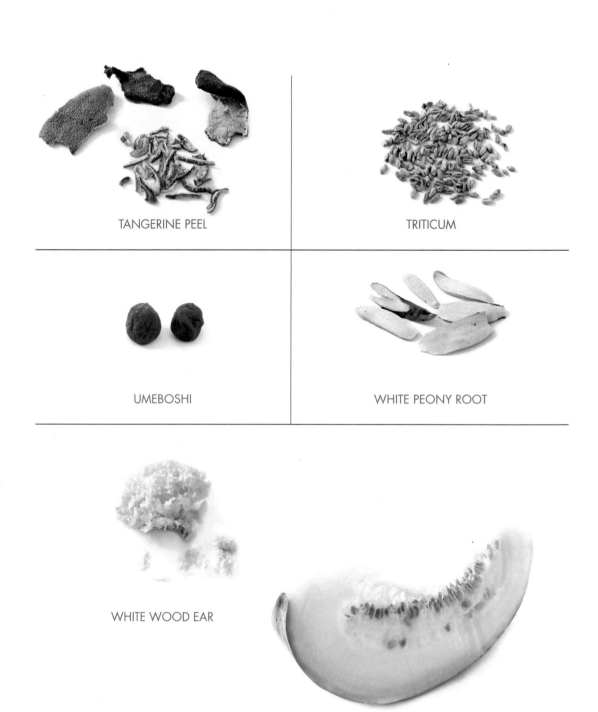

TANGERINE PEEL

TRITICUM

UMEBOSHI

WHITE PEONY ROOT

WHITE WOOD EAR

WINTER MELON

THEMES AND VARIATIONS

This dish is perfect to use up leftover rice. Other mouthwatering toppings for this dish include avocado, perilla leaves, or smoked salmon.

If you are in a hurry, it is possible to combine most of the steps and boil the ingredients in the tea; this method is not for purists or high-quality tea, but it is super quick and easy.

ESPECIALLY GOOD FOR

General health or anyone who wants to calm their emotions, reduce symptoms of menopause, reduce irritability, or help ward off such conditions as cancer or skin rashes.

Mika Says

I make a large pot of brown rice on weekends and freeze portions in freezer bags, so I have brown rice handy whenever I need it for this dish or other quick meals. Frozen brown rice is now available in some stores as a convenience food, but you can easily make it yourself for a fraction of the price.

FOR THOSE FAMILIAR WITH TRADITIONAL CHINESE MEDICINE

This dish strengthens the qi, clears Heat, and drains Dampness.

SESAME-MUSHROOM SOBA NOODLES

MAKES 3 TO 4 SERVINGS

This delicious combination draws on a host of healthy ingredients. Don't count on having leftovers!

INGREDIENTS

3 tablespoons black sesame seeds

8 ounces dried soba noodles

2 tablespoons vegetable oil, such as canola or olive oil

1 small onion, cut into ¼-inch strips

4 cloves garlic, peeled and minced

22 (1 pound) fresh shiitake mushrooms, sliced, stem discarded if desired

½ cup *dashi* or other stock (For stock recipes, see "Mixed and Sundry.")

¼ cup mirin or dry sherry

3 tablespoons soy sauce

1 to 2 tablespoons powdered kudzu, arrowroot, cornstarch, or other thickener

3 to 4 tablespoons water, plus water for boiling the noodles

3 tablespoons black sesame seeds

2 green onions, chopped into ¼-inch pieces, roots and tough tips discarded

DIRECTIONS

1. If your sesame seeds aren't already roasted, toast the sesame seeds by putting them in a wide skillet over medium heat, shaking the pan occasionally. Continue frying until fragrant, 3 to 5 minutes. Remove the seeds from the hot skillet so they don't overcook, and set aside.

2. Bring a pot of water to a boil, then add the soba noodles and cook for about 5 minutes, until al dente or according to the package directions. Drain, rinse under cold running water, and set aside.

3. Heat the oil in a pan over medium-high heat. Add the onions and garlic and sauté for a minute, until fragrant.

4. Add the mushrooms and sauté for 5 to 10 minutes, or until soft. Add the *dashi* stock, mirin, and soy sauce.

5. In a small bowl, mix the kudzu with a few tablespoons of cold water and stir well to remove any lumps. Add the kudzu mixture to the pan and cook for another minute.

6. Toss the soba noodles and vegetables together, and sprinkle with black sesame seeds and green onions before serving.

Helpful Hints about Soba Noodles

A common offering in Japanese cuisine, soba noodles are made in part or in whole from buckwheat (*soba* is the Japanese word for buckwheat), which has been linked to a variety of health benefits and can be consumed as a tea. Soba noodles are available in varieties that include wild yam (*jinenjo soba*), tea (*cha soba*), mugwort (*mugi soba*), and seaweed (*hegi soba*). (For more information on soba noodles, see "One Hundred Healthful Asian Ingredients.")

ESPECIALLY GOOD FOR

Supporting general nutrition; serving to anyone who is feeling under the weather, or who wants to soothe the stomach, help memory, or retard the graying of hair.

FOR THOSE FAMILIAR WITH
TRADITIONAL CHINESE MEDICINE

This dish strengthens the Spleen and Stomach, eliminates Dampness, strengthens the Liver and Kidneys, and augments essence.

SOBA NOODLES WITH MISO-SESAME SAUCE

MAKES 2 TO 3 SERVINGS

These noodles make a quick and satisfying lunch or dinner, which we recommend serving with extra vegetables, such as stir-fried mushrooms and/or bok choy.

INGREDIENTS

1 medium-size cucumber

1 sheet nori seaweed (optional)

8 ounces dried soba noodles

⅓ cup water, plus extra for cooking the noodles

4 tablespoons white miso

3½ tablespoons tahini or other sesame paste

2 tablespoons lemon juice

1 tablespoon mirin wine

1 (½-inch) piece fresh ginger, peeled and grated

1 medium-size carrot, peeled and sliced into matchstick-shape pieces

2 green onions, chopped into ¼-inch pieces, roots and tough tips discarded

Fast Facts about Mirin

Mirin is a sweet Japanese cooking wine that has a lower alcohol content than most wines. Made from glutinous rice, mirin can be used to add a hint of sweetness and a pleasant golden sheen to a dish. If you don't have any mirin on hand, sherry can be substituted.

DIRECTIONS

1. Peel the cucumber. Slice it in half lengthwise and scoop out and discard the seeds. Cut the cucumber into matchstick-shape pieces.

2. Toast the nori seaweed (if using) by holding the sheet by one corner and passing it briefly over a lighted burner on your stove, about an inch above, several times, being careful not to burn the seaweed. With a pair of scissors, cut the nori into ¼ by ½-inch pieces and set aside.

3. Cook the soba in boiling water for 4 to 5 minutes, until al dente or according to the package directions, then drain, rinse under cold running water, and set aside.

4. Warm the water.

5. In a small bowl, mix together the miso, tahini, lemon juice, mirin, grated ginger. Add the warm water a little at a time until the mixture is the desired consistency for your sauce (don't worry if there is water left over).

6. Place the noodles, cucumber, carrot, and green onions in a serving dish, and toss with the sauce. Garnish with the shredded nori.

THEMES AND VARIATIONS

Soba noodles can also be served in a soup or with a simple dipping sauce on the side (see Japanese Noodle Dipping Sauce, page 275), traditionally garnished with green onion, shredded nori seaweed, toasted sesame seeds, and/or wasabi.

ESPECIALLY GOOD FOR

Providing general nutrition or helping those who want to feel more calm, relieve symptoms of menopause or premenstrual syndrome, or prevent atherosclerosis.

FOR THOSE FAMILIAR WITH TRADITIONAL CHINESE MEDICINE

This dish strengthens the qi and nourishes the Blood.

FIVE-ELEMENT STIR-FRY

MAKES 4 SERVINGS

This tasty and satisfying dish combines ingredients that balance each other in a healthy ensemble.

INGREDIENTS

8 medium-size (1 ounce, or 30 grams dried; ⅓ pound fresh) dried or fresh shiitake mushrooms
2 tablespoons vegetable oil, such as canola or olive oil
1 (½-inch) piece fresh ginger, peeled and minced
2 ounces ground turkey or chicken
1 tablespoon tomato paste
2 to 3 tablespoons soy sauce
1 (19-ounce) package soft tofu, chopped into 1-inch cubes
1 medium-size green onion, chopped into ¼-inch pieces, roots and tough tips discarded
Salt and pepper

DIRECTIONS

1. If you are using dried shiitake mushrooms, soak them in cold water for about 30 minutes or until soft, then drain. (If you are using fresh shiitakes, simply rinse.) Slice the mushrooms into ½-inch pieces, removing and discarding the touch stems, if desired.
2. Heat the oil in a pan over medium-high heat, then add the ginger. Cook for about 30 seconds, or until the ginger becomes fragrant.
3. Crumble the ground turkey into small pieces in the pan, then add the mushrooms and sauté for about 3 minutes.
4. Stir in the tomato paste and soy sauce. Add the tofu and stir well to coat it in the sauce. Cook, covered, over medium-low heat for another 5 minutes, or until the tofu is heated through.
5. Add salt and pepper to taste. Garnish with the green onions before serving with rice.

ESPECIALLY GOOD FOR

Supporting general health and nutrition; serving to anyone recovering from an illness or cancer.

FOR THOSE FAMILIAR WITH
TRADITIONAL CHINESE MEDICINE

This dish supplements the qi, nourishes the Blood, and harmonizes the five yin organs.

About the Five Elements

Observing the natural world, early Chinese philosophers developed a way to explain the world's constant transformations, through an approach known as the five-element theory. In the theory, the natural world can be grouped into five categories—Wood, Fire, Earth, Metal, and Water—that support or restrain one another in continuous patterns. These relationships are mirrored in the five tastes (sour, bitter, sweet, spicy, and salty), the five colors (blue-green, red, yellow, white, and black), and the five yang organs (Liver, Heart, Spleen, Lung, and Kidney).

LONGEVITY MUSHROOMS WITH *HE SHOU WU*

MAKES 3 TO 4 SERVINGS

This tasty recipe uses mushrooms, one of our top ten herbs (see the introduction), and he shou wu, one of the most popular herbs in traditional Chinese medicine, used to increase longevity, promote health, and heal various conditions.

INGREDIENTS

1 small handful (0.35 ounces, or 10 grams) *he shou wu*

8 Chinese dates (red, *hong zao*, or black, *da zao*)

1 cup water

2 tablespoons vegetable oil, such as canola or olive oil

1 (1-inch) piece fresh ginger, peeled and minced

2 medium-size green onions, chopped into ¼-inch pieces, roots and tough tips discarded

½ pound pork, chicken, or tofu, cut into 1-inch pieces

¾ to 1 pound fresh mushrooms, cut into ¼-inch slices

2 tablespoons rice wine

1 cup chicken or vegetable stock (For stock recipes, see "Mixed and Sundry.")

1 tablespoon powdered kudzu, arrowroot, cornstarch, or other thickener

2 tablespoons water

Salt

DIRECTIONS

1. In a pot, combine the *he shou wu* and the Chinese dates with 1 cup of water. Bring to a boil, then lower the heat and simmer, covered with the lid slightly ajar, for 30 minutes, to make a concentrate. Strain out the herbs and set the concentrate aside. (Alternatively, you can tie the herb and red dates in cheesecloth or place them in a gauze bag before immersing in the water, for easy removal when this step is done.)

2. Heat the oil in a large pan or wok, then add the ginger, the white part of the green onions, and the meat, and brown on all sides (if you are using the tofu, it won't actually turn brown). Transfer the entire mixture to a bowl and set aside.

3. Place the mushrooms, wine, and chicken broth in the pan. Bring to a boil, then lower the heat and simmer, covered, for 15 minutes.

4. Pour in the herb concentrate, return the meat mixture to the pan, and cook for another 5 minutes, or until the meat is done.

5. In a small bowl, mix the kudzu with about 2 tablespoons of cold water to avoid clumping. Stir the kudzu mixture into the pot to thicken the liquid.

6. Add salt to taste, garnish with the green parts of the green onions, then serve with rice.

Helpful Hints about He Shou Wu

You can purchase *he shou wu* (a.k.a. fleeceflower or *fo-ti*) as whole or sliced roots (older, larger, and darker roots are considered the highest grade). You may also see the herb in tablet form, as some studies have suggested that *he shou wu* has antitumor and antibacterial properties, lowers blood pressure, and increases circulation. (For more information on *he shou wu*, see "One Hundred Healthful Asian Ingredients.")

Legend Has It

An emperor in the Qing dynasty was visiting a region in Sichuan Province in a boat, traveling along a long river. There, he saw a big house with a beautiful yard filled with green trees and flowers, landscaped with little streams and bridges.

"How beautiful!" said the emperor to the governor, who was accompanying him.

But as they drew closer, they noticed a sign on the house that said, "First Family Under Heaven." The governor was horrified. Surely, the emperor would punish him severely for permitting such gall in his territory.

"Who owns this house, governor?" asked the emperor sternly.

When he received no satisfactory reply from the terrified governor, the emperor proposed, "Let us go closer, then, and see if this family has any reason to speak of itself in such lofty terms."

They pulled up their boat to the green bank and disembarked to the sound of many birds singing. When they knocked on the door of the house, a well-dressed young couple came to the door.

"We are here to ask why you call yourselves the first family under heaven," the governor stated.

The couple looked perplexed for a moment and then replied, "We're not sure. We'll have to go ask our parents."

They brought the officials into a courtyard, where there was another couple, as healthy and well dressed as the first.

"Parents, these officials would like to know why we call ourselves first family under heaven."

The second couple looked at each other for a moment, then said, "We're not sure, we have to go ask our parents."

The second couple led the officials into another courtyard, where a third good-looking couple was sitting in the garden.

"Parents, why do we call ourselves the first family under heaven?" they inquired.

"We're not sure," came the reply. "We'll have to ask our parents."

They led the officials into a fourth courtyard, where a fourth couple was enjoying some tea.

"Parents, why do we call ourselves first family under heaven?" This couple did not know either, and once more said they would have to ask their parents.

For the fifth time, the emperor and governor were led into another courtyard, where they found yet another couple.

"Parents, why do we call ourselves first family under heaven?"

"Ah," said the couple. "It is because we eat *he shou wu*, which keeps us strong, fit, and healthy."

The emperor, seeing the longevity that the herb had provided to family members, conceded that the family had just reason to call itself first family under heaven and accepted a gift of some of the herb from them.

ESPECIALLY GOOD FOR

Anyone who wants to increase longevity, or who is suffering from poor memory, insomnia, tinnitus, premature graying of the hair, or hair loss.

FOR THOSE FAMILIAR WITH TRADITIONAL CHINESE MEDICINE

This warming dish strengthens the Liver and Kidney, and nourishes the Blood and essence.

What's in a Name?

The story goes that *he shou wu* got its name when, sometime in the Tang Dynasty, a man named Mr. He had not been able to father a child because he was impotent. One day he was so depressed about this situation he drank himself into a stupor. When he woke up he noticed two intertwining herbs. Curious about them, he took them to a monk, who advised Mr. He to consume this root for its restorative powers. Mr. He boiled the root in water and started drinking the decoction every day. Mr. He found his virility was restored. He fathered several children, his hair never turned gray, and he lived to be well over one hundred. After that, the herb was referred to as *he shou wu*, or "black-haired Mr. He."

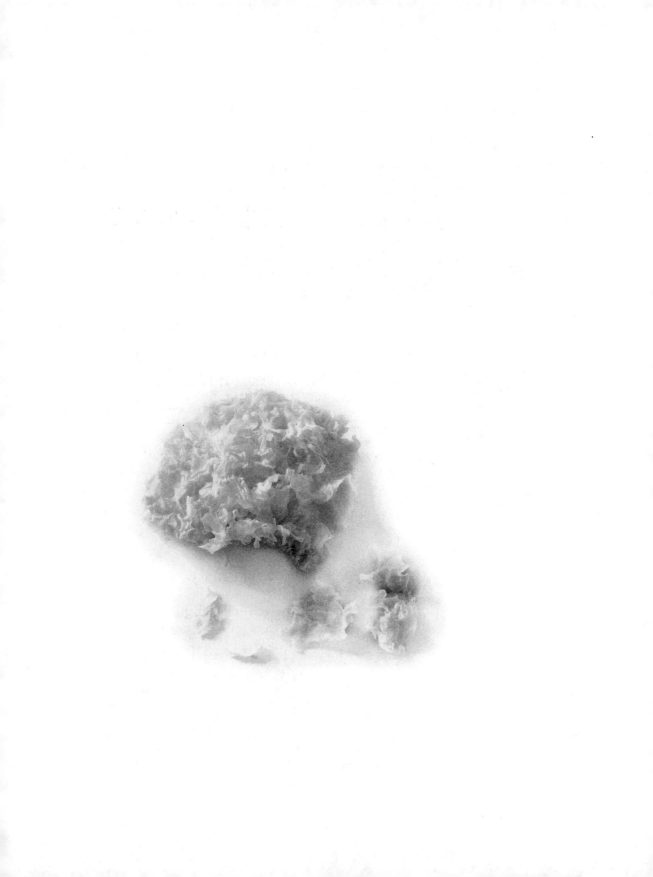

HERE, THERE, ANYWHERE—BREAKFAST, SNACKS, DESSERT

热则寒之 ，寒则热之。

If there's too much heat, cool it.
If there's too much cold, heat it.
If there's too much fullness, empty it.
If there's too much emptiness, fill it.
—THE YELLOW EMPEROR'S CLASSIC OF INTERNAL MEDICINE

BREATHE-EASY FRITILLARIA PEAR

MAKES 1 SERVING

This is a classic Asian recipe, easy and delicious, which builds on pears' reputation for soothing dry coughs.

INGREDIENTS

About 1 tablespoon (10 grams)
   fritillaria (*chuan bei mu*)
1 large ripe pear, any variety
2 teaspoons honey, or to taste

Helpful Hints about Fritillaria

There's a wide range of grades (and prices) of this herb; medium-grade is fine for most purposes. Ask the herb shop to grind it into a powder for you, or use a coffee grinder at home. (For more information on fritillaria, see "One Hundred Healthful Asian Ingredients.")

DIRECTIONS

1. Place the fritillaria in a coffee mill, spice grinder, or food processor and whir into a powder (this may take some time).
2. Wash but don't peel the pear. Cut off the top third and reserve. Cut out the core of the bottom part of the pear, making a hole but leaving the bottom and outside intact.
3. Place the fritillaria powder in the hole, then add the honey. Replace the top of the pear.
4. Transfer the pear to a steamer and cook, covered, for about 40 minutes, or until soft. (If you don't have a steamer, steam the pear in a glass or ceramic bowl, placed in a covered pot containing an inch of water.)
5. Serve warm as a dessert or snack.

THEMES AND VARIATIONS

The pears can be baked instead of steamed. Preheat the oven at 350°F and bake for about 40 minutes, or until soft. Try this dish with a ripe Asian pear—a delicious variation.

Legend Has It

Once there was a poor farmer who had many children. One of them had severe breathing difficulties, and even the doctors thought the child would die. But the father said, "Just because you are sick, doesn't mean you can't be useful around here. I want you to keep an eye on the pear garden." One day, a strong wind came and blew many unripe pears off the tree. The father saw an opportunity to save money on rice and insisted the family pick up the pears and eat them day in and day out. A few months later, the child ran into one of the doctors. "What happened to you?" the doctor asked, surprised. "You look much healthier! Have you been taking a special medicine?" "No," said the child. "All I have been eating is pears." The doctor came to the farmer's house the next day to pick up some of the pears to bring back to patients with lung problems. All were amazed at how the pears helped their recovery. Since then, pears have been used for their special healing properties for respiratory problems.

ESPECIALLY GOOD FOR

Anyone suffering from a dry or chronic cough, dry throat, bronchitis, asthma, or allergies. If you are consuming this dish therapeutically, we recommend eating this dish once a day for three to seven days.

FOR THOSE FAMILIAR WITH TRADITIONAL CHINESE MEDICINE

This dish moistens the Lungs, clears Heat, and transforms phlegm.

GINGER-HONEY PEAR

MAKES 2 SERVINGS

This is a delicious dish, fit to be served to guests or to baby yourself when you want to soothe a dry throat.

INGREDIENTS

2 medium-size pears, peeled
2 tablespoons honey
2 teaspoons grated fresh ginger
3 tablespoons water

Warren Says

When our region in California had raging wildfires a few years ago, many people suffered from coughs and throat irritation from the smoke. I recommended eating baked pears and drinking pear juice to my patients, who found them helpful.

DIRECTIONS

1. Preheat the oven to 350°F.
2. Cut off the top third of each pear and reserve. Cut out the core of the bottom part of the pear, making a hole but leaving the bottom and outside intact. Place the pears and their tops on a glass or ceramic dish.
3. In a small bowl, combine the honey, ginger, and water. (Heat the mixture to encourage the honey to dissolve, if necessary.)
4. Place the ginger mixture inside the pears. Now replace the top on each pear, restoring its original shape, and brush the sauce on the outside of the pear as well. Save 2 teaspoons or so of the sauce for later.
5. Bake the pears for 10 to 12 minutes, until they have begun to soften.
6. Take the pears out of the oven for a moment and drizzle with the remaining sauce, then return the pears to the oven and broil at a high setting for 3 to 5 minutes, until the glaze has caramelized. Serve warm.

THEMES AND VARIATIONS

If you want more flexible portion sizes, slicing the pears into wedges rather than cooking them whole also works well. In this case, there's no need to peel the pears. Bake for about 7 minutes, or until the pear pieces begin to soften, then broil at a high setting for 3 to 5 minutes, until the glaze has caramelized.

ESPECIALLY GOOD FOR

Anyone suffering from a dry cough, dry throat, bronchitis, asthma, upset stomach, or nausea.

FOR THOSE FAMILIAR WITH
TRADITIONAL CHINESE MEDICINE

This dish addresses Lung yin deficiency, dry Heat, and fluid deficiency, and harmonizes the Middle Burner.

TAKE-A-DEEP-BREATH BAKED LIME APPLE

MAKES 1 TO 2 SERVINGS

This simple, wholesome treat is especially good in the fall, when apples are in season.

INGREDIENTS

1 medium-size apple, any variety,
   cored (leave the skin on)
Juice of ½ lime

A Word from the Ancients

See simplicity in the complicated.
Achieve greatness in little things.
—LAO ZI, DAO DE JING
(TAO TE CHING)

DIRECTIONS

1. Preheat the oven to 350°F.
2. Pour the lime juice over the apple.
3. Bake for 30 to 40 minutes, or until the apple is the desired softness.

ESPECIALLY GOOD FOR

Preserving youthful skin, soothing all types of cough, calming irritability, quenching thirst.

FOR THOSE FAMILIAR WITH
TRADITIONAL CHINESE MEDICINE

This dish clears Heat, generates fluids, and moistens the Lungs.

Fast Facts about Apples

Apples are an ancient fruit that probably originated in central and southwestern Asia. Early historical records from Egypt, Babylon, and China mention apples, which were probably mostly small and sour, not the large, cultivated varieties we encounter at the supermarket today. In China, apples symbolize peace and apple blossoms represent women's beauty.

OUTSTANDING OATMEAL

MAKES 1 TO 2 SERVINGS

Warren created this easy, healthy fusion dish by combining Chinese herbs and good old-fashioned oatmeal.

INGREDIENTS

3 medium-size pieces (½ ounce, or 15 grams) astragalus root (*huang qi*)

2 cups water

½ cup rolled oats

A small handful of coarsely chopped walnut pieces

2 tablespoons (30 grams) goji berries (*gou qi zi*)

A pinch of salt

Honey or other natural sweetener (optional)

DIRECTIONS

1. Place the astragalus root and water in a small saucepan. Bring to a boil, then turn down the heat and simmer, covered with the lid slightly ajar, for about 20 minutes.

2. Remove the astragalus root from the liquid with a slotted spoon.

3. Add the rolled oats, walnuts, goji berries, and salt to the liquid and simmer for another 10 minutes, stirring occasionally, until cooked to the desired consistency.

4. Serve warm, drizzled with a small amount of honey, if desired.

Helpful Hints about Astragalus Root

Astragalus root, which is a popular herb available from Chinese herb shops and many Asian supermarkets, is sliced before it is completely dried, producing a product that somewhat resembles a tongue depressor. In addition to its use in cooking, astragalus root can be boiled in water and served as a tea; you might also be able to find it packaged with herbal teas in a natural food store. (For more information on astragalus root, see "One Hundred Healthful Asian Ingredients.")

THEMES AND VARIATIONS

For a thicker oatmeal, use less water; for a thinner texture, use more. You can make this dish with rice instead of oatmeal to make it into a congee, although this requires a longer cooking time.

ESPECIALLY GOOD FOR

Anyone who wants to increase vitality. Astragalus is particularly good for individuals who are concerned about preventing a cold or other illness, who are experiencing tiredness or fatigue, or who are recovering from surgery or childbirth.

FOR THOSE FAMILIAR WITH
TRADITIONAL CHINESE MEDICINE

This dish supplements the Spleen qi and the Kidney yang, and nourishes the Blood.

Warren Says

Too much sweet food is one of the villains of the typical Western diet, contributing to our current epidemic of diabetes and obesity. It's no secret that high-fructose corn syrup, whose use as an inexpensive sweetener skyrocketed in North American packaged food and sodas between 1975 and 1985, is suspected of detrimental health effects. (Highly refined white sugar is also on my personal hit list.) Try using only small amounts of natural sweeteners, such as honey, maple syrup, or unrefined natural sugars, and avoiding any product containing high-fructose corn syrup. If you cut back on sweet foods, you'll find your tastes will change and a little sweetener will start going a long way; the less you consume, the more sensitive you'll be. You'll probably also find yourself feeling more energetic and grounded.

GO-TO GINGER AND JUJUBE PORRIDGE

MAKES 3 TO 4 SERVINGS

Here is a soothing and delicious congee—an Asian-style porridge that often uses a rice base—with the fragrant tang of ginger and the sweetness of Chinese red dates. Eat it for breakfast or have it for a snack.

INGREDIENTS

1 (½- to 1-inch) piece fresh ginger, peeled and minced

10 dried Chinese red dates (jujube or *hong zao*), seeded and diced

½ cup uncooked short-grain rice, rinsed and drained

4 to 5 cups water

A pinch of salt (optional)

Honey or other natural sweetener

Cooking Tip

If you find your porridge is getting too thick halfway through the cooking process, add more water. Alternatively, if it is too runny, remove the lid and boil off the excess water. These tricks will help you troubleshoot if you use different varieties of rice in your congees, as the water requirements and cooking times will vary greatly.

DIRECTIONS

1. Place the ginger, Chinese red dates, rice, and water in a medium-size saucepan and bring to a boil.
2. Lower the heat to low and simmer gently, covered with the lid slightly ajar, for 45 to 60 minutes, stirring occasionally. Add extra water if the porridge is drying out and/or threatening to stick to the bottom of the pot.
3. Add a pinch of salt, if desired, to bring out the flavors.
4. Serve warm, with honey to taste.

THEMES AND VARIATIONS

Vary the amount of water to get the consistency—soupier with more water or firmer with less—that you prefer. If you are lucky enough to have a high-tech rice cooker, there may be a "porridge" setting that you can use to produce perfect congees every time.

We encourage you to experiment with different types of rice—brown, mixed, jasmine—for variety, but keep in mind you'll have to adjust the amount of water and cooking times accordingly. If you prefer brown rice, use ⅓ cup of rice and 5 to 6 cups of water, and cook for 1¾ to 2 hours, slightly mashing the grains against the edge of the pot while stirring, to release the inner starches. If you use long-grain rice instead of short-grain rice (as many people do), the porridge will come out with a less creamy consistency. If you start with leftover rice (a great way to stretch your food dollar), the dish will require less cooking time and less water (a ratio of about one part cooked rice to four parts water).

Fast Facts about Congees

Asian porridge is also known as a congee (from the Chinese *congee-zhou*) or *juk* (from the Korean), a dish mentioned in the *Shang Han Lun* (*Treatise on Cold Disease*) written almost two thousand years ago. Although congees are usually made with rice, they can also be cooked with other grains, including barley, millet, coix, and sorghum. Congees come in literally hundreds of varieties—sweet or savory, with fruit, fish, eggs, and/or vegetables—and are served as a breakfast, snack, late dinner, or side dish. In China, congees are often served with a steamed bun or egg roll. Condiments can include honey (for a sweet congee), or soy sauce, green onions, and/or sesame seeds (for a savory congee).

Cooking styles for congee vary greatly across Asia. The ratio of water to rice varies from 5:1 (Japanese congees called *okayu*) to 12:1 (Cantonese varieties), and cooking times range from 30 minutes to several hours. Stock is sometimes used instead of water for a heartier flavor. Coconut milk appears in some Southwest Asian congees.

In general, congees are great for anyone in a weakened condition, and are often the first solid food fed to babies. If you are recovering from the stomach flu or other illness, congees offer an easy-to-digest dish that can help increase energy. Congees are also used make traditional herbs that are cold, bitter, or harsh easier to digest; in this case, the herb is usually boiled first, then the concentrate is used in the cooking of the congee.

ESPECIALLY GOOD FOR

Anyone with an impaired digestive system, upset stomach, or reduced appetite; also, women who are experiencing painful menses or who are weak after menstruation.

FOR THOSE FAMILIAR WITH
TRADITIONAL CHINESE MEDICINE

This dish warms the Stomach and strengthens the Spleen.

BLACKBERRY BOOST CEREAL

MAKES 2 SERVINGS

We've adapted this recipe using brown rice cereal—which is simply finely ground brown rice and easily found in supermarkets aisles with other hot cereals—for a quicker-cooking meal than a traditional congee.

INGREDIENTS

About 8 pieces (12 grams) dried Chinese red dates (*hong zao*), seeded and diced

2 tablespoons chopped walnut pieces

2 tablespoons (15 grams) goji berries (*gou qi zi*)

2 tablespoons (15 grams) mulberries (*sang shen*)

3 cups water

A pinch of salt (optional)

A handful of fresh blackberries (about 10 large berries)

½ cup uncooked brown rice cereal

Honey or other natural sweetener (optional)

DIRECTIONS

1. In a medium-size saucepan, combine the Chinese red dates, walnuts, goji berries, mulberries, water, and salt (if using), and bring to a boil. Lower the heat and simmer, covered with the lid slightly ajar, for 10 minutes.
2. Add the blackberries, then add the rice cereal. To prevent clumping, slowly sprinkle the cereal into the pot while stirring constantly.
3. Simmer, stirring occasionally, for another 3 to 5 minutes, or until the rice cereal is cooked. Serve with honey to taste.

THEMES AND VARIATIONS

Feel free to vary the amount of water to get the consistency—soupier with more water or firmer with less—that you prefer. Try it with rice or soy milk on top—yum!

This cereal is delicious with oatmeal instead of rice cereal. Use 2 cups of water and 1 cup of oatmeal, simmering for 5 to 10 minutes for regular oatmeal (less for the quick-cook variety).

If you would like to make this dish as a traditional, slower-cooking rice congee, use ½ cup of short-grain white rice and 4 to 5 cups of water, cooking for a total of 45 minutes to 1 hour; add the walnuts at the beginning, and the berries 10 minutes before the dish is done. In this case, consider adding a handful of lily bulb to the mix when you start the congee.

ESPECIALLY GOOD FOR

Anyone who wants a warm, nourishing breakfast or snack to strengthen the body; also, women experiencing itchy skin during menopause.

FOR THOSE FAMILIAR WITH
TRADITIONAL CHINESE MEDICINE

This dish treats conditions caused by Blood deficiency or Kidney deficiency.

CINNAMON-CHESTNUT CONGEE

MAKES 3 TO 4 SERVINGS

This warm, nutty cinnamon cereal takes advantage of the flavors and health benefits of chestnuts. In northern China, chestnuts are dubbed "the king of dried fruits" (gan guo zhi wang).

INGREDIENTS

6 fresh, unshelled chestnuts
¼ cup chopped walnuts
½ cup uncooked short-grain rice, rinsed and drained
¼ teaspoon salt (optional)
4 to 5 cups water
1 teaspoon ground cinnamon, or to taste
1 to 2 teaspoons honey or other natural sweetener, or to taste (optional)

DIRECTIONS

1. Boil the chestnuts in a pot of water for ½ hour. Remove the chestnuts from the water and cut them in half (a serrated knife is helpful). Scoop out the firm flesh with a spoon, discarding the skins and shells. Chop the chestnuts into ¼-inch pieces.
2. Combine the walnuts, chestnuts, rice, salt (if using), and water in a pot.
3. Bring to a boil, then lower the heat and simmer, covered with the lid slightly ajar, for 45 to 60 minutes, stirring occasionally. Add a little extra water if the congee is drying out and/or threatening to stick to the bottom of the pot.
4. Add the cinnamon and cook for 2 to 3 more minutes.
5. Add the honey, if desired, then serve.

ESPECIALLY GOOD FOR

Anyone with cold extremities, weakness, impotence, diarrhea, low back pain, poor memory, insomnia, or frequent nighttime urination.

FOR THOSE FAMILIAR WITH
TRADITIONAL CHINESE MEDICINE

This dish harmonizes the Heart and Kidneys, augments Kidney essence, and strengthens the Spleen qi.

PINING FOR PINE NUT PORRIDGE

MAKES 2 TO 3 SERVINGS

This Korean dish, jat juk, *used to be reserved for the elite, for the sick, and for special occasions, as pine nuts were so expensive and hard to find. Today, we are lucky we aren't faced with such constraints.*

INGREDIENTS

1 cup uncooked short-grain white rice
2 Chinese red dates, seeded
½ cup pine nuts
3 cups water, plus extra for soaking
Salt (optional)
Honey or other natural sweetener (optional)

Legend Has It

In Asia, pine nuts are associated with long life. One story tells of Taoist hermits living in the mountains in ancient China who noticed that during the cold, snowy winters, pine trees stood out as among the only signs of vitality. The hermits developed ways to use many parts of the pine tree in their diet, including the nutritious pine nut.

DIRECTIONS

1. Soak the rice and the Chinese red dates in water for 30 minutes. Drain the rice and finely chop the dates.
2. In a blender or food processor, combine the rice, pine nuts, and 1 cup of water. Whir until smooth, then add another cup of water and whir some more. (If you have a small food processor, you can do this in two batches.)
3. Transfer the mixture to a medium-size pot, add the chopped Chinese red dates and the third cup of water, and bring to a boil.
4. Lower the heat to medium-low and cook, stirring constantly, for about 10 minutes. (Add more water if the mixture gets too thick.)
5. Season with salt (if using) and serve with honey, if desired. Placing a few extra pine nuts on top as a garnish adds a nice touch.

THEMES AND VARIATIONS

Recipes for Korean pine nut porridge vary widely. Some use more pine nuts, some use less. Some recommend starting with rice, some with rice flour. Others advise straining a pine nut–water mixture through cheesecloth to remove the "eyes," or adding the pine nuts at the end of the cooking process. Luckily, pine nuts and rice are a delicious pair, however they are combined.

Feel free to add ginger to your pine nut porridge, especially if you are experiencing the first signs of a cold.

ESPECIALLY GOOD FOR

Anyone with a poor appetite, a craving for sweets, a persistent sensation of dryness and thirst, dry cough, or some types of constipation.

FOR THOSE FAMILIAR WITH
TRADITIONAL CHINESE MEDICINE

This dish strengthens the Spleen and Stomach, addresses pain or thirst due to Stomach yin deficiency, moistens the Lungs, and moistens the Large Intestine.

SMOOTH BLACK SESAME CEREAL

MAKES 2 SERVINGS

This dark, rich mixture can be served as a breakfast porridge or dessert soup. Thanks to Jen Lau for sharing this wonderful recipe, passed down from her grandmother.

INGREDIENTS

2 tablespoons black sesame seeds, preferably roasted

¼ cup white or brown short-grain rice

2 cups water

A pinch of salt, or to taste (optional)

Honey or other natural sweetener

Rice milk or soy milk

Sliced fresh fruit, such as strawberries (optional)

Yuan Says

In China, black foods are believed to possess special qualities for health. Whenever I talk to my patients about this, they have a hard time thinking of many foods eaten regularly in the Western diet.

DIRECTIONS

1. In a food processor or blender, grind the sesame seeds and rice together as finely as possible to form a black powder.
2. In a small saucepan, bring the water to a boil, then add the rice mixture a little at a time, stirring constantly to keep mixture from clumping. Add the salt (if using).
3. Lower the heat to a simmer, and continue to stir for another 10 to 15 minutes, until the rice is cooked. The mixture should be creamy and smooth; if the texture is still grainy, wait until it cools, then pop the mixture back into your food processor or blender and whir until creamy.
4. Add honey to taste. Top with rice milk and sliced fresh fruit, if desired.

THEMES AND VARIATIONS

Add dried tangerine peel (½ tablespoon, soaked until soft), goji berries (2 tablespoons), or ginger (a ½-inch piece, grated). Also, other kinds of rice or milk may be substituted.

ESPECIALLY GOOD FOR

Individuals who are concerned with longevity or who want to darken gray hair; anyone recovering from a serious illness; nursing mothers who want to increase lactation; and people suffering from dry constipation.

FOR THOSE FAMILIAR WITH
TRADITIONAL CHINESE MEDICINE

This dish nourishes and strengthens the Liver and Kidneys, builds Blood, and moistens the Intestines.

SWEET BLACK RICE PUDDING

MAKES 2 SERVINGS

This delicious, dark, sweet porridge uses a whole-grain variety of sticky rice.

INGREDIENTS

½ cup black sticky rice (a.k.a. black glutinous rice or black sweet rice), rinsed

1 (½-inch piece) ginger, grated or minced

2 tablespoons (20 grams) dried longan fruit (*long yan rou*)

6 pitted, dried Chinese red dates (*hong zao*)

4 cups water

A pinch of salt (optional)

Ground cinnamon (optional)

DIRECTIONS

1. Place the rice, ginger, longan fruit, and Chinese red dates in a medium-size pot with the water and salt (if using).
2. Bring to a boil, then lower the heat, cover, and simmer for 1½ to 2 hours, stirring occasionally, until the rice is the desired consistency. Add more water if the mixture is threatening to dry out or is becoming too thick for you.
3. Add cinnamon to taste, if desired.

ESPECIALLY GOOD FOR

Promoting energy and longevity; serving to anyone facing postpartum recovery, menopause, insomnia, or irritability.

FOR THOSE FAMILIAR WITH
TRADITIONAL CHINESE MEDICINE

This dish is good for nourishing the yin and Blood, supplementing the qi, and calming the spirit.

ALWAYS-ON-CALL *OCHAZUKE*

MAKES 1 SERVING

Japanese ochazuke—*any variety of ingredients with rice and tea—is a versatile dish. It can be served at the end of an elaborate Japanese meal or as a simple snack. It acts as a first-line home remedy for colds or hangovers, drawing on one of our favorite herbs, green tea. And it's a great way to use up leftover rice!*

INGREDIENTS

¾ cup cooked rice
A small handful of leafy greens,
    such as spinach, chrysanthemum
    leaves, mizuna, or watercress,
    cut into 2-inch pieces
2 to 3 *umeboshi* (pickled plums)
1 teaspoon wasabi paste
⅔ cup hot brewed green tea
¼ sheet nori seaweed, cut into
    1 by ¼-inch stripes
Soy sauce

Words of Wisdom

There is luck in the leftovers.
—JAPANESE PROVERB

DIRECTIONS

1. Place the rice in a bowl, then arrange the greens, *umeboshi*, and wasabi on top.
2. Pour the hot tea over the rice. The greens will cook in the bowl.
3. Sprinkle the nori on top as a garnish, and add soy sauce to taste.

THEMES AND VARIATIONS

Endless. All the ingredients except the rice and tea are optional. Try a salmon fillet, egg, or bonito flakes on top (see Mouthwatering Meal in a Minute, page 178, for another version.) To make *ochazuke* even easier, most Asian food stores sell ready-made *ochazuke* packets, in such flavors as *umeboshi*, salmon, or wasabi.

ESPECIALLY GOOD FOR

Anyone with edema, urinary problems, small nodules (such as fibroids), or the feeling of having a lump in the throat.

FOR THOSE FAMILIAR WITH
TRADITIONAL CHINESE MEDICINE

This dish helps regulate qi, resolve phlegm, and drain Dampness.

HEALING LILY BULB CONGEE

MAKES 3 TO 4 SERVINGS

Here is another easy-to-digest congee. This one uses lily bulb, whose texture and taste is similar to a potato when cooked, and the famous longevity herb, goji berries.

INGREDIENTS

½ cup uncooked short-grain rice, rinsed and drained

¼ cup (30 grams) lily bulb (*bai he*)

4 to 5 cups water

¼ cup (30 grams) goji berries (*gou qi zi*)

1 to 2 teaspoons honey or other natural sweetener, or to taste (optional)

DIRECTIONS

1. Combine the rice, lily bulb, and water in a medium-size pot. Bring to a boil, then lower the heat and simmer, covered with the lid slightly ajar, for about 30 minutes, stirring occasionally.
2. Add the goji berries, then cook for another 15 to 30 minutes, stirring occasionally. Don't be shy about adding a little extra water if the congee is drying out and/or threatening to stick to the bottom of the pot.
3. Add the honey to taste, if desired, then serve.

Legend Has It

A long time ago, a gang of pirates lived on an island in the East China Sea. One day, the pirates' pillaging took them to a fishing village along the coast. There, they stole provisions and kidnapped women and children, bringing them back to their island.

A few days later, the pirates left to go on another pillaging expedition. By chance, a great storm came up. "Please let the pirate boat sink!" the women and children on the island asked the gods. "Let the boat sink and help us return to our village." Their prayers were answered and the pirates were lost at sea, never to return.

The women and children rejoiced, but as time went on provisions on the island became scarce and they needed to find food to eat. They turned to the land, gathering eggs, fruit, fish, and anything else they could find. One of the plants they collected was similar to garlic—tasty, sweet, and filling—and they ate it instead of rice.

A year later, a group of people gathering herbs came to the island. The women and children were very glad. "How did you survive? And how did you come to look so healthy?" the newcomers asked them. The women and children showed them the herb that they ate in place of rice. When the people went home together, they brought back some samples of the plant and started to cultivate it. Because the women and children on the island numbered about one hundred, the lily plant was called *bai he*, meaning "one hundred together."

THEMES AND VARIATIONS

Instead of dried whole lily bulb, you can use powdered. Most herb stores have grinders, so you can take care of this ahead of time.

As with other congees, you can vary the amount of water to get the consistency—soupier with more water, or firmer with less—that you prefer. If you prefer brown rice, use ⅓ cup of rice and 5 to 6 cups of water, and cook for 1¾ to 2 hours, slightly mashing the grains against the edge of the pot while stirring to release the inner starches. If you use long-grain instead of short-grain rice (as many people do), the porridge will have a less creamy consistency. If you start with leftover rice, the dish will require less water and less cooking time.

Lily bulb and goji berries can also be combined in an easy therapeutic tea. Simmer 1 tablespoon (8 grams) of lily bulb and 1 tablespoon (8 grams) of goji berries in 1½ cups of water, covered with the lid slightly ajar, for 30 minutes. Strain out the herbs, sweeten the liquid with honey or other natural sweetener if desired, and drink 1 to 2 times a day for the tea's therapeutic effects.

ESPECIALLY GOOD FOR

Anyone with a dry cough, insomnia, depression, irritability, menopause, breathing troubles, or concerns about protecting his or her eyesight.

FOR THOSE FAMILIAR WITH TRADITIONAL CHINESE MEDICINE

This dish moistens the Lungs, clears Heat, nourishes the Liver yin and Stomach yin, and calms the spirit.

YIN-YANG CUSCUTA SEED CONGEE

MAKES 2 TO 3 SERVINGS

This congee is prepared with a method that can be used for many therapeutic herbs—the herbs are first simmered in water, then this liquid is used to cook the rice. This congee features cuscuta seeds, small brown seeds used in traditional Chinese medicine to restore balance, improve vision, or counteract impotence, incontinence, or back pain.

INGREDIENTS

6 cups water

2 rounded tablespoons (30 grams) cuscuta seeds (*tu si zi*), rinsed and drained

⅓ cup uncooked brown rice

A pinch of salt (optional)

1 teaspoon honey or other natural sweetener, or to taste (optional)

DIRECTIONS

1. Place the 6 cups of water in a pot. Secure the cuscuta seeds in an empty tea bag for easy handling. Add the bag of cuscuta to the water. Boil, then lower the heat and simmer, covered, for about 20 minutes. Remove the bag of cuscuta seeds.

2. Add the brown rice and salt (if using) to the water and bring to a boil. Lower the heat and simmer, covered with the lid slightly ajar, for 1¾ to 2 hours, stirring occasionally and checking the water level frequently toward the end (add more water, if needed, so the mixture doesn't stick to the bottom of the pot or burn). You'll improve the texture of the congee, making it creamier, by mashing the grains against the side of the pot, releasing the inner starches.

3. Drizzle with honey, if desired, and serve.

> ### Legend Has It
>
> A farmer hired a young man to look after his rabbits. "Look after them well," the farmer said. "If any of them dies, the loss will come out of your paycheck."
>
> One day, though, the young man dropped a stick directly on the back of one of the rabbits. Afraid of what the farmer would say if he saw the injured rabbit, the young man hid the animal in a field of soybean plants. But a few days later, the farmer noticed that one of his rabbits was missing.
>
> "Where is the other rabbit?" he asked.
>
> The young man went to the field to see if the rabbit was still there. Surprisingly, the rabbit was not only alive, but running and jumping with ease.
>
> "I wonder if the rabbit recovered because of something it ate in the field," thought the young man.
>
> To test this idea, he dropped a stick on another rabbit's back and put it in the field—but this time he watched the animal carefully. Indeed, he saw that the second rabbit ate the seeds of a vine growing on the soybean plants. Soon this rabbit, too, recovered.
>
> Intrigued, the young man picked the seeds of this plant and brought them home to his father, who was suffering from terrible back pain. Soon afterward, his father was cured. Ever since, the herb has been used as a herbal medicine and known as *tu si zi*, or "rabbit thread."

THEMES AND VARIATIONS

If you don't have an empty tea bag, but do have a fine strainer, you can boil the cuscuta seeds directly in the water and then strain them out to create the concentrate in the first steps of this recipe.

You can substitute white rice if you are experiencing digestive problems or are in a weakened state; in this case, use ½ cup of short-grain white rice to about 5 cups of water and cook for 45 to 60 minutes.

Whether you use brown or white rice, add more or less water according to taste. Some people prefer their congees firm; others like them soupy.

As with many congees, this one can be made sweet or salty. If you prefer a salty version, omit the honey and add soy sauce to taste.

ESPECIALLY GOOD FOR

Anyone with lower back pain, impotence, frequent urination, or fertility concerns.

FOR THOSE FAMILIAR WITH TRADITIONAL CHINESE MEDICINE

This dish strengthens the Kidneys.

POWER-OF-TEN PORRIDGE

MAKES 3 TO 4 SERVINGS

This recipe creates a ten-grain congee—but feel free to use what you have on hand. The easiest way to shop for this dish is to buy a packet of rice mixed with other grains—available in Asian and natural food stores—and add whatever other ingredients you'd like. Other options for your mixture include purple barley, red rice, and azuki beans (if you are starting with dried azuki beans, soak them overnight before using).

INGREDIENTS

1 tablespoon uncooked brown rice

1 tablespoon uncooked black glutinous rice

1 tablespoon uncooked buckwheat groats

1 tablespoon cracked wheat

1 tablespoon rye berries

1 tablespoon rolled oats

1 tablespoon (15 grams) coix (Job's tears, *yi yi ren* in Chinese, or *hato mugi* in Japanese) or pearl barley

1 tablespoon (10 grams) lotus seeds (*lian zi*)

1 tablespoon (12 grams) fox nuts (*qian shi*)

2 medium-size pieces (6 grams) dried Chinese yam (*shan yao*), broken into ¼- to ½-inch pieces

4 cups water

A pinch of salt (optional)

Soy sauce or honey

DIRECTIONS

1. Combine the brown rice, black glutinous rice, buckwheat, cracked wheat, rye berries, rolled oats, coix, lotus seeds, fox nuts, and Chinese mountain yam, rinse, and drain. Place the mixed grains in a medium-size pot along with the 4 cups of water and the salt (if using).

2. Bring to a boil, then lower the heat and simmer, covered, for about 1½ hours, until soft. Add a little extra water if the congee is drying out, threatening to stick to the bottom of the pot, or becoming too thick for your taste.

3. Serve warm, with soy sauce for a savory congee or honey for a sweet one.

Warren Says

One of the results of the mass production of our food has been the reduction in the variety of grains we eat. High-yielding species of corn, soy, and wheat are especially prominent in Western diets. This porridge counteracts this trend with a variety of grains to provide your body with diverse sources of nutrients.

Fast Facts about the Number Ten

In East Asia, the number ten is often linked with the idea of completion. With ten, you'll have everything you need.

THEMES AND VARIATIONS

Poria (*fu ling*; ⅓ ounce, or 10 grams), broken into small pieces, can be a good addition in this mixture.

Add extra water if you like a thinner porridge; less if you like it firmer. You can halve the amount of fox nuts if you prefer the taste this way.

ESPECIALLY GOOD FOR

Anyone who wants sustained energy, or who has problems with poor digestion, loose stools, or chronic diarrhea.

FOR THOSE FAMILIAR WITH TRADITIONAL CHINESE MEDICINE

This dish strengthens the Spleen and treats diarrhea and unwanted weight loss due to Spleen deficiency.

GROUNDING GINGER AND GREEN ONION CONGEE

MAKES 2 TO 3 SERVINGS

This dish is a classic Asian home remedy. Ginger and green onion can also be boiled together as a tea.

INGREDIENTS

1 (1-inch) piece fresh ginger, peeled and grated or minced

¼ cup sticky rice (a.k.a. "sweet rice" or "glutinous rice")

2½ to 3 cups water

3 green onions, sliced into small pieces (less than ¼ inch)

Condiments: rice vinegar, soy sauce, salt, and/or sesame oil for a savory congee; honey or other natural sweetener for a sweet congee

DIRECTIONS

1. Combine the ginger, sticky rice, and water in a medium-size pot, bring to a boil, then lower the heat to low and simmer, covered with the lid slightly ajar, for 30 to 40 minutes, until the congee is the desired consistency. Add a little extra water if the congee is drying out, threatening to stick to the bottom of the pot, or becoming too thick for your taste.

2. Turn off the heat and add the green onion to the congee.

3. Season with the condiment(s) of your choice and serve warm.

ESPECIALLY GOOD FOR

Anyone fighting off a cold or cough.

FOR THOSE FAMILIAR WITH
TRADITIONAL CHINESE MEDICINE

This dish helps treat an attack of exterior Wind-Cold.

Voice of Experience

I will not forget the instinctive wisdom of the friend who, every day for those first few weeks [after my husband died], brought me a quart container of scallion-and-ginger congee from Chinatown. Congee I could eat. Congee was all I could eat. —Joan Didion, *The Year of Magical Thinking*

SUSTAINING PUMPKIN CONGEE

MAKES 2 SERVINGS

This is a sweet and flavorful pumpkin rice dish, perfect for a snack, late dinner, or side dish, which we suggest with brown rice for its more moderate effect on blood sugar levels than white rice.

INGREDIENTS

10 to 12 ounces pumpkin or winter squash (any variety, such as kabocha or butternut squash) (about 2 cups when peeled and cut into 1-inch cubes)

1 tablespoon dark sesame oil

½ small onion, diced

2 teaspoons curry powder (optional)

4 medium-size pieces (20 grams) dried Chinese yam (*shan yao*), broken into ½-inch pieces

⅓ cup uncooked short-grain brown rice

3½ cups water

A pinch of salt

Soy sauce

THEMES AND VARIATIONS

For those in a weakened condition, this dish can be made with white rice; use ½ cup of short-grain white rice to 4 to 5 cups of water and simmer for about 45 minutes.

Whether you use brown or white rice, add more or less water according to taste. Some people prefer their congees firm, others like them soupy.

DIRECTIONS

1. Seed, peel, and chop the pumpkin into 1-inch cubes. (An efficient way to chop a pumpkin is to cut it into wedges, cut off the skin if desired, then cut the wedges into cubes. A large, sharp cleaver can be a useful tool here, as the raw vegetable can be tough. Another handy trick is to place the pumpkin in the microwave for 5 minutes to soften it before cutting and peeling.) Set aside.

2. Heat the sesame oil in a medium-size saucepan over medium-high heat, then add the onion and cook, stirring occasionally, until it starts to turn golden brown (about 3 minutes).

3. Add the curry powder (if using) and cook for another minute.

4. Add the rest of the ingredients to the saucepan—pumpkin, Chinese yam, brown rice, water, and salt—and stir. Bring the mixture to a boil, then lower the heat to low and simmer, covered with the lid slightly ajar, for 1¾ to 2 hours, until the rice is done. Stir occasionally so the mixture doesn't stick to the bottom of the pot. Add a little extra water if you see the congee is drying out, threatening to stick to the bottom of the pan despite stirring, or becoming too thick for your taste.

5. Serve warm.

ESPECIALLY GOOD FOR

Diabetics and anyone who wants sustained energy.

FOR THOSE FAMILIAR WITH TRADITIONAL CHINESE MEDICINE

This dish aids digestion and strengthens Spleen qi.

ENHANCE-THE-QI MOUNTAIN YAM CONGEE

MAKES 3 TO 4 SERVINGS

This simple breakfast or snack is a classic way to enjoy the subtle taste and gentle, healthful effects of Chinese yam (not to be confused with the sweet potatoes commonly sold as "yams" in the West). If you opt for a congee that's not sweet, consider serving this dish with pickled vegetables or kimchi.

INGREDIENTS

½ pound fresh Chinese yam (*shan yao*)

½ cup uncooked short-grain white rice

4 to 5 cups water

A pinch of salt (optional)

Condiments: rice vinegar, soy sauce, salt, and/or sesame oil for a savory congee; a small amount of honey or other natural sweetener for a mildly sweet congee

DIRECTIONS

1. Peel the Chinese yam and cut it lengthwise into halves or quarters, then widthwise into ⅛-inch slices. (The fresh yam will have a slimy texture; don't worry, it will disappear with cooking.)
2. Combine the Chinese yam, rice, water, and salt (if using) in a medium-size pot and bring to a boil. Lower the heat and simmer, covered with the lid slightly ajar, for 45 to 60 minutes, stirring occasionally. Add a little extra water if you see the congee is drying out or becoming too thick for your taste.
3. Serve warm, with your condiments of choice.

Yuan Says

While Chinese yam (*shan yao*) is one of the premier herbs in traditional Chinese food therapy, related varieties of yam are also gaining a reputation for their health-giving properties. One striking variety of yam is the purple yam (also known as *Dioscorea alata*, water yam, or winged yam, *ube/ubi* in the Philippines, *uhi* in Hawaii), which—true to its name—is a striking violet color inside. Like the Chinese yam, these yams can also be cooked in congees and soups; purple yam is also made into a sweet dessert. I like to simply place a whole, washed yam on top of my rice when I cook it and enjoy the way the textures and flavors blend.

THEMES AND VARIATIONS

A variation of this congee is to use 2 ounces (50 grams) of powdered dried Chinese mountain yam (which you can powder yourself by putting the crumbled pieces of about nine dried slices of Chinese yam in a coffee mill or spice grinder), ½ cup of short-grain white rice, and 5 cups of water. Stir regularly, as this mixture has a tendency to stick to the bottom of the pot.

As with other congees, you can experiment with using different varieties of rice—including brown, black, and mixtures. If you use short-grain brown rice, use ⅓ cup of rice to 3½ cups of water and cook for 1¾ to 2 hours. If you use long-grain instead of short-grain rice (as many people do), the porridge will come out with a less creamy consistency. If you start with leftover rice, the dish will require less water and less cooking time.

Also, vary the amount of water to get the consistency—soupier with more water or firmer with less—that you prefer.

ESPECIALLY GOOD FOR

Anyone who is suffering from poor appetite, fatigue, loose stools or diarrhea, or (especially when made with brown rice and no sweetener) diabetes.

FOR THOSE FAMILIAR WITH
TRADITIONAL CHINESE MEDICINE

This dish addresses Spleen qi deficiency.

Legend Has It

In the days when China was made up of many competing countries, two armies faced off in a battle. The larger, stronger army won handily, chasing soldiers and horses from the weaker army high up into a mountain. For a while, the stronger army remained vigilant, making a blockade to ensure members of the losing army could not come down the mountain to get food. Months passed, winter came, and finally the victorious soldiers concluded that their opponents must have died from starvation. One year later, however, a band of strong, healthy soldiers and their horses charged down the mountain, took the previously victorious group completely by surprise, and drove them away. One of the villagers asked, "How did you survive all winter on the mountain?" One of the strong, healthy soldiers replied, "At first we had nothing to eat. We were so hungry we started digging up roots. We found that a plant with white flowers had a large, sweet, nourishing root. We started eating it and feeding it to the horses. That root is what sustained us and made us so strong." The Chinese yam is today known in China as *shan yao*, or "mountain medicine."

RESTORATION PORRIDGE

MAKES 3 TO 4 SERVINGS

This nutty-tasting and easy-to-digest breakfast or snack will be particularly soothing for anyone suffering from diarrhea or an upset stomach.

INGREDIENTS

3 to 4 medium-size (10 to 15 grams) pieces dried Chinese yam (*shan yao*), broken into ½-inch pieces

1 tablespoon (10 to 15 grams) coix (Job's tears, *yi yi ren* in Chinese, or *hato mugi* in Japanese)

1 heaping tablespoon (10 to 15 grams) lotus seeds (*lian zi*)

½ cup uncooked short-grain white rice

4 to 5 cups water

A pinch of salt (optional)

Honey or other natural sweetener

Warren Says

In the clinic, I recommend this dish to my Spleen-deficient patients all the time, with great results. This congee usually helps patients get over their diarrhea and digestive distress within a few days.

DIRECTIONS

1. Combine the Chinese yam, coix, lotus seeds, rice, water, and salt (if using) in a medium-size pot and bring to a boil. Lower the heat and simmer, covered with the lid slightly ajar, for 45 to 60 minutes, stirring occasionally. Add a little extra water if you see the congee is drying out or becoming too thick for your taste.

2. Serve warm, drizzled with honey.

THEMES AND VARIATIONS

Poria (*fu ling*, ⅓ ounce, or 10 grams), broken into small pieces, can be another helpful addition to this porridge. One tablespoon (⅓ ounce, or 10 grams) of fox nuts can also be added.

As with other congees, you can vary the amount of water to get the consistency—soupier with more water or firmer with less—that you prefer. If you use long-grain instead of short-grain rice (as many people do), the porridge will come out with a less creamy consistency. If you start with leftover rice, the dish will require less water and less cooking time.

ESPECIALLY GOOD FOR

Anyone with diarrhea or poor appetite can try eating this porridge two to three times a day until he or she is feeling better. (If you suspect an infection, though, skip the porridge and see your doctor.)

FOR THOSE FAMILIAR WITH
TRADITIONAL CHINESE MEDICINE

This dish strengthens the Spleen to aid digestion and astringe diarrhea.

MILD MUNG BEAN–KUDZU CONGEE

MAKES 2 TO 3 SERVINGS

Mung bean congee is a classic Chinese food therapy dish. This congee has a pleasant puddinglike texture with the kudzu powder, which is often used as a thickener. Like many congees, this can be served as a savory dish (which can be garnished with black sesame seeds or green onions and served with vegetables or meat) or a sweet one.

INGREDIENTS

¼ cup mung beans
¼ cup short-grain white rice
A pinch of salt (optional)
5 cups cold water
3 to 4 tablespoons (50 grams)
   powdered kudzu (*ge gen*)
Soy sauce (for a savory congee) or
   honey (for a sweet congee)

DIRECTIONS

1. Combine the mung beans, rice, and salt (if using) in a large pot.
2. Add 4¾ cups of the water and bring to a boil, then lower the heat and simmer, covered with the lid slightly ajar, for about 1 hour. Add a little extra water if you see the congee is drying out or becoming too thick for your taste.
3. Mix the kudzu with about ¼ cup cold water to make it into a paste, then stir the mixture into the pot.
4. Cook the ingredients together for another 2 to 3 minutes, and serve.

ESPECIALLY GOOD FOR

Eating in the summer; managing high cholesterol or diabetes; clearing up skin problems.

FOR THOSE FAMILIAR WITH
TRADITIONAL CHINESE MEDICINE

This dish clears Heat, drains Dampness, and benefits the Spleen and Stomach.

SWEET FRUIT AND NUT RICE

MAKES 4 TO 6 SERVINGS

In Korean, this sweet dish is known as yaksik/yakshik or yakbap, which translates as "medicinal food" or "medicinal rice." It is traditionally served on the holiday Jeongwol Daeboreum, which celebrates the first full moon after the New Year. The Chinese enjoy a similar dish called ba bao fan, *or "eight treasures," common for holidays or the Chinese New Year.*

INGREDIENTS

1 cup sticky rice (a.k.a. "sweet rice" or "glutinous rice")
1 teaspoon soy sauce
1 tablespoon rice wine
1 tablespoon dark sesame oil
¼ cup honey
½ cup Chinese red dates (*hong zao*), pitted
½ cup shelled walnuts or chestnuts, chopped into ¼-inch pieces
1 tablespoon pine nuts
1½ teaspoons ground cinnamon

THEMES AND VARIATIONS

If you are lucky enough to have a rice cooker, you can make a simplified version of this dish. Place the sticky rice, walnuts, pine nuts, soy sauce, rice wine, honey, dark sesame oil, Chinese red dates (pitted), and ground cinnamon, and the amount of water called for by the cooker's manufacturer's instructions into the rice cooker and press the START button. When the rice is done, let it sit on the KEEP WARM setting for at least 10 minutes before serving.

DIRECTIONS

1. Soak the rice in warm water for about 1 hour. Drain through a fine strainer.
2. Place the rice grains in the top half of a stovetop steamer, fill the base with an inch of water, and wrap a piece of cheesecloth or a clean dish towel around the lid to absorb some of the steam and keep the rice firm. Cover and cook for 30 minutes over medium heat.
3. Combine the soy sauce, rice wine, ½ tablespoon of the sesame oil, and honey in a large saucepan. Warm the mixture for a minute to dissolve the honey, then turn off the heat.
4. Add the Chinese red dates, all but a teaspoon of walnut pieces and a teaspoon of pine nuts, and the cinnamon, and stir. Add the hot rice from the steamer and mix well.
5. Brush a casserole dish or bread pan with the remaining ½ tablespoon of sesame oil. Scoop the rice mixture into the dish and pack it down. Place the dish into a larger pot with some water in the bottom. The water should come about halfway up the outside of the dish.
6. Cover the large pot (so the rice mixture steams in its dish) and cook for about 1 hour. Turn off the heat and let the dish rest for 15 minutes. Garnish with the reserved walnut pieces and pine nuts before serving.

ESPECIALLY GOOD FOR

Substituting for highly processed or sugar-laden desserts; also, serving to those recovering from childbirth or having chronically cold hands and feet.

FOR THOSE FAMILIAR WITH TRADITIONAL CHINESE MEDICINE

This dish is good for qi and Blood deficiency.

STICKY SESAME AND WALNUT BALLS

MAKES 4 TO 6 SERVINGS

A sweet, nutty treat made of healthy ingredients. Why eat junk food when you can indulge like this?

INGREDIENTS

⅓ cup (about 2 ounces) black sesame seeds

⅓ to ½ cup (about 2 ounces) chopped walnut pieces

3 to 4 tablespoons honey

Color Counts

From the perspective of traditional Chinese medicine, the color of food provides an important clue to some of its properties for health. (Interestingly, scientific evidence has supported the view that certain phytonutrients, organic compounds often associated with naturally colored fruits and vegetables, can fight disease—for instance, the lycopene in red tomatoes and grapefruit, or the lutein in leafy greens such as kale and spinach.) In Chinese medicine, black foods are thought to nourish the Kidneys, supporting the reproductive systems, strengthening bones, increasing libido, and favoring longevity. Black sesame seeds, black wood ear, black beans, seaweed, and black dates are common in Asian cuisine.

DIRECTIONS

1. If your sesame seeds aren't already roasted, toast them in a wide skillet over medium heat, shaking the pan occasionally. Continue frying until fragrant, 3 to 5 minutes. When they are done, transfer the seeds from the hot skillet to a bowl so they don't overcook, and let cool for at least 1 minute.
2. In a food processor, whir together the sesame seeds, walnuts, and 3 tablespoons of the honey.
3. Roll into ¾-inch balls. If the balls don't stick together at first, add a little more honey and whir the mixture some more.
4. Serve—and don't tell anyone how easy this dish was to make!

THEMES AND VARIATIONS

If you aren't in the mood for something sweet, the black sesame seeds and walnuts can be consumed as a powder, either in spoonfuls or sprinkled on another dish.

ESPECIALLY GOOD FOR

Anyone suffering from insomnia or who wants to slow the onset of gray hair or hair loss. For insomnia, eat two sesame and walnut balls (or 1 tablespoon of the powder) an hour or two before bedtime.

FOR THOSE FAMILIAR WITH TRADITIONAL CHINESE MEDICINE

This dish addresses Kidney deficiency.

Yuan Says

At the clinic, I recently had a patient who was complaining about chronic insomnia. I recommended this dish in a powdered form to be taken before bedtime. She came back the next week and said she still couldn't sleep. I told her to just stick with it. After two or three months, she began noticing an improvement. Now she tells me she wakes up in the morning after a good sleep and says, "Thanks to Dr. Wang for this recipe!"

PORIA–BLACK SESAME BISCUITS

MAKES ABOUT 6 SERVINGS

These biscuits are a tasty snack or dessert, and are especially good when served warm with tea.

INGREDIENTS

¼ cup black sesame seeds
4 ounces (100 grams) poria mushrooms (*fu ling*)
1 cup water
2 tablespoons honey
2½ tablespoons sweet rice flour
A pinch of salt (optional)
2 to 3 tablespoons vegetable oil,
   such as canola or olive oil

Helpful Hints about Poria

Poria (*fu ling*), a type of oval, light-colored fungus that grows on pine tree roots, is sold in Asian markets sliced and dried, often as part of an herbal mixture. You may also be able to find it in powdered form. (For more information on poria, see "One Hundred Healthful Asian Ingredients.")

DIRECTIONS

1. If your sesame seeds aren't already roasted, toast them in a wide skillet over medium heat, shaking the pan occasionally. Continue frying until fragrant, 3 to 5 minutes. When they are done, transfer the seeds from the hot skillet to a bowl so they don't overcook. Set aside.

2. If you have poria in a form that is not yet powdered, break it into small pieces, then whir it in a spice mill, coffee grinder, or food processor until it is powdered. Set aside.

3. Warm ½ cup of the water and add the honey to it. Stir until the honey dissolves.

4. In a medium-size bowl, mix together the poria powder, black sesame seeds, rice flour, and salt (if using). Stir in the honey mixture. Add the remaining water, a little at a time, until a smooth dough is formed (this will take about ½ cup more water).

5. Roll the dough into small balls, then press into ¼ by 1-inch circles.

6. Heat a skillet over medium heat, pour in the oil and allow it to heat, then cook the biscuits until both sides are browned and the center is warm, about 5 minutes.

Legend Has It

A Korean legend about poria concerns an aristocratic young woman, Ki-ryeong, and a servant, Ki-bok, who fell in love. Because such a union was strictly forbidden, they decided they would elope. Ki-ryeong, however, fell ill. Ki-bok wandered the countryside looking for an herb to cure her. During his search, he shot an arrow at a rabbit. The arrow missed the rabbit and landed in a hole in the ground near a pine tree. There, in what Ki-bok believed to be divine intervention, he discovered a type of fungus he had never seen before. Ki-bok boiled it in water to make a drink for Ki-ryeong. When she drank the decoction, she was cured. Since then, poria has been called *bok-ryeong* after the couple.

ESPECIALLY GOOD FOR

Anyone who wants to increase energy, or women going through menopause.

FOR THOSE FAMILIAR WITH TRADITIONAL CHINESE MEDICINE

This dish strengthens the Spleen and addresses Blood deficiency.

SWEET DECORATED RICE BALLS

MAKES 4 TO 6 SERVINGS

A quick and tasty dessert. We were surprised to find sweet rice flour available in the Asian food section of our local supermarket.

INGREDIENTS

1 cup sweet rice flour

A pinch of salt

⅓ cup hot water, plus extra for boiling

½ cup ground cinnamon, toasted black sesame seeds, and/or chopped pine nuts, for coating the balls

Honey or other natural sweetener

DIRECTIONS

1. In a bowl, combine the sweet rice flour and salt, and mix well.
2. Add the hot water a little at a time, stirring constantly.
3. Knead the mixture into a crumbly dough and shape into 15 to 18 balls. (There should be barely enough water to hold the mixture together.)
4. In a medium-size saucepan, bring about 6 cups of water to a boil. Drop the balls into the boiling water one by one.
5. Cook for 6 to 7 minutes, until the balls float to the top of the water and become slightly translucent.
6. Remove the balls from the boiling water with a slotted spoon, and place them in a bowl of cold water to stop the cooking.
7. Roll the balls thoroughly in the coating of your choice and serve with honey on the side as a dip.

Yuan Says

In China, sweets are not traditionally part of the everyday diet but are reserved for special occasions, such as holidays and festivals. Thanks to this approach, sweets stay a treat rather than becoming a habit.

THEMES AND VARIATIONS

Plain rice balls can be added to Sweet Red Bean Soup (see page 222), right before serving. Some people like to add *matcha* (green tea powder) to the dough, about 1 teaspoon per cup of rice flour.

A related dish that features Chinese red dates, which are believed to promote energy, involves stuffing the dates with sweet rice flour dough, then steaming them. In this case, mix together ½ cup of sweet rice flour with 2 tablespoons of water. Split each red date down one side, remove the seed if necessary, and stuff with the dough. Fry briefly in oil to caramelize the outside of the dates, if desired, then steam them for 10 minutes. Thanks to Jeff Tien for sharing this variation—and his delicious stuffed dates when Warren was hungry!

ESPECIALLY GOOD FOR

Substituting for highly processed or sugar-laden desserts.

A cinnamon topping is good for those who want to increase vitality or address reduced appetite, diarrhea, and some types of abdominal pain. Black sesame seeds are considered a longevity herb especially appropriate for those who want to help darken gray hair, address some types of headaches, dizziness, or numbness, or counteract dry constipation. Pine nuts, which are used as an antiaging tonic, are also good for those who want to sooth a dry throat and cough, counteract constipation, or address conditions involving dizziness, drowsiness, or rheumatism.

FOR THOSE FAMILIAR WITH TRADITIONAL CHINESE MEDICINE

Cinnamon is considered pungent, sweet, and hot, entering the Heart, Kidney, Liver, and Spleen channels. Black sesame seeds, sweet in flavor and neutral in temperature, nourish the yin, for yin deficiency; nourish the Blood and extinguish Wind; and moisten the Intestines. Pine nuts, which are considered sweet in flavor and neutral to warm in temperature, increase Kidney energy.

SIMPLE PEACH *KANTEN*

MAKES 6 SERVINGS

The Japanese make sweets from agar-agar, a white translucent seaweed product that can be transformed into a vegetarian, jiggly gelatin. Here, we provide a basic recipe for kanten, *which can be adapted endlessly by varying the fruit (fresh or dried) and fruit juice in the mixture. Fruit can also be served on top of the* kanten *rather than inside the dessert. The traditional Japanese dish* anmitsu *features a* kanten *made with sweetened water and a touch of lemon juice, with fresh fruit and sweet red bean paste on top.*

INGREDIENTS

1 (¼ ounce) bar agar-agar, torn into pieces

1½ cups fruit juice, such as apple or peach

¾ cup water

A pinch of salt (optional)

2 to 3 peaches, pitted, peeled, and diced (1½ cups when diced)

Helpful Hints about Agar-Agar

You might encounter agar-agar sold in several different forms— in flakes, strands, or powder as well as bars. All of these will work; however, powder some- times contains unwanted addi- tives. Flakes do not need to be soaked; 2 rounded tablespoons of flakes are approximately equal to one bar. (For more information on agar-agar and seaweed in general, look under "seaweed" in "One Hundred Healthful Asian Ingredients.")

DIRECTIONS

1. Place the agar-agar, fruit juice, water, and salt (if using) in a saucepan. Let soak for 30 minutes.

2. Bring to a boil over medium heat. Lower the heat and simmer, stirring occasionally, until the agar-agar has dissolved, 5 to 10 minutes.

3. Place the diced peaches in the bottom of a jelly mold or 8 by 8-inch dish.

4. Pour the hot liquid over the peaches. Set aside in a cool place for 1 to 1½ hours to let the dessert gel (if you are in a hurry, you can put it in the refrigerator after it cools at air temperature for 30 minutes, but this is not necessary).

5. Cut the jelly into pieces or spoon it into dessert bowls.

Legend Has It

In Asia, the peach is seen as symbol of hope, long life, and immortality. One Chinese legend tells of the fabled Peach Tree of the Gods, which blossoms once every three thousand years, producing fruit that grants health and immortality to all who eat it. Birthday celebrations in China still often feature peaches. In Japan, one famous folktale chronicles the adventures of Momotaro, a hero who was born from an enormous peach.

THEMES AND VARIATIONS

For a firm jelly, add more agar-agar; for a softer jelly, add less. For a sweeter dessert, omit the water and add more juice; for a less sweet dessert, try a mixture of half water and half juice.

Try sprinkling some roasted sesame seeds or other seed or sliced nut on top.

In addition to using different types of fruit and fruit juice, variations of this recipe include using green tea or chrysanthemum tea as the liquid base that is gelled with the agar-agar. A similar jelly made with sweetened coconut milk is also popular in Southeast Asia. In general, the more acidic the liquid, the more agar-agar you will need for the mixture to set.

ESPECIALLY GOOD FOR

Eating in the summer; quenching thirst; or serving to anyone suffering from constipation or who is concerned about soft masses such as goiter, ovarian cysts, breast lumps, fibroids, or lymph node swelling.

FOR THOSE FAMILIAR WITH TRADITIONAL CHINESE MEDICINE

This dish moistens the Intestines, softens hardness, and counteracts Summer Heat.

SWEET RED BEAN SOUP

MAKES 3 TO 4 SERVINGS

Red bean soup is a popular dish in East Asia, where folk wisdom has it that the soup contributes to health and beauty. In China and Japan, it is often served at celebrations such as New Year, weddings, and birthdays, as the color red is associated with luck and happiness. In Korea, red bean soup (called pat juk) is especially prominent on the winter solstice holiday, when it is believed the dish drives away spirits bringing bad luck and epidemics.

INGREDIENTS

½ cup dried azuki beans

2 to 3 tablespoons dried lotus seeds (*lian zi*) (optional)

1 tablespoon (4 grams) dried tangerine peel (*chen pi*), shredded

3½ cups water, plus extra for soaking

3 tablespoon-size pieces rock sugar or other natural sweetener, or to taste

Coconut milk or coconut cream (optional)

Helpful Hints about Rock Sugar

Rock sugar, a clear, hardened form of cane sugar composed of crystallized sugar and water, can be found in most Asian markets.

DIRECTIONS

1. Soak the azuki beans in about 2 cups of water for at least 8 hours or overnight.
2. In a separate container, soak the lotus seeds (if using) in about ½ cup of water for at least 3 hours, or overnight.
3. Soak the tangerine peel in warm water for 15 minutes to soften. Drain and dice.
4. Drain the beans and lotus seeds.
5. Pour the 3½ cups of fresh water into a medium-size pot and bring to a boil.
6. Add the beans, lotus seeds, and tangerine peel, bring the water back to a boil, then lower the heat and simmer, covered with the lid slightly ajar, for about 1 hour and 15 minutes, until the beans and lotus seeds are soft.
7. Add the rock sugar, stir to dissolve, then simmer for another 5 minutes.
8. Spoon the bean soup into bowls and garnish with a swirl of coconut milk, if desired.

THEMES AND VARIATIONS

Red bean soup can be served hot in the winter and fall, or chilled in the warm summer months. Some recipes call for longan fruit, lotus root, or lily bulb. In Japan, red bean soup (called *shiruko*) often contains *mochi* (pounded rice cake), chestnuts, or small rice balls (see Sweet Decorated Rice Balls, page 218; don't roll in the coating and add them before serving); in some versions of the soup, the beans are crushed and strained to make a paste. In Vietnam, coconut cream (the thick part of the milk that floats to the top) or coconut milk is sometimes used as a garnish, swirled into the soup right before serving, which we think is an attractive and delicious touch.

A smaller amount of granulated sugar can be substituted for rock sugar if necessary, although in terms of traditional Chinese medicine, white sugar is used only with caution because it may injure the Spleen and Stomach. Other, natural sweeteners are preferred over processed sugars.

ESPECIALLY GOOD FOR

Eating warm in the fall or winter; serving to anyone who wants to increase energy or reduce water retention or puffy skin.

FOR THOSE FAMILIAR WITH
TRADITIONAL CHINESE MEDICINE

This dish strengthens the Spleen and Kidneys, helps to drain Dampness, and eliminates toxicity.

REJUVENATING WOOD EAR AND RED DATE DESSERT SOUP

MAKES 3 TO 4 SERVINGS

Dessert soups are quite popular in Asia. This one brings together the firm texture of wood ear with the sweet accent of Chinese dates. Although in the West, mushrooms and related fungi are associated with savory dishes, wood ears, with their neutral flavor and firm texture, are also often found in Eastern sweet dishes, especially sweet soups.

INGREDIENTS

½ cup (¾ ounce, or 20 grams) dried black wood ear (*hei mu er* in Chinese, *kikurage* in Japanese)

6 dried Chinese red dates (*hong zao*), seeded

2 teaspoons rock sugar or honey, to taste

3 cups water, plus extra for soaking

2 to 3 teaspoons pine nuts (optional)

DIRECTIONS

1. Rinse the wood ear and soak it for half an hour in warm water, where it will expand to two to five times its original size. Drain and cut off any fibrous material/stem adhering at the base of the wood ear, as this will be tough. Cut the remainder of the wood ear into ¼-inch slices.

2. Combine the wood ear, Chinese red dates, and rock sugar with the water in a glass bowl or ovenproof dish.

3. Place the bowl onto a steamer tray or rack within a lidded wok or pot that has water in the bottom. (If you happen to have an appropriately sized double boiler, by all means use this instead). Cover, bring the water to a boil, then lower the heat and steam the soup (replacing the pot's water as necessary) for about 1 hour, or until the wood ear is tender.

4. Sprinkle the soup with pine nuts as a garnish, if desired, before serving.

Helpful Hints about Chinese Dates

Don't be misled by the name—the Chinese red date, an oval fruit that comes in red, black, and wild varieties, is a different species than the fruit of the date palm that goes by the common name of "date" in many Western supermarkets. (For more information on Chinese dates, see "One Hundred Healthful Asian Ingredients.")

THEMES AND VARIATIONS

Here, we call for a traditional method of steaming or "double boiling" the soup, which results in a clear broth and intense flavor. If you don't have the patience or the equipment for double boiling, don't worry. You can gently simmer the ingredients together in a pot directly on a stove burner.

Cloud ear (*Auricularia polytricha*) can be substituted for wood ear, although cloud ear tends to be slightly more expensive. Both varieties are sold dried and can be used interchangeably in the kitchen—and are often confused in common usage.

ESPECIALLY GOOD FOR

Anyone recovering from injury or surgery, and women feeling drained after menstruation or childbirth.

FOR THOSE FAMILIAR WITH TRADITIONAL CHINESE MEDICINE

This dish helps treat Blood deficiency.

FIVE-FRUIT DESSERT POTAGE

MAKES 4 TO 6 SERVINGS

A fruit salad in a soup! From the perspective of traditional Chinese medicine, cooking makes foods easier to digest.

INGREDIENTS

- 1.4 ounces (40 grams) dried white wood ear (*bai mu er* or *yin er* in Chinese, *hakumokuji* or *shiro kikurage* in Japanese)
- 4 cups water
- 1 medium-size pear or apple, peeled, cored, and cut into 1-inch pieces
- 1 medium-size kiwi, peeled and cut into 1-inch pieces
- 1 medium-size peach, orange, or star fruit (carambola), peeled, seeded, and cut into 1-inch pieces (if using star fruit, cut instead into ¼-inch slices to show off its pretty shape)
- 1 cup diced and seedless/seeded watermelon
- ½ cup blackberries, black raspberries, black seedless grapes, or blueberries
- 1 tablespoon rock sugar or other sweetener, or to taste

DIRECTIONS

1. Rinse and soak the wood ear in warm water until soft, about 30 minutes. Cut off and discard the fibrous base of the wood ear, then cut the remainder into ¼-inch slices.
2. Place the water and wood ear in a pot and bring to a boil. Lower the heat, cover, and simmer for about 20 minutes.
3. Add the fruit and rock sugar to the pot, and bring back to a boil.
4. Turn down the heat and simmer for about 5 minutes, or until the fruit is soft and the rock sugar is dissolved, then serve as a snack or dessert.

THEMES AND VARIATIONS

You have a pretty free hand in substituting other fruits in this basic recipe, which comes in many variations. Here, we chose five different-colored fresh fruits to represent the five elements.

In many traditional recipes, the white wood ear is cooked in a steamer or double boiler for 1 to 2 hours before the fruit is added.

ESPECIALLY GOOD FOR

Anyone who is weak or recovering from an illness, or who wants to improve the complexion.

FOR THOSE FAMILIAR WITH TRADITIONAL CHINESE MEDICINE

This dish clears Heat in the Lungs, supplements the Spleen and Stomach, and relieves toxicity.

Good Inside and Out

As well as providing a succulent fruit, watermelon offers a rind that can be used topically for its soothing effects. If you are suffering from itchy skin in the summer, perhaps a heat rash, try applying watermelon rind to your skin.

CHESTNUT-LOTUS DESSERT SOUP

MAKES 4 SERVINGS

This dessert soup combines the benefits and flavors of chestnuts with other healthful ingredients, including the warming and fragrant spices nutmeg and cinnamon.

INGREDIENTS

6 to 8 medium-size fresh, unshelled chestnuts (1 cup)

1 small lotus root (*ou* in Chinese, *renkon* in Japanese) (about 1 cup)

1 rounded tablespoon (5 grams) dried tangerine peel (*chen pi*), shredded

5 cups water

¼ cup chopped walnut pieces

8 dried Chinese red dates (*hong zao*), seeded

¼ teaspoon salt (optional)

½ teaspoon ground nutmeg

¼ teaspoon ground cinnamon

2 tablespoons rock sugar or other sweetener, or to taste

DIRECTIONS

1. To shell the chestnuts, boil them in a pot of water for ½ hour. Remove the chestnuts from the water and cut them in half (a serrated knife is helpful). Scoop out the firm flesh with a spoon, discarding the skins and shells. Chop the chestnuts into ¼-inch pieces.
2. Peel and slice the lotus root, discarding the ends. Place the slices in a bowl of cold water to prevent discoloration, and set aside.
3. In a saucepan or pot, combine the tangerine peel and water and bring to a boil.
4. Drain the lotus root and add it to the soup. Also add the chestnut pieces, walnuts, Chinese red dates, and salt (if using).
5. Lower the heat, cover, and simmer for 1 hour.
6. Add the nutmeg, cinnamon, and rock sugar, and cook a few minutes longer, until the rock sugar has dissolved. Serve.

THEMES AND VARIATIONS

To substitute peeled, dried chestnuts for fresh ones, soak them for 2 to 3 hours before adding to the soup.

ESPECIALLY GOOD FOR

Anyone who is feeling tired, cold, or lacking in energy, or who is recovering from chronic illness.

FOR THOSE FAMILIAR WITH TRADITIONAL CHINESE MEDICINE

This dish strengthens the Kidney and Spleen.

LOQUAT HERBAL SOUP

MAKES 6 SERVINGS

This dessert soup combines a number of commonly used Chinese herbs with loquat, a popular ingredient in Asia for soothing the throat and easing coughs.

INGREDIENTS

- 1 ounce (30 grams) dried white wood ear (*bai mu er*)
- 10 fresh loquats, cut in half and seeded (peel if desired)
- 6 dried Chinese red dates (*hong zao*), seeded
- 3 tablespoons goji berries (*gou qi zi*)
- 1 tablespoon (10 grams) apricot kernels (*xing ren*, preferably sweet), crushed or ground finely
- 4 to 6 cups water
- 1 to 2 teaspoons rock sugar or honey, or to taste

Helpful Hints about Loquats

Loquats can be difficult to find in supermarkets, as they bruise easily and aren't ideal for commercial production. If you live in California, Hawaii, or Florida, however, in the spring look out for loquats at your local farmers' market, Asian grocery, or on your or your neighbor's tree! Loquats are also sold canned in syrup, sometimes available at Mexican groceries. (For more information on loquat, see "One Hundred Healthful Asian Ingredients.")

DIRECTIONS

1. Soak the white wood ears in water for 20 minutes. Drain, cut off and discard the fibrous base, and cut the remaining wood ear into ½ by 2-inch pieces.
2. Combine the wood ear, loquats, Chinese red dates, goji berries, apricot kernels, and water in a pot and bring to a boil. Lower the heat, cover tightly, and simmer for 30 minutes, stirring occasionally so the wood ear doesn't stick to the bottom of the pot.
3. Stir in the rock sugar to taste, until dissolved, and serve warm.

THEMES AND VARIATIONS

If you can't find loquats, apricots or pears can be substituted.

This soup can be cooked in a double boiler, steamed for 1 to 2 hours.

ESPECIALLY GOOD FOR

Anyone with a cough (dry or phlegmy), dry throat, hiccoughs, or nausea. Don't overdo the apricot kernels, though, as large doses can be toxic.

FOR THOSE FAMILIAR WITH
TRADITIONAL CHINESE MEDICINE

This dish is good for moistening the Lungs, clearing Lung Heat, and redirecting Lung qi downward.

CELESTIAL PAPAYA DESSERT

MAKES 2 SERVINGS

This sweet, smooth, and attractive dish is famous in China, where it is traditionally made with swallow's nest, an expensive delicacy harvested from the sea caves of the South China Sea.

INGREDIENTS

½ cup (¾ ounce, or 20 grams) dried white wood ear (*bai mu er* or *yin er* in Chinese, *hakumokuji* or *shiro kikurage* in Japanese)

1 medium-size papaya, cut in half and seeded

2 tablespoons honey, or to taste

DIRECTIONS

1. Soak the white wood ear in warm water for 30 minutes. It will expand a lot. When the white wood ear is done soaking, cut off and discard the fibrous base, then cut the remaining wood ear into ½ by 2-inch strips.

2. In a small pot, bring water to a boil. Add the wood ear and simmer for 30 minutes. Drain.

3. Place the papaya in a steamer whose base is filled with about an inch of water, and cook for 30 minutes.

4. When both the papaya and the wood ear are done, place the wood ear into the scooped-out cavity of the papaya halves.

5. Drizzle with honey before serving.

ESPECIALLY GOOD FOR

Restoring a youthful tone to skin; supporting cancer treatment.

FOR THOSE FAMILIAR WITH
TRADITIONAL CHINESE MEDICINE

This dish addresses yin deficiency.

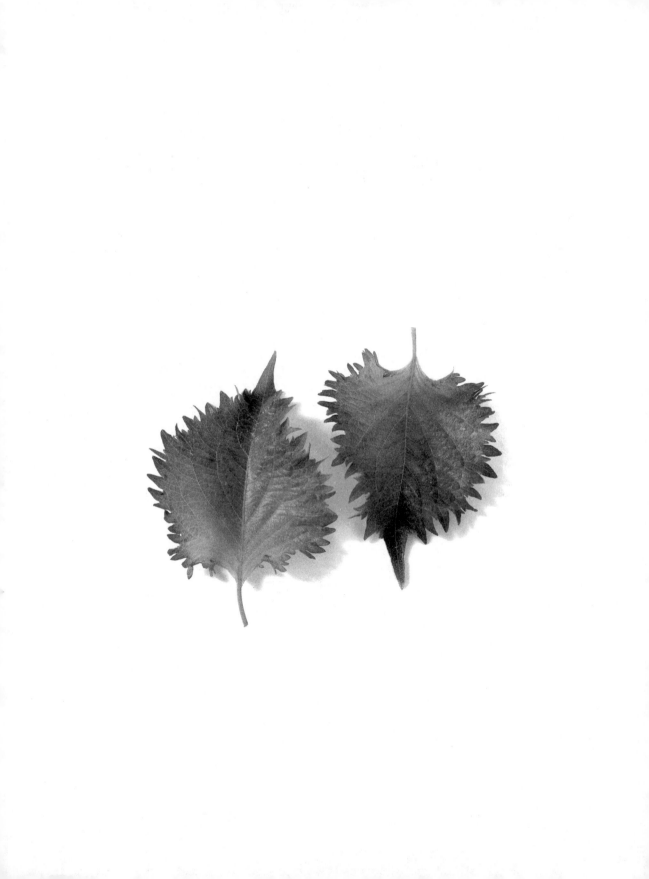

COMFORT IN A CUP

健康之液，灵魂之饮

It is better to drink green tea than to take medicine.

—CHINESE PROVERB

GOT-TO-HAVE-IT GREEN TEA

SERVES 2

We include this recipe here not because you don't know how to make tea—of course you do!—but because you might be interested in subtle details such as water temperature and reusing tea leaves. It's hard to overemphasize the importance of green tea—as a ubiquitous beverage, a cultural touchstone, and a therapeutic herb—in Asia.

INGREDIENTS

2 cups water
1 tea bag green tea, or 1
    tablespoon loose leaves

Words of Wisdom

Better to be deprived of food for three days, than tea for one.
—CHINESE PROVERB
If man has no tea in him, he is incapable of understanding truth and beauty.
—JAPANESE PROVERB

DIRECTIONS

1. Heat the water to 160° to 180°F. This can be accomplished by bringing the water to a boil, then letting it sit for 1 minute, or heating the water until steam clearly starts to rise (but before it boils), then removing the kettle from the burner.

2. Pour the water over the tea. You can use a teapot, or, if you prefer loose tea leaves in a cup; it is handy to have a steel mesh infuser for the leaves so you can remove them easily. Let the tea steep for 30 seconds to 5 minutes, depending on your taste and the strength of the tea leaves. Remove the tea bag or leaves so the tea doesn't become too strong.

3. Serve and savor.

Yuan Says

In China, tea—called the "beverage of health"—is everywhere. Any time you go to someone's house, you are offered tea. Making excellent tea has evolved to an art form. Not only do people examine the different sorts of tea leaves, their shapes, and varieties, they also pay attention to the water they use. A particular spot in a stream, for example, can get a reputation for providing fresh, clear, water for the best-tasting tea. People also say the kind of teapot makes a difference to the taste of the tea; Yixing, in the Jiangsu province of China, is an area reputed to have the best clay to hold tea—a smooth, purple earth that is especially good at keeping tea warm. These teapots are often left unglazed to enhance the flavor of the tea.

THEMES AND VARIATIONS

Endless, given the many varieties of teas (there are some three thousand to choose from) and possible combinations with other herbs (see additional recipes in this section). Experiment and see what you like!

In Asia, tea leaves are traditionally reinfused with water several times for additional servings of the beverage. Each reinfusion coaxes a slightly different flavor from the leaves. Those who are sensitive to caffeine might find it helpful to know that much of the caffeine from tea is released in the first infusion, so to reduce caffeine, pour hot water over the tea, let it steep, then discard this cupful (or serve it to a less sensitive friend or family member) and brew again. Some people like to start a pot of tea in the morning and keep adding water throughout the day; by the time the evening comes, the caffeine is long gone, so the last cup of tea doesn't interfere with a good night's sleep.

ESPECIALLY GOOD FOR

Tea is a staple to quench thirst, raise the spirit, help digestion, increase urination, suppress coughs, sharpen vision, assist clear thinking, reduce inflammation, and clear toxicity.

Legend Has It

One popular story credits the invention of tea to Emperor Shen Nong, a.k.a. the Divine Farmer, a legendary figure who is said to have founded agriculture and herbal medicine in China some five thousand years ago. As the tale goes, one day, as was his custom, Shen Nong boiled his water to make it safe to drink. During the process, the wind blew a few tea leaves into his bowl. Curious, he sampled the brew and found that he not only enjoyed the new beverage's flavor, but the drink also helped him stay alert. Some stories go on to add that the emperor later found another use for tea. As he liked to test the effects of various herbs on himself, sometimes he would fall ill when his experiments went awry. When they did, the emperor found tea helped restore him to health.

FOR THOSE FAMILIAR WITH TRADITIONAL CHINESE MEDICINE

Green tea, which is considered bitter and cold, is an herb that harmonizes the Stomach, directs rebellious Stomach qi downward, dispels Dampness, and assists in clear thinking.

SOOTHING GINGER-HONEY DRINK

SERVES 1

Although a classic Asian recipe, this soothing brew could also be from your grandmother's kitchen. In Japan, this drink is called shoga-yu *and is considered an excellent way to respond to the first signs of a cold.*

INGREDIENTS

1½ cups water
1 (1-inch) piece fresh ginger, cut
    into ¹⁄₁₆-inch slices
1 teaspoon honey, or to taste

THEMES AND VARIATIONS

You can vary the strength of the tea, adding more or less ginger and leaving it on the stove for more or less time, according to your tastes and needs.

ESPECIALLY GOOD FOR

Anyone suffering from stomach upset, morning sickness, or a cough with profuse, clear phlegm. Also, this beverage is good for those with a cold, flu, cough, hangover, poor circulation, or general debility.

DIRECTIONS

1. In a small saucepan, boil the water, then add the ginger slices.
2. Lower the heat and simmer at a low boil for 5 to 10 minutes.
3. Remove the ginger pieces from the tea with a slotted spoon or strainer.
4. Add honey to taste.

FOR THOSE FAMILIAR WITH TRADITIONAL CHINESE MEDICINE

For those suffering from a cough from an exterior attack of Wind-Cold, or from nausea and vomit from rebellious qi in the stomach. Ginger is especially appropriate in the autumn and winter.

Helpful Hints about Ginger

When shopping for ginger, look for plump, firm specimens and avoid those that look as if they have begun to dry out around the edges. (For more information on ginger, see "One Hundred Healthful Asian Ingredients.")

EXPANDING-HORIZONS CHRYSANTHEMUM AND GOJI BERRY TEA

SERVES 2

This tea is a classic herbal mixture to improve vision and protect eyesight, as well as to improve general health. The taste might remind you of chamomile.

INGREDIENTS

2 tablespoons (about 10 grams) chrysanthemum flowers (*ju hua*)

2 tablespoons (30 grams) goji berries (*gou qi zi*)

2 to 3 cups water

1 teaspoon honey, or to taste (optional)

DIRECTIONS

1. Combine the chrysanthemum flowers, goji berries, and water in a small pot and bring to a boil.
2. Lower the heat, and simmer, partially covered, for about 5 minutes. Turn off the heat and let the tea steep for another 5 minutes.
3. Strain the tea to remove the berries and flowers.
4. Add honey to taste, if desired.

THEMES AND VARIATIONS

This tea can be made with ginseng, or without the goji berries as a simple chrysanthemum flower tea. Simple chrysanthemum flower tea is a popular and fragrant beverage available in many Asian restaurants and, in packaged form, at Asian grocery stores. In Chinese tradition, once a pot of chrysanthemum tea is finished, you add more boiling water to the pot to produce another brew, which is slightly less strong.

ESPECIALLY GOOD FOR

Anyone who is concerned about his or her vision, or who is recovering from influenza. Also, this dish is good for serving during the cold and flu season, and for supporting general health.

FOR THOSE FAMILIAR WITH
TRADITIONAL CHINESE MEDICINE

This sweet, cooling herbal tea helps clear Heat, improve eyesight, and prevent sore throats.

MULBERRY-CHRYSANTHEMUM TEA

SERVES 2

This sweet and flowery tea includes the fruit of the mulberry tree, which has a long history in China. Almost all parts of the tree—from fruit to leaves and twigs—play a role in traditional Chinese medicine. Mulberry fruit contains significant amounts of resveratrol, a substance that has recently received a lot of press about its health benefits, especially through consumption of red wine.

INGREDIENTS

2 tablespoons dried mulberries
2 slightly rounded tablespoons
    (about 10 grams) chrysanthe-
    mum flowers (*ju hua*)
3 cups water

DIRECTIONS

1. Combine the mulberries, chrysanthemum, and water in a small pot and bring to a boil.
2. Lower the heat and simmer, covered, for about 5 minutes. Turn off the heat and let the tea steep for another 5 minutes.
3. Strain the tea to remove the berries and flowers.

THEMES AND VARIATIONS

Mulberry tea can also be consumed as a single-ingredient tea (as, of course, can chrysanthemum).

ESPECIALLY GOOD FOR

Serving to anyone who wants to improve his or her vitality or eyesight; drinking in hot weather.

FOR THOSE FAMILIAR WITH
TRADITIONAL CHINESE MEDICINE

This beverage nourishes the Kidneys, clears Heat, and improves eyesight.

LEGENDARY GINSENG TEA

SERVES 1

This herbal infusion is perhaps the simplest way to take this famous sweet and slightly bitter herb—one of the few herbs from the traditional Chinese pharmacopeia to be commonly prescribed as a single ingredient. Since the dried root is quite hard, to acquire ground ginseng we recommend you ask the herb shop to grind it for you, or buy it in a powdered form. You may also be able to find prebagged ginseng tea, although connoisseurs of ginseng may find it more difficult to determine quality this way.

INGREDIENTS

1 teaspoon (5 grams) ground
    ginseng (*ren shen*)
1 cup water
Honey (optional)

DIRECTIONS

1. Combine the ground ginseng and water in a small pot, cover, and bring the mixture to a boil.
2. Turn off the heat and steep the mixture for 5 to 10 minutes.
3. Strain out the ginseng through a fine-mesh strainer.
4. Add honey to taste, if desired.

THEMES AND VARIATIONS

Although ground ginseng makes the most of the herb's surface area for a tea, it is fine to make your brew from a whole, dried ginseng root or slices of it. However, you will need a longer cooking time—an estimated 45 minutes depending on the size of the pieces—to extract its benefits.

Numerous traditional Chinese medicinal formulas call for ginseng. For two simple combinations, see Pulse-of-Life Tea, page 242, and Boost-the-Qi Tea, page 244.

ESPECIALLY GOOD FOR

Anyone who wants to increase strength and immunity.

FOR THOSE FAMILIAR WITH
TRADITIONAL CHINESE MEDICINE

This beverage strengthens the qi of the Lungs and Spleen.

HARMONIZING GINGER-PERILLA GREEN TEA

SERVES 1 OR 2

This delicious beverage combines some of our favorite flavors. All three of the herbs—ginger root, perilla leaves, and, of course, tea—make terrific stand-alone beverages.

INGREDIENTS

1 (½-inch) piece fresh ginger, peeled and minced

3 fresh or dried perilla leaves (*zi su ye* in Chinese, *shisoyo, akajisō, aoba, aojiso,* or *ōba* in Japanese)

1 bag green tea, or 1 rounded teaspoon of loose leaves

2 cups water

1 teaspoon honey, or to taste (optional)

DIRECTIONS

1. Combine the ginger, perilla leaves, tea, and water in a small pot and bring to a boil.
2. Turn off the heat and let the mixture steep for about 2 minutes.
3. Strain out the herbs and remove the tea bag, if necessary.
4. Add honey to taste, if desired.

THEMES AND VARIATIONS

Also consider brewing a single-ingredient tea featuring perilla leaf, which offers a distinct but minty flavor and anti-inflammatory properties. This tea can be consumed before bedtime to calm and warm you, or to help fight off some types of common cold and nausea.

ESPECIALLY GOOD FOR

Anyone coming down with a cold with runny nose, headache, chills, upset stomach, and body aches, or suffering from nausea and vomiting. This beverage also helps with poor circulation.

FOR THOSE FAMILIAR WITH
TRADITIONAL CHINESE MEDICINE

This decoction treats an exterior attack of Wind-Cold and harmonizes the Stomach.

SCINTILLATING CINNAMON TEA

SERVES 1 TO 2

This fragrant Korean tea enlivens your palate with ginger, the spicy rhizome, and cinnamon, an ancient and aromatic herb from the inner bark of a small evergreen tree. Some scientists suggest that cinnamon can help control blood sugar, making it potentially useful in the management of diabetes, and the spice may also have antibacterial activity.

INGREDIENTS

1 stick (5 grams) cinnamon
1 (1-inch) piece fresh ginger,
  peeled and cut into 1/16-inch
  slices
2 cups water
3 or 4 pine nuts
Honey (optional)

DIRECTIONS

1. Combine the cinnamon stick, ginger, and water in a pot, cover, and bring to a boil.
2. Lower the heat and simmer for about 15 minutes, or until the desired strength.
3. Strain out the ginger and cinnamon or remove the pieces with a slotted spoon.
4. Add honey, if desired, and garnish with a few pine nuts before serving.

ESPECIALLY GOOD FOR

Anyone with diabetes; individuals who are concerned about atherosclerosis, tend to run cold or have poor circulation, or desire to increase pain tolerance.

FOR THOSE FAMILIAR WITH
TRADITIONAL CHINESE MEDICINE

This tea is warming and helps open the channels.

GINGER BLACK TEA

SERVES 4 TO 5

Black tea and ginger meet to create a healthy, tasty brew. Black tea is from the same plant as green tea, but processed differently. For green tea, the leaves are heated soon after harvest by steaming (common for Japanese teas) or dry cooking (common for Chinese teas). The heat stops the oxidation process that turns the leaves dark. For black tea—commonly referred to as "red tea" in Asia—the tea leaves are allowed to oxidize completely and turn a darker shade.

INGREDIENTS

1 (2-inch) piece fresh ginger, peeled and cut into ⅛-inch slices

6 cups water

1½ tablespoons black tea, or 2 to 3 tea bags

1 teaspoon honey, rock sugar, or other natural sweetener, or to taste (optional)

DIRECTIONS

1. Place the ginger slices and water in a pot and bring to a boil.
2. Lower the heat and simmer, covered with the lid slightly ajar, for 5 to 10 minutes. Turn off the heat.
3. Add the tea and let the brew steep for about 5 minutes, or to taste. Strain out the ginger and tea.
4. Add sweetener to taste, if desired, and drink throughout the day.

ESPECIALLY GOOD FOR

Those who have a tendency to run cold, or who are concerned about water retention, weight control, or constipation.

FOR THOSE FAMILIAR WITH
TRADITIONAL CHINESE MEDICINE

This tea warms the Interior and helps drain Dampness.

Yuan Says

Harvesting and drying tea leaves are considered an art in Asia. The Chinese have a saying that the quality of tea leaves depends on heaven (weather and climate), earth (soil and location, with high elevations particularly prized as growing areas), and people (correctly tending, harvesting, and processing the tea leaves, buds, or twigs).

FIVE-FLAVOR BERRY TEA

SERVES 1 TO 2

This tea is particularly popular in Korea, where teas are also made from a variety of leaves (such as dried mulberry or persimmon leaves, or pine needles), grains (such as barley, corn, or rice), and fruit (such as goji berries, citron, or Chinese red dates). This tea feels wonderful washing over a sore throat.

INGREDIENTS

2 tablespoons (15 grams) schisandra berries (*wu wei zi*)
2 cups water
2 teaspoons honey, or to taste
2 to 6 pine nuts (optional)

What's in a Name?

The pinkish berries we know as schisandra berries are called *wu wei zi* ("five-flavor seed") in Chinese, because they are thought to possess all five of the flavors recognized in traditional Chinese medicine: sweet, salty, bitter, spicy, and especially sour. (For more information on schisandra berries, see "One Hundred Healthful Asian Ingredients.")

DIRECTIONS

1. Combine the schisandra berries and water in a small pot and bring to a boil.
2. Simmer for 3 to 5 minutes. Do not overcook, as the berries will become bitter.
3. Strain out the berries.
4. Flavor with honey to taste (the drink will be quite sour if you don't), then garnish with a few pine nuts, if desired.

THEMES AND VARIATIONS

Some people like to add licorice root (10 to 12 pieces, or ⅓ ounce) and/or fresh ginger (a couple of ⅛-inch slices) to this tea for a mixture of flavors.

ESPECIALLY GOOD FOR

Anyone with a cough, night sweats, insomnia, or physical exhaustion.

FOR THOSE FAMILIAR WITH
TRADITIONAL CHINESE MEDICINE

This tea helps contain leakage of Lung qi, strengthen the Kidneys, and calm the spirit.

PULSE-OF-LIFE TEA

SERVES 1

This is the recipe for a classic therapeutic formula, first described by physician Li Dong Yuan (Li Gao) in a book published in 1247, which is still widely used in China today. Called sheng mai san—*literally "to generate the pulse"—the formula is used in medical settings for patients who have suffered illnesses such as heart attack, congestive heart failure, severe bronchitis, or a sudden drop in blood pressure due to septic shock. It is also useful for asthma.*

INGREDIENTS

½ teaspoon (1.5 grams) ground ginseng root (*ren shen*)
½ teaspoon (1.5 grams) ophio-pogon tuber (*mai men dong*)
15 seeds (1 gram) schisandra fruit (*wu wei zi*)
1 cup water

DIRECTIONS

1. Combine the ginseng root, ophiopogon tuber, schisandra fruit, and water in a small pot and bring to a boil.
2. Immediately lower the heat and simmer for at least 10 minutes.
3. Strain out the herbs before serving.

ESPECIALLY GOOD FOR

Addressing a chronic dry cough, shortness of breath, fatigue, spontaneous sweating, or dry mouth. The recommended dose is three times a day for these conditions.

FOR THOSE FAMILIAR WITH TRADITIONAL CHINESE MEDICINE

This drink augments the qi, generates fluids, preserves the yin, stops excessive sweating, and strengthens the pulse, but should be used with caution in the case of high fever or when a disease has not yet resolved.

MEDITATIVE MINT, GINGER, AND TANGERINE TISANE

SERVES 1 TO 2

Your grandmother might have served this terrific tea if she had only thought of it.

INGREDIENTS

1 to 2 cups water

2 tablespoons fresh mint, chopped coarsely, or 1 mint tea bag

1 (½-inch) piece fresh ginger, minced

1 teaspoon dried or fresh tangerine or orange peel

Honey (optional)

DIRECTIONS

1. In a small pot, boil the water.
2. Place the mint, ginger, and tangerine peel in the hot water, then lower the heat and simmer, covered, for about 3 minutes.
3. Turn off the heat and let the brew steep for another 3 minutes.
4. Remove the herbs by pouring the mixture through a strainer.
5. Add honey, if desired, then serve.

THEMES AND VARIATIONS

This tea can also be made with ginger and tangerine peel only. For morning sickness, try combining the ginger and tangerine peel with two Chinese red dates.

ESPECIALLY GOOD FOR

Anyone with stomach upset or hangover, or those who love the taste of tangerine, ginger, and mint—yum!

FOR THOSE FAMILIAR WITH
TRADITIONAL CHINESE MEDICINE

This beverage is good for calming the Stomach and eliminating food stagnation.

BOOST-THE-QI TEA

SERVES 2

This famous formula has been recommended for centuries, appearing in a book called Formulas to Aid the Living (Ji Sheng Fang), *written in 1253 CE.*

INGREDIENTS

1 (1-inch) piece (6 to 9 grams) fresh ginger, peeled and cut into ¹⁄₁₆-inch slices

5 shelled walnuts, crushed

2 teaspoons (6 to 9 grams) ground ginseng root (*ren shen*), or 2 ginseng tea bags

2½ cups water

Honey

ESPECIALLY GOOD FOR

Anyone suffering from general weakness or from wheezing, coughing, or asthma.

FOR THOSE FAMILIAR WITH TRADITIONAL CHINESE MEDICINE

This classic formula strengthens the Lungs and Kidneys.

DIRECTIONS

1. Combine the ginger, walnuts, ginseng, and water in a medium-size pot and bring to a boil.
2. Lower the heat and simmer, covered with the lid slightly ajar, for 10 minutes.
3. Strain the herbs through a piece of cheesecloth or a fine-mesh strainer (you may have to clean out the strainer during the process if the herbs clump).
4. Add honey to taste.

Legend Has It

One story tells of two brothers who went to the mountains for a hunting trip. When they were there, a huge snowstorm hit the region. After it had raged on for two days and two nights, the brothers found that the snow had covered their tracks and had made going down the mountain impossible.

To survive, they took shelter in a hollow tree and continued hunting for game. On clear days, they also dug for roots to eat. That's how they discovered a root shaped like a human form, whose root fibers looked like legs and arms. Sampling the root, the brothers found it slightly sweet and very nourishing. They continued to dig for it and eat it throughout the long, cold winter.

When spring came and melted the snow, the brothers returned to the village, where people were astonished to learn they had survived: "What did you eat to stay alive? How come you are so full of energy?" The brothers showed the villagers the root, which no one had seen before. "Look at that," the villagers said. "The root is shaped like a man."

The word for *ginseng* in Mandarin, *ren shen*, means "man root." Today, the roots with the closest resemblance to the human body are still the most valuable.

ROASTED CASSIA SEED TEA

SERVES 1 TO 2

This tea's flavor is slightly reminiscent of roasted chicory or roasted barley tea. Cassia seeds, which have been used as a medicinal herb for centuries, can be found in Asian markets and herb shops.

INGREDIENTS

1 tablespoon (20 grams) cassia
  seeds (*jue ming zi*)
2 cups water
Honey or other natural sweetener
  and/or milk or soy milk
  (optional)

DIRECTIONS

1. Toast the cassia seeds in a dry skillet over medium-high heat until they pop and you smell their coffee-like aroma, 4 to 5 minutes.
2. Combine the cassia seeds and water in a small pot and bring to a boil.
3. Lower the heat and simmer, covered with the lid slightly ajar, for 5 to 10 minutes, until the desired strength.
4. Strain out the cassia seeds.
5. Add honey and/or milk to taste, if desired, and stir well.

THEMES AND VARIATIONS

If you like, you can combine hawthorn (1 rounded tablespoon) with the cassia seeds in this tea.

ESPECIALLY GOOD FOR

Those with high blood pressure, high cholesterol, or dizziness. Drink twice a day for these conditions.

FOR THOSE FAMILIAR WITH
TRADITIONAL CHINESE MEDICINE

This tea clears Liver Heat, brightens the eyes, and lubricates the Intestines.

RESTFUL HONEYSUCKLE AND MINT GREEN TEA

SERVES 1 TO 2

This tea offers crisp, floral overtones. In traditional Chinese medicine, honeysuckle is considered a therapeutic herb that relieves Heat and resolves toxicity.

INGREDIENTS

2 teaspoons (2 grams) honeysuckle flower (*jin yin hua*)

2 cups water

1 teaspoon dried peppermint leaves, 1 peppermint tea bag, or 1 rounded tablespoon of chopped fresh peppermint leaves

1 teaspoon green tea, or 1 tea bag

Honey or other natural sweetener (optional)

THEMES AND VARIATIONS

Spearmint or any variety of mint may be substituted for peppermint.

DIRECTIONS

1. Combine the honeysuckle flower and water in a small pot, and bring to a boil.
2. Simmer for 10 minutes, covered with the lid slightly ajar. Turn off the heat, and add the peppermint and green tea. Let the mixture steep for 5 minutes.
3. Strain out the herbs.
4. Add honey or other natural sweetener to taste, if desired.

ESPECIALLY GOOD FOR

Anyone with high fever, irritability, thirst from the flu, sore throat with a burning sensation, thirst, or indigestion; anyone with throat or lung problems; anyone who tends to run warm.

FOR THOSE FAMILIAR WITH TRADITIONAL CHINESE MEDICINE

This sweet, acrid, cool tea clears Heat, replenishes body fluids, and relieves toxicity.

Legend Has It

Long ago, twin girls were born and their proud parents named them Golden Flower and Silver Flower. As the girls grew, they did everything together. They especially loved embroidery and made wonderful creations with their skillful hands. By the time they were eighteen, they were as pretty as flowers and many suitors came to call. But the twins had no interest in marriage. "We were born together, and want to be buried together," they said.

One day, Golden Flower suddenly fell ill. She developed a fever and broke out in red spots. She was bedridden. The girls' parents called the doctor. "There is nothing I can do," he said. "No medicine can save this young lady." Silver Flower was distraught and refused to leave her sister's side. Before long, she, too, fell ill.

"We hope that after we die we turn into a plant that cures fever," the sisters said. "That way, people like us won't face certain death."

After they died, the twins were buried side by side. One year later, a vine began to grow from their grave. When it blossomed with silver, then golden flowers, the townspeople remembered the girls' dying wish and picked the flowers to brew into an herbal tea. From then on, whenever one of the townspeople came down with a fever, they drank the beverage and the fever soon vanished. The plant was named Golden-Silver Flower, *jin yin hua* (honeysuckle), after the girls.

LULLABY LONGAN TEA

SERVES 1 TO 2

This sweet and nutty-flavored beverage is gentle and soothing. Longan fruit, which is reputed to add luster to the skin, can also be brewed as a single-ingredient tea.

INGREDIENTS

8 pieces dried longan fruit (*long yan rou*)
10 lotus seeds (*lian zi*)
2 cups water

ESPECIALLY GOOD FOR

Anyone who has trouble falling asleep.

DIRECTIONS

1. Combine the longan fruit, lotus seeds, and water in a small pot and bring to a boil.
2. Lower the heat and simmer, covered with the lid slightly ajar, for about 10 minutes.
3. Strain out the herbs and serve.

FOR THOSE FAMILIAR WITH TRADITIONAL CHINESE MEDICINE

This beverage clams the spirit and treats insomnia.

KUDZU TEA

SERVES 1 TO 2

This mild, slightly earthy, therapeutic tea can be taken once a day. Kudzu tea is especially popular in Korea, where it is sold in open markets. Although kudzu is commonly sold powdered to be used as thickener, this recipe calls for larger pieces of the root, which will be available from a Chinese herb shop.

INGREDIENTS

6 or 7 thick pieces (1 ounce, or 30 grams) dried kudzu root (*ge gen*), cut into small pieces
2 cups water

ESPECIALLY GOOD FOR

Anyone with headache and dizziness from high blood pressure, or who wants to cool down.

DIRECTIONS

1. Combine the kudzu and water in a small pot and bring to a boil.
2. Lower the heat and simmer for 30 minutes.
3. Strain out the kudzu root.
4. Let the tea cool before serving.

FOR THOSE FAMILIAR WITH TRADITIONAL CHINESE MEDICINE

Kudzu root dispels Wind from the Exterior, releases muscles, clears Heat, and generates fluids.

CALM-THE-SPIRIT TEA

SERVES 2

In China, this sweet tea is nicknamed "Happy Tea." This formula dates back the Han Dynasty, when it was developed by Zhang Zhong Jing (circa 150–220 CE), one of the most famous physicians in Chinese history. The formula has been passed down through the centuries and is still in common use by traditional Chinese medicine practitioners today.

INGREDIENTS

10 to 12 pieces (9 grams) licorice root (the herb, not the candy; *gan cao* in Chinese)
1 tablespoon (12 grams) triticum (*fu xiao mai*)
10 Chinese red dates (*hong zao*)
2½ cups water

Helpful Hints about Triticum

Triticum, which is a kind of wheat common throughout China, is available from Chinese herb stores under the name *fu xiao mai*.

DIRECTIONS

1. Combine the licorice root, triticum, Chinese red dates, and water in a small pot and bring to a boil.
2. Lower the heat and simmer, partially covered, for about 30 minutes.
3. Strain out the herbs and serve.

THEMES AND VARIATIONS

Some people like to put the herbs in a tea bag, which you can buy empty at many natural food stores, to remove the herbs easily and to make a clearer beverage.

ESPECIALLY GOOD FOR

Anyone suffering from emotional distress, including mild depression; also, women coping with symptoms of premenstrual syndrome, menopause, and postpartum recovery.

FOR THOSE FAMILIAR WITH TRADITIONAL CHINESE MEDICINE

This beverage treats restless organ disorder, called *zang zao* in Chinese, which includes disorientation, unexplained crying, and emotional outbursts and distress.

NO-MORE-COUGH MULBERRY LEAF TEA

SERVES 1

This sweet, mild herbal tea features leaves from the famous mulberry tree, whose parts are widely used in Chinese medicine.

INGREDIENTS

1½ cups water

2 tablespoons (5 grams) mulberry leaves (*sang ye*)

1 rounded teaspoon (5 grams) goji berries (*gou qi zi*)

1 teaspoon honey (optional)

DIRECTIONS

1. In a small pot, boil the water.
2. Add the mulberry leaves and goji berries, then lower the heat and simmer for 5 minutes. Turn off the heat and let the herbs steep for another 5 minutes.
3. Strain out the berries and leaves from the tea.
4. Add honey to taste, if desired.

THEMES AND VARIATIONS

This tea can be made without the goji berries, if desired. Another combination matches mulberry leaves with chrysanthemum flowers.

ESPECIALLY GOOD FOR

Anyone suffering from dry cough or general debility, or who wishes to strengthen eyesight and hearing. Slowly sip one cup twice a day for best results.

FOR THOSE FAMILIAR WITH
TRADITIONAL CHINESE MEDICINE

This tea relieves cough from Lung Heat or Dryness, and improves vision and addresses eye problems.

SOOTHING SIPPING BROTH

SERVES 1 OR 2

This nutty herbal broth features sour date seeds—small, reddish-brown seeds frequently used in Chinese medicine for their calming properties, and celery, which in China is considered a therapeutic herb as well as a food.

INGREDIENTS

1 rounded tablespoon (about 12 grams) sour date seed (*suan zao ren*)

3 stalks celery, cut into 3- to 4-inch lengths

3 cups water

Yuan Says

One mother brought her little boy, who had been diagnosed with attention-deficit disorder, into my clinic. I mentioned how calming sour date seed could be. The mother found a creative way to feed it to her son, who had picky tastes—she ground it up, mixed it with peanut butter, and spread it on his sandwiches! She found that the herb helped her son stay more grounded.

DIRECTIONS

1. Toast the sour date seeds in a pan over medium-high heat until they crackle and pop and release a nutty fragrance, 3 to 5 minutes. Let the seeds cool, then crush them lightly with a rolling pin to further crack them open.

2. Boil the water in a small pot, then add the sour date seed and celery. Lower the heat and simmer for 20 to 30 minutes.

3. Strain out the celery and seeds.

4. Serve the broth warm.

ESPECIALLY GOOD FOR

Anyone who has insomnia or irritability, particularly those who are experiencing restless sleep with excessive, vivid dreams, and women who suffer insomnia due to anemia. Drink a cup one to two times a day, especially before bedtime, to stay calm and get a good night's sleep.

FOR THOSE FAMILIAR WITH
TRADITIONAL CHINESE MEDICINE

This broth nourishes the Heart yin, augments the Liver Blood, and calms the spirit.

HEART-HEALTHY TEA

SERVES 2 OR MORE

This tea takes advantage of the hawthorn berry, an herb used in both Eastern and Western traditions. In European herbalism, hawthorn berries—a tart, bright red fruit—have been associated with improving cardiovascular function, an effect supported by some scientific studies.

INGREDIENTS

2¼ cups water

1 teaspoon (2 grams) green tea leaves

2 tablespoons (5 grams) chrysan-themum flowers (*ju hua*)

1 rounded tablespoon (10 grams) hawthorn berries (*shan zha*)

Honey or other natural sweetener (optional)

DIRECTIONS

1. In a small pot, boil the water.
2. Combine tea, chrysanthemum flowers, hawthorn berries, and boiled water in a saucepan or teapot.
3. Steep for 5 to 10 minutes, until the desired strength, then strain.
4. Add honey to your cup, if desired.
5. Keep filling the pot or teapot with hot water throughout the day, making new cups of tea to drink to quench your thirst.

THEMES AND VARIATIONS

Hawthorne berries (fresh or dried) can be brewed as a heart-healthy single-ingredient tea that tastes slightly reminiscent of hibiscus.

ESPECIALLY GOOD FOR

Anyone concerned about high cholesterol, preventing cardiovascular disease, or warding off cancer. Caution: Large doses of hawthorn berries should be avoided during pregnancy.

FOR THOSE FAMILIAR WITH
TRADITIONAL CHINESE MEDICINE

This tea drains Dampness, helps counteract food stagnation (especially the digestion of fat), clears Heat, and moves the Blood.

Yuan Says

One of my patients, a woman in her fifties, came to me with the disturbing news that a blood test during her last physical had revealed she had high cholesterol. She was looking for a simple way to bring her cholesterol down. I gave her the recipe for this tea. She was skeptical, but agreed to try it for a few months. At first, she thought the tea was a bit sour, but she grew to like its flavor. When she went back to the doctor for a follow-up visit and new tests after about three months, her "bad" cholesterol levels had dropped dramatically. She attributed the improvement to the tea and now makes a batch of this tea every morning and carries it around in a thermos so she can drink it throughout the day. She also tells her friends they should be drinking it, too!

CLASSIC COLD CURE

SERVES 2

This fragrant, spicy, and sweet beverage might remind you of chai. The recipe is a classic Chinese medical formula known as "Cinnamon Twig Decoction," one of the most famous and ancient remedies for the common cold, attributed to Zhang Zhong Jing of the late Han Dynasty, around 200 CE. The dried ingredients, including honey-prepared licorice root, can be found at Chinese herb stores.

INGREDIENTS

3 tablespoons (9 grams) small slices of cinnamon twig (*gui zhi*)

3 (2-inch) pieces (6 grams) white peony root (*bai shao*)

4 slices (3 grams) honey-prepared licorice root (*zhi gan cao*)

3 Chinese dates (*da zao* or *hong zao*)

3 to 5 thin slices of fresh ginger

2½ cups water

According to Legend

According to a Chinese proverb, a woman who consumes peony root regularly becomes as beautiful as the peony flower.

DIRECTIONS

1. Combine the cinnamon twig, white peony root, licorice root, Chinese dates, fresh ginger, and water in a small pot, cover, and bring to a boil.
2. Quickly lower the heat and simmer, covered with the lid slightly ajar, over low heat for 20 minutes. Do not overcook.
3. Strain the liquid to remove the herbs, then serve.

THEMES AND VARIATIONS

Throughout the ages, this basic formula has been modified to treat a variety of conditions, from arthritis to menstrual irregularities. To treat indigestion and stomach cramping, for example, double the amount of white peony root and serve with barley malt as a sweetener.

ESPECIALLY GOOD FOR

Drinking at the first sign of a cold if your symptoms include chills, fever, slight sweat, runny nose, fatigue, stiff neck, joint pain, and body aches; serving to people with weakened immune systems and those with arthritis or poor circulation. Sip two cups a day for the best results. (See "Recipes for Common Health Concerns," page 298, for more information on Chinese medicine and the common cold.)

FOR THOSE FAMILIAR WITH TRADITIONAL CHINESE MEDICINE

If you know about Chinese medicine, you'll probably know about this formula, which addresses an external attack of Wind-Cold. Variations on this formula treat other illnesses as well.

CORNSILK TEA

SERVES 1

This tea tastes like corn on the cob without the cob—or the corn. Cornsilk, the silky threads that grow between the husk and the golden grains, can be found in fresh ears of corn sold with the husk still on.

INGREDIENTS

1½ cups water

¾ ounce (20 grams, or the amount from 2 cobs) fresh cornsilk (*yu mi xu*), rinsed and trimmed of any brown tips

Fast Facts about Cornsilk

The literal translation of *yu mi xu* is "jade rice whiskers," as corn is known as "jade rice" and the silk resembles fine hair. (For more information on cornsilk, see "One Hundred Healthful Asian Ingredients.")

DIRECTIONS

1. Boil the water in a small pot.
2. Place the cornsilk in the boiled water and steep, covered, for 10 minutes.
3. Strain out the cornsilk and serve.

THEMES AND VARIATIONS

If necessary, you can also buy dried cornsilk from a Chinese herb shop; in this case, use ⅓ ounce (5 to 6 grams). Fresh cornsilk, however, is preferred for both strength and taste.

ESPECIALLY GOOD FOR

Anyone who has high blood pressure, is experiencing water retention, or tends to bruise easily can drink this tea several times a day.

FOR THOSE FAMILIAR WITH
TRADITIONAL CHINESE MEDICINE

This tea drains Dampness, reduces edema, and promotes urination.

LIGHTENING LOTUS LEAF TEA

SERVES 1 TO 2

This tea uses staples from Asian cuisine, including lotus leaves, which are available dried from Chinese herb shops and may be available fresh in the summer from Asian grocery stores.

INGREDIENTS

½ teaspoon dried mung beans

1½ cups water

½ teaspoon dried lotus leaf (*he ye*), crumbled into small pieces

½ teaspoon green tea leaves

Legend Has It

Lotus leaves come from the famed lotus plant, which in many Asian traditions symbolizes immortality, purity, and enlightenment. The Buddha is often depicted sitting on a lotus leaf, and lotus flowers were said to bloom wherever he walked.

DIRECTIONS

1. Crush the mung beans into bits. You can accomplish this by whirring the beans in a coffee/spice mill or simply by putting the beans between two sheets of waxed paper and crushing them with a rolling pin.
2. Boil the water in a small pot.
3. Place the mung beans, lotus leaf, and green tea in an empty tea bag, tea ball, or strainer.
4. Pour the boiled water into a large cup or teapot, and steep the tea bag in the water for 5 minutes.
5. Remove the tea bag and serve.

THEMES AND VARIATIONS

Lotus leaf can be made into a single-ingredient tea with similar effects.

ESPECIALLY GOOD FOR

Drinking in the summer to cool down and quench thirst; also, serving to anyone who is concerned about weight control, high cholesterol, high blood pressure, fluid retention, certain types of constipation, or his or her complexion.

FOR THOSE FAMILIAR WITH
TRADITIONAL CHINESE MEDICINE

This beverage helps cool internal Heat with signs of fever or thirst, as well as helping to drain Dampness.

Warren Says

If weight loss is your goal, our recommendation is to focus on changing your lifestyle rather than dieting, which is often a futile approach over the long term. Instead, avoid processed food and refined sugars and flours, and eat a balanced diet of vegetables, whole grains, fruit, and small amounts of meat or fish (if you're not already a vegetarian). The importance of exercise can't be underestimated, not only for burning calories but also for boosting your metabolism. Find exercise you enjoy—walking, dancing, swimming—and do it regularly. Simple good habits will take you far.

CONQUER-YOUR-COUGH PEAR JUICE

MAKES 1 SERVING

This simple, sweet beverage is a common home remedy for dry coughs in Asia. Pear juice also has a formal place in traditional Chinese medicine, included in a formula in the classic 1798 text Systematic Differentiation of Warm Diseases. *This formula, called "five-juice beverage" (pear juice with lotus root, ophiopogon tuber (mai men dong), phragmitus (lu gen), and water chestnut juice) is recommended for Heat in the Stomach and Lungs, and was commonly used to provide sustenance to critically ill patients before the introduction of intravenous fluids.*

INGREDIENTS

2 to 3 medium-size pears, preferably Asian or Anjou, cored

Fast Facts about Juices

Although pear juice for cough is probably the most popular therapeutic juice in Asia, other juices are also used as home remedies, including:

- Watermelon juice for replenishing fluids, reducing fever, promoting urination, or calming restlessness in the hot summer months
- Loquat juice for soothing coughs and quenching thirst
- Kiwi juice for cooling down, replenishing body fluids, and reducing irritability
- Star fruit juice for soothing a sore throat or drinking in hot, dry weather
- Orange juice for quenching thirst and counteracting restlessness

DIRECTIONS

1. Place the pears in a juicer and process. (If you don't have a juicer, whir the cored pears in a blender or food processor. You can then strain out the pulp by squeezing the puree through a piece of cheesecloth. Squeeze gently, though, or you'll get splattered.)
2. Pour your refreshing beverage into a cup.

THEMES AND VARIATIONS

If you have a phlegmy cough or are suffering from asthma, try including ½ pound of lotus root and ½ pound (about 2 cups) of daikon radish with two pears, for a spicy-sweet drink to clear your chest.

ESPECIALLY GOOD FOR

Serving to anyone with a dry cough; drinking in dry weather.

FOR THOSE FAMILIAR WITH TRADITIONAL CHINESE MEDICINE

This beverage clears Heat, moistens Dryness, generates body fluids, and transforms phlegm.

WALNUT-ALMOND MILK

MAKES ABOUT 2 SERVINGS

Similar to the almond milk you can buy in a health food store, this delicious beverage is easy to make in your own kitchen.

INGREDIENTS

¼ cup walnuts
¼ cup raw almonds
2 to 3 cups water
Honey (optional)

THEMES AND VARIATIONS

Some people like to soak their nuts for a few hours or overnight before blending.

ESPECIALLY GOOD FOR

Anyone who is interested in facial rejuvenation, or who wants to counteract poor memory.

DIRECTIONS

1. Combine the walnuts, almonds, and water in a food processor or blender. Blend together well.
2. Strain the liquid through a strainer or piece of cheesecloth to remove the solids. You may need to clean your strainer during the process, and strain the mixture twice to achieve the desired consistency.
3. If desired, place the liquid in a pot, bring to a boil, and simmer for a minute or two, stirring frequently.
4. Add honey to taste, if desired, before serving warm.

FOR THOSE FAMILIAR WITH TRADITIONAL CHINESE MEDICINE

This beverage strengthens the Kidneys.

ALMOND SOY MILK

MAKES ABOUT 4 SERVINGS

This homemade beverage combines two health food staples, soy milk and almond milk.

INGREDIENTS

1 cup dried soybeans
6 raw, unsalted almonds
4 to 5 cups water
1½ tablespoons honey, or to taste

Yuan Says

Soy milk and similar beverages are traditional in China. These days, you can buy a soy milk–maker appliance for your kitchen, to blend, strain, and boil such drinks for you. If you're interested, look in your local Asian food store or search online (try "soy milk maker" and "soymilk maker"). Several models are available through Amazon.com. Like using a coffee maker, you can place the ingredients in the machine the night before and in the morning your steaming beverage will be ready. In addition, many Asian markets sell prepared bags, similar to tea bags, with which you can make bean or nut drinks.

DIRECTIONS

1. Soak the soybeans and almonds for at least 10 hours or overnight at room temperature. Drain.
2. Place the soybeans, almonds, and fresh water into a blender or food processor, and whir together until smooth.
3. Strain the mixture through a strainer or piece of cheesecloth to remove the solids. You may need to clean your strainer during the process, and strain the mixture twice to achieve the desired consistency.
4. Transfer the liquid in a heavy pot and bring to a boil, stirring frequently. Lower the heat to a simmer and cook for another 5 to 10 minutes, stirring frequently.
5. Add the honey to taste, stir, and serve warm.

THEMES AND VARIATIONS

You can freeze this beverage in serving-size portions for later use. Like other drinks of this kind, if stored in the refrigerator this beverage will last several days; we recommend rewarming before serving.

ESPECIALLY GOOD FOR

Anyone experiencing menopausal symptoms, high blood pressure, constipation, or problems with insufficient lactation.

FOR THOSE FAMILIAR WITH
TRADITIONAL CHINESE MEDICINE

This beverage supplements the Spleen and Kidneys, and counteracts dryness.

MEMORY DRINK

MAKES 4 TO 6 SERVINGS

You can make your own special blend of nutty-tasting soy milk, which provides the added satisfaction of coming fresh from your own kitchen.

INGREDIENTS

⅓ cup (about 2 ounces) dried soy-beans

¼ cup (about 1 ounce) walnuts

3 tablespoons (about 1 ounce) black sesame seeds (roasted preferred)

6 to 8 cups water

2 tablespoons honey or other natural sweetener, or to taste

THEMES AND VARIATIONS

A nice variation for a more roasted flavor is to toast the walnuts beforehand in your oven at 350°F for 7 to 8 minutes, or until fragrant.

You can freeze any leftovers of this drink in serving-size portions.

DIRECTIONS

1. Soak the soybeans for at least 10 hours or overnight at room temperature. Drain.
2. Place the soybeans, walnuts, black sesame seeds, and fresh water in a blender or food processor, and blend well.
3. Strain the mixture through a fine strainer or piece of cheesecloth to remove the solids. You may need to clean your strainer during the process, and strain the mixture twice to achieve the desired consistency.
4. Transfer the liquid to a heavy pot and bring to a boil, stirring frequently. Lower the heat to a simmer and cook for another 7 to 8 minutes, continuing to stir frequently.
5. Stir in the honey and serve warm.

ESPECIALLY GOOD FOR

Anyone concerned with preserving good memory or youthful hair color.

FOR THOSE FAMILIAR WITH TRADITIONAL CHINESE MEDICINE

This drink strengthens the Kidneys.

LOTUS ROOT DRINK

MAKES 4 SERVINGS

This subtle, slightly floral tasting drink offers soothing refreshment.

INGREDIENTS

1 fresh lotus root (*ou* in Chinese, *renkon* in Japanese), cut into ¼-inch-wide pieces

2 teaspoons rock sugar or other natural sweetener, or to taste

Water, 4 cups

DIRECTIONS

1. Combine the lotus root slices, rock sugar, and water in a small pot and bring to a boil.
2. Turn off the heat and let the ingredients steep for about 10 minutes. Stir.
3. Remove the lotus root slices.
4. Serve the beverage at room temperature.

THEMES AND VARIATIONS

Instead of adding rock sugar, you can sweeten this beverage by boiling a piece of sugarcane with the lotus root slices. If you want to enhance lotus root's cooling effects, avoid honey, which has more warming properties. Some health food stores sell powdered lotus root (sometimes with ginger) to make into a lotus root beverage, even if they don't happen to stock whole lotus root.

ESPECIALLY GOOD FOR

Drinking in the summer; serving to anyone who runs warm, wants to improve digestion, or suffers from nose bleeds.

FOR THOSE FAMILIAR WITH
TRADITIONAL CHINESE MEDICINE

Lotus root, which is cooling, harmonizes the Spleen and Stomach.

PLEASANT PERSIMMON PUNCH

MAKES 3 TO 4 SERVINGS

This fragrant, fruity beverage (known as su jeong gwa in Korean) is often served cold as a dessert (hwachae) at special gatherings, such as weddings. This is an "old-style" version of the recipe that suggests honey as a sweetener, rather than sugar that has become widespread in the preparation of this dish. Centuries ago, sugar was not available and the natural sweetness of the persimmon carried the day.

INGREDIENTS

1 (2-inch) piece fresh ginger, cut into 1/16-inch slices

2 cinnamon sticks

4 cups water

1 tablespoon honey or other natural sweetener, or to taste

6 to 8 slices dried persimmon

2 tablespoons pine nuts

What's in a Name?

In ancient times, sweet foods were a rarity in Korea. Persimmons were a welcome exception and the Korean word for persimmon, *gam*, means sweet. (For more information on persimmons, see "One Hundred Healthful Asian Ingredients.")

DIRECTIONS

1. Combine the ginger, cinnamon sticks, and water in a medium-size pot, then bring to a boil. Simmer for about 30 minutes.
2. Remove the ginger slices and cinnamon sticks, using a slotted spoon or strainer.
3. Add honey to taste while the water is warm, and stir to help it dissolve.
4. Add the dried persimmon slices and let the brew steep for 2 to 3 hours (or up to three days in the refrigerator) to allow the dried fruit to soften and give off its sweet flavor. Remove the persimmons or leave them in the punch bowl for decoration.
5. Add the pine nuts as a garnish before serving.

THEMES AND VARIATIONS

Ginger tea bags can be substituted for fresh ginger if you find it more convenient.

ESPECIALLY GOOD FOR

Anyone who wants to aid digestion and increase immunity.

FOR THOSE FAMILIAR WITH
TRADITIONAL CHINESE MEDICINE

This beverage is warming and good for the digestion, helps Kidney energy, and revitalizes Blood.

CHEERFUL CHERRY-BERRY BEVERAGE

MAKES 1 SERVING

This bright red, sweet, fruity herbal tea includes cherries, which are sometimes called the "fruit of fire" in China, as they are believed to generate heat in the body and increase energy.

INGREDIENTS

8 fresh cherries
1 tablespoon (10 grams) longan fruit (*long yan rou*)
1 tablespoon (10 grams) goji berries (*gou qi zi*)
1 to 2 cups water

DIRECTIONS

1. Combine the cherries, longan fruit, goji berries, and water in a small pot and bring to a boil.
2. Lower the heat and simmer for 5 to 10 minutes, stirring occasionally and crushing the cherries against the side of the pot to help coax the juice out.
3. Strain out the fruit, if desired (or leave it in and eat it with a spoon).

THEMES AND VARIATIONS

If fresh cherries aren't available, try dried cherries, cut in half.

ESPECIALLY GOOD FOR

Anyone with dizziness, palpitations, or memory or vision problems, or who is in a weakened state.

FOR THOSE FAMILIAR WITH TRADITIONAL CHINESE MEDICINE

This herbal drink is good for Liver Blood deficiency, dizziness, and palpitations. Longan fruit acts on the Heart and Spleen to nourish Blood, calm the spirit, and treat problems such as insomnia, palpitations, and poor memory. Traditionally, cherries are used to warm the body, strengthen the Spleen-Stomach to counteract fatigue, and generate fluids. Goji berries nourish the Blood and the yin, increase the essence, and improve vision.

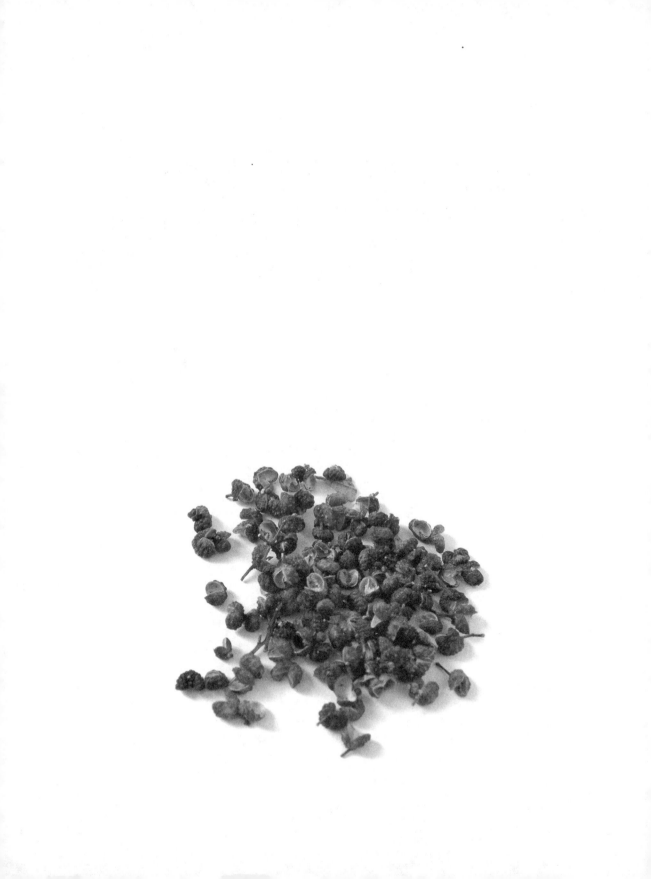

MIXED AND SUNDRY: STOCKS, SAUCES, AND TOPPINGS

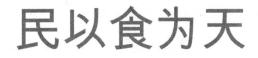

Eating is heaven.

—KOREAN PROVERB

QUICK KOMBU *DASHI* STOCK

MAKES 3½ CUPS

This vegetarian, mineral-rich stock is the simplest form of dashi, *traditional Japanese soup stock. Dashi is a staple in Japanese cuisine, adding a light yet complex flavor to dishes such as Basic Miso Soup (page 67), Mushroom Medley–Miso Soup (page 74), and Japanese New Year's Soup (page 80).*

INGREDIENTS

1 (8 by 4-inch piece) dried kombu
   seaweed
3½ cups water

DIRECTIONS

1. Place the seaweed and water in a medium-size pot and let the kombu soak for 20 minutes (longer won't hurt). The kombu will have a powdery white coating; this is normal and adds valuable trace minerals to the soup, so there's no reason to wipe it off.
2. Heat the mixture over medium heat until just before it boils (the water will be steaming but not actively bubbling), 5 to 10 minutes. Turn off the heat.
3. Remove the seaweed (which can be reserved for other dishes or reused to make more stock).
4. The stock can now be used for cooking. Most stocks keep well in the refrigerator for about a week and can be frozen in small portions for later use.

THEMES AND VARIATIONS

Lightly scoring the kombu with a knife will help release the seaweed's flavors and other attributes. Add mushrooms—or the water you soaked your dried mushrooms in—to add a different twist.

ESPECIALLY GOOD FOR

Vegetarians looking for a delicious, nutritious, and quick soup base; or anyone who wants to help cleanse his or her system of swelling or masses, or who may suffer from hypothyroidism or goiter.

FOR THOSE FAMILIAR WITH
TRADITIONAL CHINESE MEDICINE

This basic stock helps counteract stagnation and drain Dampness.

DASHI OF THE SEA

MAKES 3½ CUPS

This is a common recipe for dashi, *a soup stock that is a building block for many dishes in Japanese cuisine—from miso soup to marinades. Luckily,* dashi *is a cinch to prepare. You can also make a large batch and freeze it smaller portions to have on hand whenever you need it.*

INGREDIENTS

1 (8 by 4-inch piece) dried kombu
  seaweed
3½ cups water
2 tablespoons dried bonito flakes
  (*katsuobushi*)

Helpful Hints about Bonito Flakes

Dried bonito flakes (*katsuobushi*) are shavings from dried, aged bonito fish. A common ingredient in Japanese cuisine, they are widely available in Asian supermarkets. (For more information on bonito flakes, see "One Hundred Healthful Asian Ingredients.")

DIRECTIONS

1. Place the seaweed and water in a medium-size pot and let the kombu soak for 20 minutes (longer won't hurt). The kombu will have a powdery white coating; this is normal and adds valuable trace minerals to the soup, so there's no reason to wipe it off.
2. Heat the mixture over medium heat until just before it boils (the water will be steaming but not actively bubbling), 5 to 10 minutes. Turn off the heat.
3. Remove the seaweed (which can be reserved for other dishes or reused to make more stock) and stir in the bonito flakes. Let the mixture sit for 5 minutes.
4. Strain the bonito flakes from the stock (a strainer lined with a paper towel works well for this purpose).
5. The stock can now be used for cooking. Most stocks keep well in the refrigerator for about a week and can be frozen in small portions for later use.

THEMES AND VARIATIONS

Some people use a cold preparation method, whereby they simply soak the kombu and bonito in water for a few hours or overnight, then strain.

Dried baby sardines (*niboshi*) can be used instead of bonito flakes. Also, shiitake mushrooms can be included with the seaweed.

ESPECIALLY GOOD FOR

Supporting general health and nutrition and using instead of high-sodium and/or MSG-containing commercial soup stocks.

FOR THOSE FAMILIAR WITH
TRADITIONAL CHINESE MEDICINE

This basic stock helps counteract stagnation, drain Dampness, and nourish yin.

I-CAN'T-BELIEVE-IT'S-THIS-EASY MUSHROOM STOCK

MAKES 3½ CUPS

This simple stock can be used anywhere a vegetarian stock or Japanese dashi is called for, including for a variety of miso soups (pages 67, 74, and 75) or Japanese New Year's Soup (page 80).

INGREDIENTS

6 (about 1 ounce) dried shiitake
    mushrooms
4 cups water

Legend Has It

In ancient times in Japan, shiitakes were so sought after that there were "shiitake wars," during which precious logs inoculated with shiitake spores were stolen from their owners.

DIRECTIONS

1. Place the mushrooms and water in a medium-size pot and set aside for several hours.
2. Remove the mushrooms (and, by all means, save them for cooking in another dish).
3. Bring the water to a boil, lower the heat, and simmer for 2 minutes.
4. The stock can now be used for cooking, stored for a few days in the refrigerator, or frozen in small portions for later use.

ESPECIALLY GOOD FOR

Enhancing immunity, supporting general health.

FOR THOSE FAMILIAR WITH
TRADITIONAL CHINESE MEDICINE

Shiitakes strengthen the Spleen and Stomach and augment qi.

CLASSIC KOREAN FISH STOCK

MAKES 3½ CUPS

Korean stocks can be made from a variety of seafood, but this is the most common version—super easy as well as flavorful and nutritious. Miso paste or red pepper paste are often added to the broth once it is done, and of course the broth is used as a base for more elaborate soups, including Classic Korean Seaweed Soup, page 72.

INGREDIENTS

½ ounce dried anchovies
4 cups water
A dash of rice vinegar or lemon juice

DIRECTIONS

1. Place the dried anchovies on a piece of cheesecloth and make a bag by tying the ends together.
2. Place the water in a pot, add the bag of anchovies, and bring to a boil.
3. Lower the heat to low, and simmer, loosely covered, for about 10 minutes (avoid overcooking, or the anchovies will become bitter).
4. Remove the pot from the heat and remove the bag of anchovies.
5. Add the rice vinegar, to eliminate any fishy taste.
6. The stock can now be used for cooking. Most stocks keep well in the refrigerator for about a week and can be frozen in small portions for later use.

ESPECIALLY GOOD FOR
Anyone with poor appetite, chronic illness, or difficulty with lactation.

FOR THOSE FAMILIAR WITH
TRADITIONAL CHINESE MEDICINE
This stock strengthens the qi and Blood, as well as the Spleen.

VEGETABLE STOCK WITH KOMBU AND GINGER

MAKES 6 CUPS

This rich vegetable stock will add flavor to any dish, such as Curry Favor Pumpkin Soup (page 70). We've omitted salt from this and many of the other stocks, to give you more flexibility when cooking with them later. Add salt as need when cooking.

INGREDIENTS

- 1 medium-size carrot, chopped into 1-inch pieces
- 1 stalk celery, chopped into 1-inch pieces
- 1 medium-size onion, chopped into 1-inch pieces
- 1 (1-inch) piece fresh ginger, cut into slices the width of a quarter
- 1 (8 by 4-inch piece) dried kombu seaweed
- 10 cups water

DIRECTIONS

1. Place all the ingredients—the carrot, celery, onion, ginger, kombu, and water—in a large pot.
2. Bring to a boil. Lower the heat and simmer, covered, for 30 to 45 minutes.
3. Strain out the vegetables.
4. You can use your vegetable stock immediately, store in the refrigerator for several days, or freeze in small portions for later use.

THEMES AND VARIATIONS

Many vegetables work well for making a vegetable stock, including chard, yellow squash, leeks, mushrooms, and parsley stems; don't hesitate to use scraps. Avoid stronger-tasting or highly colored vegetables, such as artichokes, beets, asparagus, fennel, and green peppers, as they will overpower the other flavors. Some people like to roast the vegetables before adding them to the stock.

ESPECIALLY GOOD FOR

Reducing small masses or nodules, gallstones, and high cholesterol.

FOR THOSE FAMILIAR WITH
TRADITIONAL CHINESE MEDICINE

This dish addresses qi stagnation, obstruction from phlegm, and Liver/Gallbladder Damp Heat.

SHIITAKE-ASTRAGALUS VEGETABLE STOCK

MAKES 5 TO 6 CUPS

This stock is so good it almost qualifies as a soup in itself. This stock can be used in any recipe that calls for vegetable stock, such as Buddhist Tofu Soup (page 66) or Gingery Pumpkin Soup (page 69).

INGREDIENTS

8 to 10 cups water
1 leek, washed well and cut into
   1-inch pieces
3 cloves garlic, peeled and crushed
8 dried or fresh shiitake mushrooms, rinsed (if fresh, cut into
   quarters)
6 dried and seeded Chinese red
   dates (*hong zao*)
3 medium-size pieces (10 grams)
   astragalus (*huang qi*)
A pinch of salt (optional)

DIRECTIONS

1. Place all the ingredients—the water, leek, garlic, shiitake mushrooms, Chinese red dates, astragalus, and salt (if using)—in a
   large pot. Bring to a boil. Lower the heat and simmer, covered,
   for 30 to 45 minutes.
2. Strain out the vegetables (or at least remove the astragalus) and
   you have your vegetable stock, which can be used right away,
   stored in the refrigerator for several days, or frozen in small portions for later use.

ESPECIALLY GOOD FOR

Anyone who wants to increase immunity or who suffers from high
blood pressure, high cholesterol, diabetes, or urinary tract infections.

FOR THOSE FAMILIAR WITH
TRADITIONAL CHINESE MEDICINE

This stock clears Heat, drains Dampness, and strengthens the qi.

IMMUNITY-BOOSTING CHICKEN STOCK

MAKES 9 CUPS

This is a great start for a soup during the flu season or anytime you're beginning to feel under the weather. Try using this stock in Flu Season Soup, page 96.

INGREDIENTS

- 1 (2-inch) piece fresh ginger, cut into ⅛-inch slices the width of a quarter
- 3 cloves garlic, peeled and crushed
- 1 medium-size leek, washed well and cut into 3-inch pieces
- 1 pound chicken bones
- 4 dried or fresh shiitake mushrooms, rinsed
- 6 medium-size pieces (about 20 grams) astragalus (*huang qi*) .
- 12 cups water

Mika Says

The easiest way to get chicken bones for your stock is to save them from a roasted or baked chicken. The bones freeze well, so you can store them in the freezer until you are inspired to make a stock. Otherwise, you might have some luck asking for bones at your local supermarket meat counter or butcher, or you can substitute bony chicken pieces, such as wings.

DIRECTIONS

1. Place all the ingredients—the ginger, garlic, leek, chicken bones, shiitake mushrooms, astragalus, and water—in a large pot and bring to a boil. Skim off the fat and oil that floats to the surface of the soup as necessary.
2. Lower the heat and simmer gently, covered, for 2 hours.
3. Strain the broth through cheesecloth or a fine-mesh strainer, removing the bones and herbs.
4. You can enjoy your stock immediately, store in the refrigerator for several days, or freeze in small portions for later use.

THEMES AND VARIATIONS

If you want to make this stock into a quick soup, add potatoes, carrots, celery, peas, mushrooms, cellophane noodles, thyme, and soy sauce. Voilà, a delicious meal and just what the doctor ordered to boost your natural protection against illnesses.

This stock cooks up in 1 hour in a pressure cooker.

ESPECIALLY GOOD FOR

Increasing immunity, fighting off the common cold, strengthening bones, or counteracting frequent colds and fatigue.

FOR THOSE FAMILIAR WITH
TRADITIONAL CHINESE MEDICINE

This dish strengthens the qi of the Spleen and Lungs and harmonizes *ying qi* and *wei qi*.

CHICKEN STOCK WITH GINGER AND WINE

MAKES 6 CUPS

The ginger and rice wine give this broth a classic Asian flavor. Try it in a soup, such as Simple Winter Melon Soup, page 84.

INGREDIENTS

1 (1- to 2-inch) piece fresh ginger, cut into slices the width of a quarter

6 green onions, chopped into 3-inch pieces, ends trimmed

1 to 2 pounds chicken bones or bony pieces (such as backs and necks)

1 cup rice wine

9 cups water

Warren Says

If you use chicken stock, I highly recommend making your own. Many commercial chicken stocks contain ingredients such as MSG and preservatives that are best avoided. If you must buy your chicken stock, look for organic varieties and don't forget to read the label to make sure it passes muster!

DIRECTIONS

1. Place all the ingredients—the ginger, green onions, chicken bones, rice wine, and water—in a large pot and bring to a boil.
2. Decrease the heat and simmer gently, uncovered, for 2 hours. Skim off the fat and oil that floats to the surface of the soup as necessary.
3. Strain the broth through cheesecloth or a fine-mesh strainer, removing the bones, ginger, and green onions.
4. Your broth is now ready to use. You can also store it in the refrigerator for several days or freeze it in small portions for later use.

ESPECIALLY GOOD FOR

Anyone with arthritis, muscle aches and pain, or prostatitis.

FOR THOSE FAMILIAR WITH
TRADITIONAL CHINESE MEDICINE

This stock strengthens the qi, nourishes Blood, and harmonizes the Spleen and Stomach.

BONE-BUILDING STOCK

MAKES 10 TO 14 CUPS

Bone stock is very popular in China. From the perspective of traditional Chinese medicine, bones in the diet help strengthen bones in the body, and bone marrow in the diet helps increase the essence, strengthening the entire body. If you want to maximize this stock's healing effects for chronic diseases such as cancer, choose large bones with plenty of marrow. This basic stock can be used in Classic Korean Seaweed Soup, page 72, or Simple Winter Melon Soup, page 84. Or, once you have made the stock, simply add ingredients you prefer: vegetables such as mushrooms, carrots, Chinese cabbage, or kale; herbs such as astragalus or dang gui (boil the herbs in the soup for 30 minutes, then remove); and/or meat such as shrimp, chicken, beef, or pork. Season with salt and/or soy sauce to taste.

INGREDIENTS

2 pounds cooked or raw beef,
   lamb, or pork bones
½ cup rice wine or white wine
16 cups (1 gallon) water
1 medium-size carrot (optional),
   chopped into 1-inch pieces
1 medium-size onion (optional),
   chopped into 1-inch pieces

THEMES AND VARIATIONS

Other vegetables, such as broccoli stems, mushrooms, and leeks, can be added or substituted, depending on what you have on hand. Avoid stronger-tasting or highly colored vegetables, such as artichokes, beets, asparagus, fennel, and green peppers, as they will overpower the other flavors. This and most other stocks freeze well for later use.

DIRECTIONS

1. Place the bones, wine, water, and vegetables (if using) in a large pot. If the bones aren't covered with the liquid, add water until they are.
2. Bring to a boil, lower the heat, and simmer, uncovered, for 5 minutes. Skim off and discard any froth that rises to the top of the stock.
3. For beef bones, simmer, covered, for 8 to 10 hours; add more water if needed. For pork or lamb bones, simmer, covered, for at least 2½ hours.
4. Remove the bones, vegetables, and ginger from the stock, using a slotted spoon, a strainer, or piece of cheesecloth.
5. Skim off any excess fat. Season the stock with salt if desired (or wait to add until you cook with the stock).
6. If you aren't using the stock immediately, you can store it in the fridge for a few days or freeze it in small portions for later use.

ESPECIALLY GOOD FOR

Eating in the wintertime. Serving to those recuperating from bone surgery, bone injury, or illness; experiencing chronic joint pain; or concerned with minimizing the effects of age.

FOR THOSE FAMILIAR WITH
TRADITIONAL CHINESE MEDICINE

Bone stock strengthens the Liver and Kidneys; fortifies bones, tendons, and muscles; and warms the yang.

SOME-LIKE-IT-HOT CHILI OIL

MAKES ¾ CUP

Chili oil demystified: Now you can make your own blend, using your choice of hot peppers and high-quality oil for use as a condiment or as an ingredient in other dishes, such as spicy dipping sauce.

INGREDIENTS

¼ cup red chili flakes (see "Themes and Variations")
A pinch of salt (optional)
⅔ cup canola or peanut oil
⅓ cup dark sesame oil

DIRECTIONS

1. Place the chili flakes and salt (if using) in a tempered glass container, such as a Pyrex bowl.
2. In a wok or heavy skillet, heat the canola and sesame oils over medium heat for about 5 minutes.
3. To test whether the oil is the correct temperature, drop a chili flake into the oil. It should be surrounded instantly by foam, but should not turn black. (If the flake turns black, let the oil cool for a few minutes and try again.) Carefully pour the hot oil over the chili flakes.
4. Let the mixture cool (it can be used immediately, but for best results, let it sit for a day), then strain out the chili flakes to get your homemade hot chili oil, which you can store in a cool, dark cupboard or refrigerator.

THEMES AND VARIATIONS

If you are starting with whole dried chili peppers, cut off the stems, remove the seeds, and chop the peppers into flakes (either by hand or in a food processor). Then follow the recipe above. Caution: You may want to wear plastic gloves to protect your hands from the spice when handling the peppers. At least avoid contact with your eyes, and wash your hands with soap and water afterward.

ESPECIALLY GOOD FOR

Anyone who tends to run cold, or who wants to help blood circulation and reduce cardiovascular disease. This condiment should be used sparingly by those who tend to run warm.

FOR THOSE FAMILIAR WITH
TRADITIONAL CHINESE MEDICINE

Chili oil helps warm the Stomach, move the qi and Blood, warm the channels, and release pain.

FIVE-SPICE POWDER

MAKES ¼ CUP

Five-spice powder, known as wu xiang fen *in Chinese, incorporates all five flavors—sour, bitter, sweet, spicy, and salty. This represents the five elements—wood, fire, earth, metal, and water. In addition to homemade varieties, five-spice powder is commonly sold in the spice aisle in supermarkets. We use it in dishes such as Five-Spice Powder Chicken, page 156.*

INGREDIENTS

2 teaspoons Sichuan peppercorns
8 whole dried star anise
½ teaspoon whole cloves
2 teaspoons fennel seeds
1 (3-inch) stick cinnamon, or
　1 tablespoon ground

DIRECTIONS

1. If your Sichuan peppercorns aren't already roasted, heat a dry skillet over low-to-medium heat and add the peppercorns. Toast until fragrant (about 3 minutes).
2. Grind the Sichuan peppercorns, star anise, cloves, fennel seeds, and cinnamon into a fine powder, using a spice mill or coffee grinder. (If you are substituting ground spices for any of the ingredients, add them after grinding the other spices, and stir.)
3. Store in an airtight container in a cool place.

THEMES AND VARIATIONS

You can substitute black peppercorns for the Sichuan peppercorns, if need be. Other possible substitutions are 4 teaspoons of ground anise for the 8 whole star anise pieces, or ⅜ teaspoon of ground cloves for the whole cloves.

ESPECIALLY GOOD FOR

Anyone with poor appetite, cold hands and feet, premenstrual syndrome, chronic pain, or low pain tolerance.

FOR THOSE FAMILIAR WITH
TRADITIONAL CHINESE MEDICINE

Five-spice powder harmonizes the Spleen and Stomach, warms the channels and collaterals, and releases pain. It addresses Cold Damp bi syndrome.

DELICIOUS DUMPLING DIPPING SAUCE

MAKES ⅔ CUP

A tasty dipping sauce for dumplings or spring rolls.

INGREDIENTS

3 to 4 medium-size cloves garlic, peeled and minced
¼ cup rice vinegar
¼ cup soy sauce
½ to 1 teaspoon chili oil, or to taste (optional)
2 teaspoons dark sesame oil

DIRECTIONS

1. Mix all the ingredients—the garlic, rice vinegar, soy sauce, chili oil, and sesame oil—together in a bowl, and serve on the side.

ESPECIALLY GOOD FOR

Supporting good general nutrition; strengthening digestion; and counteracting some types of nausea, diarrhea, and food poisoning.

FOR THOSE FAMILIAR WITH TRADITIONAL CHINESE MEDICINE

This dipping sauce harmonizes the Spleen and Stomach, and can clear Heat and toxic Heat.

JAPANESE NOODLE DIPPING SAUCE

MAKES ABOUT 4 SERVINGS

This dipping sauce can be served on the side to as a dip for cold Japanese noodles, such as soba noodles garnished with green onion, shredded nori seaweed, toasted sesame seeds, and/or wasabi. The sauce can also be served warm, as a broth containing noodles and other ingredients, such as fish cake.

INGREDIENTS

2 cups *Dashi* of the Sea (page 265)
⅓ cup mirin or dry sherry
⅓ cup soy sauce

DIRECTIONS

1. Place all the ingredients—*dashi*, mirin, and soy sauce—in a small saucepan and bring to a boil.
2. Turn off the heat and let the sauce cool.

ESPECIALLY GOOD FOR

Supporting general health and helping to resolve conditions involving small masses, such as fibroids.

FOR THOSE FAMILIAR WITH TRADITIONAL CHINESE MEDICINE

This basic stock helps resolve Damp phlegm.

DO-IT-YOURSELF DUMPLING WRAPPERS

MAKES ABOUT 80

Here is a recipe for homemade dumpling wrappers to accompany homemade dumplings or pot stickers. Be prepared: making the wrappers is trickier than making the filling. For traditional meat dumplings, a good rule of thumb for how much dough to make is to use 2 cups of flour for every pound of meat in the filling.

INGREDIENTS

5 cups (1⅔ pounds) all-purpose flour, plus extra to flour the work surface
½ teaspoon salt (optional)
1¼ cups water

DIRECTIONS

1. Mix the flour and salt (if using) together, adding the water a little at a time until you achieve the right consistency for a soft dough—it should be smooth and silky.

2. Knead the dough for about 15 minutes, then cover with a wet paper towel and leave the dough to "rest" for another 30 minutes (during which time you can make the dumpling filling).

3. Roll the dough into about twelve even "logs" (cylinders) 1¼ inch in diameter.

4. Using a knife, cut each log into ¾-inch slices.

5. On a floured surface, flatten a slice with your palm. Using a floured rolling pin or bottle, roll each slice into a circle about 3 inches in diameter (it should be thin, but not so thin as to develop holes), slightly thicker in the center than at the edges (which will require you to roll an extra pass around the edges).

6. *Do not stack the dumpling wrappers.* Keep them floured while you continue rolling out the other slices, so the wrappers don't stick together and become unusable. If the wrappers start to dry out, cover them with a damp paper towel. Once you fill the wrappers with filling, pinch the edges to make dumplings. Keep their bottoms floured. Fresh dumpling wrappers are best used immediately.

A Note on Wheat

Although most Westerners think of rice when they think of East Asian grains, wheat is also an ancient and important crop, especially in northern China, where noodles, buns, steamed breads, and dumplings are popular. The concept of grinding wheat into flour was probably introduced to China from the West in the Han dynasty more than two thousand years ago. Like rice, wheat (and other grains such as barley, millet, and corn) are considered *fan*—the more fundamental, main, or primary food, necessary to any meal. Ideally, *fan* is accompanied by *cai*—meats, fruits, and vegetables that make the meal more tasty and balanced.

ESPECIALLY GOOD FOR

Making into dumplings or pot stickers (see page 170) by those with the time and patience to try their hand at the art of making dumpling wrappers from scratch.

THEMES AND VARIATIONS

Some people like to add an egg yolk to the dough. If you do this, use about 3 tablespoons less water, so there's not too much liquid.

FOR THOSE FAMILIAR WITH TRADITIONAL CHINESE MEDICINE

Wheat, which is considered cool and sweet, strengthens qi and Blood.

CREAMY UMEBOSHI DRESSING

This simple, interesting dressing livens up a salad or vegetables such as broccoli or asparagus.

INGREDIENTS

3½ ounces (¼ package) tofu, soft or medium varieties of firmness preferred

3 *umeboshi* (pickled plums), pitted if necessary

2 tablespoons mirin or dry sherry

1 tablespoon lemon juice

DIRECTIONS

1. Place all the ingredients—the tofu, *umeboshi*, mirin, and lemon juice—in a food processor or blender.
2. Whir until smooth.

ESPECIALLY GOOD FOR

This dressing is good for eating on a hot day, and serving to promote digestion.

FOR THOSE FAMILIAR WITH TRADITIONAL CHINESE MEDICINE

This dressing strengthens Spleen qi, harmonizes the Stomach, and clears Heat.

UMEBOSHI-SESAME DRESSING

MAKES 2 TO 3 SERVINGS

A tasty dressing for salads or cooked vegetables, such as broccoli, asparagus, or green beans. This dressing will keep for several days in your refrigerator.

INGREDIENTS
1 *umeboshi* (pickled plum), or
   1 tablespoon *umeboshi* paste
1 clove garlic, peeled and minced
2 tablespoons tahini or other
   sesame paste
1 teaspoon dark sesame oil
4 teaspoons lemon juice
2 to 4 tablespoons water

Warren Says
Whereas salads are popular as a health food in the West, traditional Chinese medicine views cold and uncooked foods as difficult to digest. This salad dressing helps promote good digestion.

DIRECTIONS
1. If you are using a whole *umeboshi*, remove and discard the pit and mince the umeboshi fruit.
2. Combine the *umeboshi*, garlic, tahini, sesame oil, and lemon juice in a small bowl and stir well. Add the water, 1 tablespoon at a time, and stir until you have the desired consistency.

ESPECIALLY GOOD FOR
Helping to promote digestion, and counteract insomnia and irritability.

FOR THOSE FAMILIAR WITH
TRADITIONAL CHINESE MEDICINE
This dressing soothes the Liver, strengthens the Liver yin, and addresses yin deficiency.

MISO-TAHINI DRESSING

MAKES 1 TO 2 SERVINGS

This dressing takes advantage of the smooth consistency of the miso and tahini for a delicious topping for salads or vegetables. We like it on top of mixed salad greens. The dressing will keep in your refrigerator for several days.

INGREDIENTS

1 clove garlic, peeled and minced
2 tablespoons tahini or other sesame paste
1 tablespoon lemon juice
1 tablespoon white miso
2 tablespoons water, or to taste

DIRECTIONS

1. Mix the garlic, tahini, lemon juice, and white miso together in a small bowl.
2. Spoon in the water and stir well. Add more water if you prefer a more runny consistency.

ESPECIALLY GOOD FOR

Helping to promote digestion, calm the emotions, and counteract insomnia.

FOR THOSE FAMILIAR WITH
TRADITIONAL CHINESE MEDICINE

This dish strengthens the Liver and Kidneys and harmonizes the Middle Burner.

GET-UP-AND-GO GARLIC SAUCE

MAKES ABOUT ⅓ CUP

This garlic-flavored sauce can be served on the side or cooked with seafood, meat, and/or vegetables. Garlic appears in ancient writings of the Chinese, Egyptians, Babylonians, and Indians, as far back as five thousand years ago.

INGREDIENTS

3 tablespoons rice vinegar

3 tablespoons soy sauce

1 tablespoon rice wine or dry sherry

½ teaspoon chili oil or chili sauce, or to taste

1 tablespoon dark sesame oil

2 teaspoons powdered kudzu, arrowroot, cornstarch, or other thickener

1½ tablespoons vegetable oil, such as olive or canola

1 tablespoon water

4 medium-size cloves garlic, minced (about 4 teaspoons)

Mika Says

Asian condiments are often served on the side so people can cater to their own tastes when flavoring their meals. Unlike many sauces in the West that rely on fats (butter, cream, mayonnaise), Asian condiments often feature herbs and spices, such as garlic, vinegar, sesame, and hot peppers.

DIRECTIONS

1. Stir together the rice vinegar, soy sauce, rice wine, chili oil, and sesame oil in a small bowl.
2. In a separate small bowl, dissolve the thickener in the water to make a slurry.
3. Heat the vegetable oil in a small saucepan over medium heat, then add the garlic. Cook, stirring, until aromatic (about 30 seconds).
4. Add the chili mixture to the pan. Cook over low heat for about a minute.
5. Add the slurry and stir, then remove from the heat.

THEMES AND VARIATIONS

If you'd like to cook your seafood, meat, and/or vegetables directly in the sauce, chop into 1-inch pieces, add them to the pan after step 3, and stir-fry for 5 minutes, or until cooked. Proceed with steps 4 and 5.

In addition, you might like to substitute white vinegar for rice vinegar, especially if you plan to use the sauce with seafood.

ESPECIALLY GOOD FOR

Anyone who wants to help blood circulation, increase appetite, or treat indigestion.

FOR THOSE FAMILIAR WITH TRADITIONAL CHINESE MEDICINE

This sauce reflects garlic's ability to warm the Stomach, strengthen the Spleen, promote the movement of qi, reduce stagnation, and relieve toxicity.

TOGARASHI TOPPING

MAKES ⅓ TO ½ CUP

This flavorful, spicy, and healthy condiment is a staple on the Japanese table, eaten with grilled meats, tempura, noodles, soups, stews, and a variety of other dishes.

INGREDIENTS

2 tablespoons powdered Sichuan peppercorn (*hua jiao* or *shanō jiao* in Chinese, *sansh* in Japanese), or about 20 whole dried Sichuan peppercorns, or 1 tablespoon black peppercorns

1 tablespoon red chili powder

2 teaspoons black sesame seeds

2 teaspoons golden sesame seeds or poppy seeds

2 teaspoons garlic powder

1 tablespoon dried and shredded tangerine peel

2 teaspoons nori seaweed, flaked or cut into ⅛- by ¼-inch strips

Helpful Hints about Sichuan Peppercorns

Sichuan peppercorns are harvested from a different species of plant than are black peppercorns or chili peppers. Sichuan peppercorns are sold in packages at Asian markets, and are often used to make Sichuan pepper–flavored oil. (For more information on Sichuan peppercorns, see "One Hundred Healthful Asian Ingredients.")

DIRECTIONS

1. Place the Sichuan peppercorn, chili powder, sesame seeds, garlic powder, and tangerine peel in a spice grinder, coffee mill, or grooved Japanese mortar (*suribachi*) and grind together.
2. Add the nori and mix.
3. Store in an airtight container. The mixture should remain fresh for a month or more.

THEMES AND VARIATIONS

The mixture is also commonly available in Asian food stores. Look for *shichimi togarashi* (*shichi* means "seven"; *togarashi* means "chili") or *nanami togarashi* (a variation that emphasizes the citrus flavor).

ESPECIALLY GOOD FOR

Eating in cold weather, or serving to anyone who tends to run cold. This topping should only be used sparingly by those who tend to run warm.

FOR THOSE FAMILIAR WITH TRADITIONAL CHINESE MEDICINE

This condiment warms the Interior.

SESAME SHAKE

MAKES 1 CUP

This handy topping, known as gomashio/gomasio *in Japanese, adds a classic Asian touch to stir-fries, soups, and rice.*

INGREDIENTS

1 cup black or brown sesame
   seeds
1 teaspoon salt

Helpful Hints about Sesame Seeds

Black and brown sesame seeds, which have been enjoyed for millennia, are available at Asian markets, herbal shops, and some natural food stores. Like many other seeds and nuts, sesame seeds do age, so when you are shopping, select a batch that looks and smells fresh and sweet. (For more information on sesame seeds, see "One Hundred Healthful Asian Ingredients.")

DIRECTIONS

1. Place the sesame seeds in a dry skillet and toast over low heat for about 5 minutes, until they become fragrant, golden, and begin to pop. Turn off the heat, transfer the seeds to a plate or a bowl, and let them cool for at least 1 minute.
2. Place the sesame seeds in a food processor or grooved Japanese mortar (*suribachi*), then grind with the salt.
3. You can use the mixture right away or store it in an airtight container in the refrigerator for up to one month.

ESPECIALLY GOOD FOR
People concerned about high blood sugar levels or high cholesterol. Black sesame seeds are associated with longevity.

FOR THOSE FAMILIAR WITH
TRADITIONAL CHINESE MEDICINE
Black sesame seeds strengthen the Liver and Kidneys and darken the hair, while both types of sesame are thought to nourish the Blood and moisten the Intestines.

KOREAN CABBAGE KIMCHI

MAKES 4 CUPS

Korean cuisine wouldn't be the same without kimchi (today more correctly transliterated as gimchi*), a spicy, fermented side dish served with almost every meal and featured as a key ingredient in soups, pancakes, and other dishes. Kimchi is often made with Chinese cabbage, as in this recipe, but daikon, turnip, cucumber, and leek are other favorite main ingredients. Both Chinese and Japanese cuisines have their own versions of pickled and/or fermented vegetables, which make excellent condiments for serving with rice, congee, or soup.*

INGREDIENTS

3 tablespoons plus 1 teaspoon salt
6 cups water
2 pounds Chinese cabbage
  (1 medium head), chopped into
  2-inch chunks
1 (2-inch) piece fresh ginger,
  minced
5 or 6 cloves garlic, minced
4 green onions, cut into ¼-inch
  slices (discard white roots)
2 tablespoons hot chili powder or
  flakes
1 teaspoon honey or sugar

DIRECTIONS

1. Dissolve 3 tablespoons of the salt in the water. Place the chopped cabbage into a large bowl, jar, or pot, then pour the saltwater over it. Cover with plastic wrap, then place a plate or other heavy object on top to weigh the cabbage down and keep it submerged under the water. Let stand overnight, or for 12 hours.

2. Pour off the water, rinse the cabbage, and squeeze dry. The cabbage will have shrunk considerably in volume.

3. Place the ginger, garlic, green onions, chili powder, and remaining 1 teaspoon of salt in a bowl and stir.

4. Wearing gloves if you want to protect your hands, mix the cabbage leaves with the spice mixture.

5. Place the mixture (including any liquid that accumulated during the mixing) in a glass jar (an old pickle jar works well), leaving at least 2 inches of space at the top. Cap the jar tightly and place it in a cool room for about 2 days. If it starts to bubble, it's ready to eat and to be stored in the refrigerator. If it isn't bubbling yet, leave it out for another day or so before refrigerating.

6. Kimchi should stay good for 3 for 4 weeks, tightly covered, in your refrigerator.

Helpful Hints about Chili Peppers (and Related Species)

Hot peppers are not only delicious for those who like spicy food, but they are also believed by Chinese traditional medical practitioners to have medicinal qualities. In the West, spicy food is often avoided in cases of stomach distress. However, in traditional Chinese medicine, chili peppers are sometimes prescribed to alleviate abdominal pain or gastric upset if the diagnosis involves too much Cold (for example, in a case when a patient experiences stomach cramping). (For more information on chili peppers, see "One Hundred Healthful Asian Ingredients.")

THEMES AND VARIATIONS

There are probably as many different versions of kimchi as there are Korean cooks, and different preparations of kimchi are favored in different seasons. Some versions known as "white kimchi" and popular in North Korea aren't even spicy. Other potential ingredients not mentioned above include anchovies, shrimp, oysters, walnuts, lemon juice, pear, mustard greens, chestnuts, pine nuts, Chinese red dates, shiitake mushrooms, and watercress.

Fast Facts about Kimchi

Kimchi, which has been eaten for thousands of years in Korea, has been an important source of vegetables in the cold season, when fresh vegetables are not available. Traditionally, a large batch of kimchi was made in the fall, placed in an earthenware pot, and buried in a shady spot in the backyard, to keep the kimchi at a constant temperature before its consumption during the winter months.

ESPECIALLY GOOD FOR

Simulating the appetite, helping circulation, and counteracting high cholesterol and high glucose levels. This condiment should be used sparingly by those who tend to run warm, need to avoid salt, or suffer from heartburn.

FOR THOSE FAMILIAR WITH
TRADITIONAL CHINESE MEDICINE

This warming dish helps clear Dampness and move the Blood.

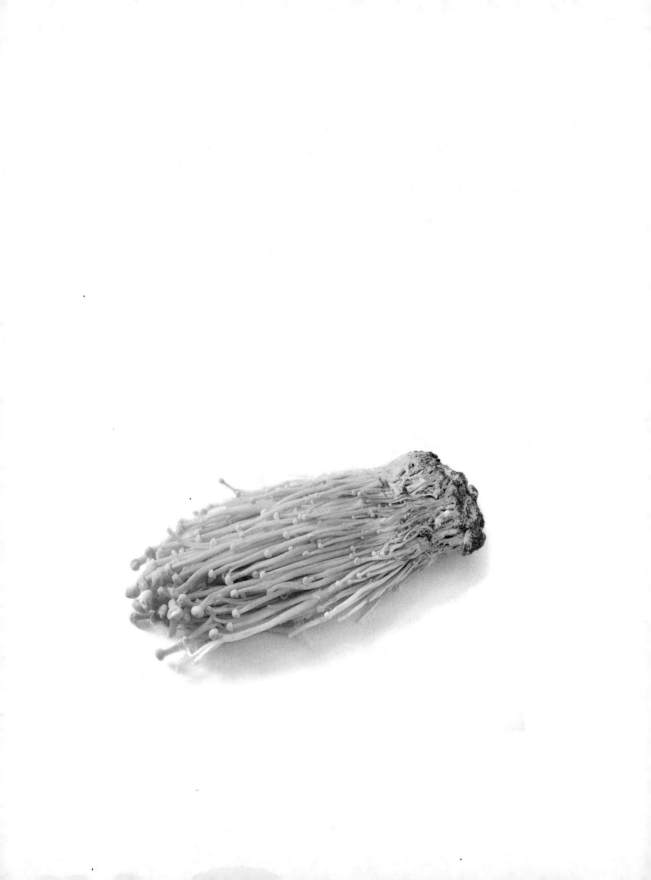

APPENDIXES

GLOSSARY
OF COMMON TRADITIONAL
CHINESE MEDICINE TERMS

BI SYNDROME. *Bi* syndrome (also called "painful obstruction syndrome") is a common pattern that may involve pain, swelling, soreness, numbness, and limited movement of muscles, tendons, and joints. It results from an invasion of Wind, Cold, Dampness, or Heat.

BLOOD. Blood—not the fluid referred to in Western medicine, but related to it—circulates through the body to nourish and moisten the organs, skin, muscles, tendons, and bones, as well as to support memory and mental activities. In the Chinese tradition, much importance is placed on replenishing blood lost due to injury, menses, or childbirth.

BLOOD DEFICIENCY. Blood deficiency is a pattern that occurs when Blood is insufficient to carry out its basic functions. Symptoms of Blood deficiency include pale complexion, dizziness, poor memory, burred vision, dry skin, anxiety, insomnia, scanty menstruation, and numbness in the hands and feet.

BLOOD STASIS. Blood stasis is a condition that occurs when Blood fails to move properly. Symptoms of this disorder include stabbing pain, fixed masses, and dark purple bleeding.

BODY FLUID. Body fluid (*jin ye*)—which includes saliva, gastric fluid, joint cavity fluid, tears, sweat, and urine—is derived from food and drink and serves to warm and nourish the muscles, moisten the skin, lubricate the joints, moisten the orifices, and surround the brain. *Jin* refers to light, clear, and watery body fluid that goes to the skin and muscles. *Ye* refers to heavy, dense fluid that moistens the joints, spine, brain, bone marrow, and sensory organs.

CHANNELS AND COLLATERALS. Channels (or meridians) and collaterals are pathways that flow through the body, enabling qi and Blood to circulate. Acupuncture uses needles on points on these pathways to help heal the body.

COLD. Like cold in the natural environment and sometimes associated with it, Cold in Chinese medicine is associated with contraction, obstruction, slower movement, and underactivity. An individual influenced by Cold will feel cold, appear pale, and will typically seek warmth with sweaters or blankets. Typical symptoms of a Cold disorder include chills, headache, loose stools, body aches, and sharp, cramping pain.

DAMP-HEAT. Damp-Heat is a union of Dampness and Heat, often resulting in infection. Damp-Heat is expressed in diseases whose symptoms include low-grade fever, headache, body aches, feelings of heaviness in the body and limbs, fatigue, abdominal distention, poor appetite, bitter taste and stickiness in the mouth, and scanty yellow urine.

DAMPNESS. Like Damp weather and sometimes associated with it, in Chinese medicine Dampness is heavy, wet, and turbid. Diseases caused by Dampness tend to linger and be difficult to cure. Like Cold, Dampness can cause pain, but Damp pain is heavy and protracted, rather than sharp and cramping. Dampness is associated with sticky secretions and tends to attack lower portions of the body. Dampness can appear in the body as water retention (edema), especially in the legs or abdomen, a sense of heaviness, lack of appetite, a feeling of distention in the chest or abdomen, urinary problems, sluggishness, or tiredness.

DEFICIENCY. Deficiency refers to cases of insufficient vital energy and lowered resistance to pathogenic factors. A number of syndromes, such as qi deficiency, Blood deficiency, yang deficiency, yin deficiency, and body fluid deficiency, fall into this category. Each type of deficiency has its own

pattern. These patterns are often made up of a specific combination of the following symptoms: fatigue, emaciation, low spirits, listlessness, sluggishness, pale complexion, shortness of breath, spontaneous sweating, night sweats, loose stools, frequent urination, insomnia, poor memory, and pain alleviated by pressure.

DRYNESS. Sometimes appearing with Heat or Cold, dryness is associated with dehydration and scant body fluids. Its symptoms can include dry nostrils, lips, and skin, hard stools, and scanty urination. Dryness can affect the Lung as a dry cough, asthma, or chest pain.

EXCESS. Excess refers to the presence of a pathogenic factor, while the body's natural resistance remains intact. The struggle between the pathogen and the body's natural resistance causes strong symptoms. Symptoms of excess syndromes can include agitation, coarse breathing, loud voice, fullness in the chest and abdomen, and pain aggravated by pressure.

EXTERIOR. Exterior refers to the relatively superficial parts of the body, such as the skin, muscles, and channels. Disorders are defined as Interior or Exterior.

FOOD STAGNATION. Symptoms of food stagnation, which occurs after overeating or eating too quickly, include stomachache, indigestion, fullness and distention of the abdomen, nausea, belching, and vomiting.

HEART. Not exactly the physical organ referred to in Western medicine but related to it, in traditional Chinese medicine the term *Heart* refers to the organ system that governs the Blood and blood vessels, as well as the consciousness and spirit.

HEAT. Heat (or in its extreme form, Fire) can take hold and produce symptoms such as fever, a red face, red eyes, dark urine, inflammation, thirst, and reddish eruptions of the skin. Heat is often associated with problems of the upper body, such as headaches, and consumes body fluids. Like Wind, Heat causes movement, but Heat's movement has a sudden and abrupt quality, associated with states like agitation, delirium, and irritability.

INTERIOR. Interior refers to the parts of the body away from the surface, including the internal organs. Disorders are defined as Interior or Exterior.

JING. Jing or essence refers to a refined and precious substance that forms the organic basis for all life. *Jing* influences our constitution, reproduction, growth, and development—and our longevity. *Jing* comes in (at least) two forms, prenatal *jing* and postnatal *jing*. Traditional Chinese medical practitioners advise you to conserve your prenatal *jing* as much as possible, approaching life's activities—including diet, work, and sexual activity—with balance and moderation. Postnatal *jing* can be enhanced by eating the proper diet.

KIDNEYS. As with other organs, the Kidneys are not the physical organs referred to in Western medicine but are related to them. In traditional Chinese medicine, the Kidneys are the system that stores essence, governs human reproduction, growth, and development, and controls metabolism, bones, hair, and the brain. Traditional Chinese medical practitioners view the Kidney as the source of the body's yin and yang.

LIVER. As with other organs, the Liver is not the physical organ referred to in Western medicine, but is related to it. In traditional Chinese medicine, the Liver ensures the smooth flow of qi throughout the body, stores and regulates the Blood, and controls the connective tissues.

LUNGS. As with other organs, the Lungs are not the physical organ referred to in Western medicine but related to it. In traditional Chinese medicine, the Lungs govern qi, control respiration, direct the passage of water, influence the defensive qi to protect against external pathogens, and control the hair, skin, and pores.

MIDDLE BURNER. The Middle Burner, which is responsible for digestion, includes the Spleen and Stomach. Located in the area above the belly button and below the diaphragm, the Middle Burner is part of the "Triple Burner" concept in traditional Chinese medicine, which also includes the Upper Burner (Heart and Lungs) and Lower Burner (Kidneys, Urinary Bladder, and Intestines).

ORGANS. The organs are often a source of confusion to those new to traditional Chinese medicine, since these terms refer to systems and functions, rather than to physical organs. For traditional Chinese medical practitioners, the five yin organs—the Liver, Heart, Spleen, Lung, and Kidney—and six yang organs—Gall Bladder, Stomach, Small Intestine, Large Intestine, Bladder, and Triple Burner—provide a method of differentiating among different types of syndromes. The five yin organs, *zang* in Chinese, which are responsible for storing vital substances, coexist with the six yang organs, *fu*, which are responsible for transportation. Together, these organ systems are called *zang fu*.

PATTERN. Traditional Chinese medical practitioners make their diagnoses based on patterns of symptoms. For example, Spleen qi deficiency is diagnosed when a practitioner observes a pattern of symptoms that include sallow complexion, tiredness, dislike of speaking, reduced appetite, abdominal distention, and loose stools. One disease, as defined in Western medicine, often has different Chinese medical patterns depending on the patient, and the same pattern may occur across different diseases.

PHLEGM. In traditional Chinese medicine, phlegm is an important concept and refers to either "substantial phlegm," which is a visible substance such as mucus or pus, or "insubstantial phlegm," which can be found in the channels, under the skin, or misting the mind. Phlegm slows and obstructs the flow of qi, and can result from problems with water metabolism as a result of a dysfunction of the Spleen, Lungs, or Kidneys.

RESTLESS ORGAN DISORDER. Restless organ disorder (*zang zao* in Chinese) is an emotional condition, more common in women, that includes disorientation, unexplained crying, insomnia, and distress. This disorder is caused by frustration (constrained Liver qi) or excessive ruminating (Spleen deficiency).

QI. Qi (pronounced "chee") is an ancient and central concept in Chinese philosophy. Although difficult to translate, qi can be understood as the life force or energy flowing through all things, including animals, minerals, and vegetables. Qi circulates in channels called meridians on the body's surface, as well as in pathways inside the body. There are many categories of qi, including *yuan qi* (original qi), *gu chi* (qi of food), *zong qi* (gathering qi), *zhen qi* (true qi), *ying qi* (nutritive qi), and *wei qi* (qi defending against external pathogenic factors, such as Wind, Cold, Heat, and Damp). According to the Chinese worldview, illnesses take hold when the flow of qi is disturbed, insufficient, or blocked. To restore health, Chinese medical practitioners seek to free, supplement, and realign the flow of qi, with such measures as acupuncture, herbs, food, exercise, or meditation.

QI DEFICIENCY. According to traditional Chinese medicine, illness can occur when there is insufficient qi. Qi deficiency can occur in specific organ systems, especially in the Spleen and the Lungs, but also the Kidneys and Heart. Symptoms of Spleen qi deficiency include sallow complexion, emaciation, tiredness, reduced appetite, abdominal distention, and loose stools. Symptoms of Lung qi deficiency include fatigue, shortness of breath, spontaneous sweating, tendency to catch frequent colds, weak cough, and soft voice. Symptoms of Kidney qi deficiency include inability to control urinary flow and soreness or weakness of the lower back. Symptoms of Heart qi deficiency include palpitations, shortness of breath, sweating, and tiredness.

QI STAGNATION. This is any cessation of the normal flow of qi, which can be caused by constrained emotions or pathogenic factors. Qi stagnation can occur in specific organs. Liver qi stagnation results in irritability, a tendency toward anger, sighing, oppression in the chest, and menstrual disorders. Middle Burner or Spleen Stomach qi stagnation results in abdominal distention with pain, nausea, vomit, belching, and acid regurgitation. Lung qi stagnation involves coughing and wheezing, difficulty breathing, and a stifling sensation in the chest.

SPIRIT. The spirit (*shen*) is housed by the Heart and is responsible for sleep, thinking, memory, consciousness, and zest for life. A calm spirit allows people to think clearly and have good concentration, memory, and sleep.

SPLEEN. As with other organs, the Spleen is not the physical organ referred to in Western medicine but is related to it. In traditional Chinese medicine, the Spleen governs digestion, helps transform food and drink to produce Blood, controls muscles and limbs, and houses the intellect.

STAGNATION. Stagnation refers to a blockage or inhibition of flow, including stagnation of the qi, phlegm, food, and body fluid.

STASIS. Stasis describes a condition of the Blood in which flow is blocked or inhibited.

SUMMER HEAT. Summer Heat occurs only in summer. It can present as two distinct patterns. Summer Heat-Heat, which occurs with exposure to extreme heat, includes symptoms such as sudden high fever, heavy sweating, and exhaustion, with aversion to heat and craving for cold beverages. Summer Heat-Damp, which occurs in conditions of high heat and humidity, includes symptoms such as heaviness, fatigue, loss of appetite, diarrhea, and a stifling sensation in the chest and abdomen.

TOXICITY. In traditional Chinese medicine, the term *toxicity* (from toxins or *du*) refers to the fever, inflammation, and other adverse affects of infectious disease.

WIND. Analogous to wind in nature, the concept of Wind in Chinese medicine embodies movement and change. Diseases caused by Wind often have migratory symptoms, sudden onset, and rapid progression, or other features associated with movement such as spasms, tremors, twitching, or dizziness. Wind, prominent in the spring but appearing in any season, often promotes the invasion of the body by one of the other pernicious influences, such as Heat, Cold, or Damp.

WIND-COLD. Wind-Cold is a common disorder of a union between Wind and Cold, whose symptoms include pronounced chills with slight fever, headache, body aches, runny nose, and neck ache.

WIND-DAMP. Wind-Damp is a union between Wind and Damp resulting in symptoms including neck pain and stiffness, headache, body aches, and swollen joints.

WIND-HEAT. Wind-Heat is a common disorder of a union between Wind and Heat, whose symptoms may be similar to Wind-Cold, but with a higher fever and less pronounced chills, as well as thirst and sweating.

YANG. Yang is the force relating to heat, exterior, dryness, movement, upward movement, and function. In the body, yang helps the body generate warmth and maintain circulation. If there's too much yang, though, an individual is susceptible to illnesses expressed with quick, forceful movement, heat, or hyperactivity.

YANG DEFICIENCY. Symptoms of yang deficiency are similar to symptoms of qi deficiency, but with signs of Interior Cold, including cold limbs, and aversion to cold. Yang deficiency occurs in specific organs, often the Kidneys or Spleen. Symptoms of Kidney yang deficiency include weakness and an aching sensation in the lumbar region and knees, aversion to cold, cold limbs, profuse, clear urination or general edema, declining libido or impotence, and female infertility. Symptoms of Spleen yang deficiency include pallor, cold limbs, poor appetite, abdominal distension exacerbated by eating, dull abdominal pain that improves with warmth and pressure, and loose stools.

YIN. In general, yin is the force associated with cold, interior, moisture, density, stillness, downward movement, and substance. In the body, yin represents the body's substance, including Blood and bodily fluids that nourish and moisten the organs and tissues. If there's too much yin in the body, though, a person will come down with an illness that involves weakness, slowness, coldness, or lethargy.

YIN DEFICIENCY. Symptoms of yin deficiency include a low-grade fever (especially in the afternoon), dry throat, and night sweats. Yin deficiency usually concentrates in specific organs, such as the Kidneys, Lungs, Liver, or Stomach. Symptoms of Kidney yin deficiency include soreness and weakness of the lumbar region and knees, dizziness, ringing in the ears, hearing problems, a dry mouth and throat, a hot sensation in the palms, soles, and chest, night sweating, constipation, and seminal emission. Symptoms of Lung yin deficiency include a dry cough (possibly blood-tinged), dryness of the mouth and throat, afternoon fever, and night sweats. Symptoms of Liver yin deficiency include dizziness, headache, ringing in the ears, blurred vision, dry eyes, insomnia, night sweats, thirst, and dry throat. Symptoms of Stomach yin deficiency include frequent hunger for small amounts of food, a burning sensation in stomach area, and thirst.

RECIPES
FOR COMMON HEALTH CONCERNS

WE ARE PROVIDING this list of recipes targeting common health concerns to help you get the most out of this book and to help bridge the divide between the Western and traditional Chinese approaches to health and healing. However, please keep in mind several caveats.

First, a diagnosis according to Western medicine can be seen as several different conditions according to traditional Chinese medicine, depending on the pattern of symptoms displayed by the individual patient. A single Western diagnosis, for example asthma, can correspond to multiple patterns in traditional Chinese medicine; for example, breathing difficulties due to Cold, Heat, phlegm, and so on. Each pattern calls for a different treatment approach. Where practical, we have indicated a few of these distinctions, sometimes as subsections of Western medical terminology. Details on the traditional Chinese medical perspective are also listed with each recipe. If you are seeking to address specific health concerns, try to

keep these differences in mind when selecting recipes. Also, don't hesitate to consult with a traditional Chinese medical practitioner who can tailor your treatment, including food therapy, to your individual needs.

In addition, none of our recipes are meant as a substitute for consulting with your physician. Some of the conditions listed below may be serious and need to be addressed promptly if you have not already done so. Here, we offer diet as a way to support the treatments you work out with your doctor—or as an approach to reducing your risk of disease in the first place.

We encourage you to integrate these recipes into your everyday diet according to your needs. We believe no one food or category of foods, either Eastern or Western, will promote maximum health. For health and wellness, seek quality, balance, and variety in food, while respecting your own unique circumstances.

Aches and Pains (including arthritis, muscle aches, inflammation)

As in Western medicine, in traditional Chinese medicine, aches and pains are thought to develop due to a variety of underlying causes. These recipes help to counteract some of these conditions, such as Blood stasis, qi stagnation, Cold or Damp stagnation, and qi and Blood deficiency.

Acne, Rashes

Red skin irritations such as acne can be a sign of Heat, Heat toxins, or Damp Heat toxins with Blood stasis, according to traditional Chinese medicine. The following recipes, which feature ingredients such as mung beans, seaweed, and bitter melon, help cool the body and drain Dampness.

Appetite (poor)

Poor appetite can be caused by Spleen qi deficiency, qi stagnation, or Damp stagnation, among a variety of other conditions according to traditional Chinese medicine. The following recipes help harmonize the Middle Burner with such ingredients as lotus seeds and stimulate the appetite with such ingredients as ginger and other spices.

Bone Weakness or Injury

According to traditional Chinese medicine, the principle of "like treats like" advises using stocks and dishes made with bones (such as the following) to help fortify bones in the body.

Circulation/Cold Hands and Feet

Poor circulation can correspond to patterns of Cold stagnation and Blood stasis in traditional Chinese medicine. Dishes with ingredients such as green onion, ginger, and other spices can help warm and invigorate the Blood.

Cold Weather/Tendency to Feel Cold

In East Asia, it is commonly believed that to optimize health people should eat according to the seasons. In the winter, warming foods and spices, such as lamb and chestnuts, help the body cope with cold weather. Individuals are also encouraged to eat according to their constitution, so people who tend to run cold also benefit from including warming foods in their diet on a regular basis.

Common Cold/Flu

In Asia, the common cold is thought of as coming in at least three varieties, which each call for a different kind of remedy. In an attack of Wind-Cold, you feel chilly and feverish and experience body aches, headache, cough, and stuffy nose with watery nasal discharge. Warming foods and beverages can help counteract this type of condition. In an attack of Wind-Heat, you have a fever or feel like you do, possibly with chills, and also experience a sore throat, thirst, yellow urine, and a stuffy nose with a thick yellow discharge. This calls for foods and beverages considered cooling, such as chrysanthemum, peppermint, or mulberry leaf. In an attack of Summer Heat and Dampness, you have a slight fever, heaviness in the head, aching in the arms and legs, thirst without a desire to drink, yellow urine, and loss of appetite or nausea. In this case, the condition calls for cooling foods that drain Dampness, such as watermelon, cucumber, and mung beans. Here are some recipes for these conditions.

WIND-COLD TYPE

WIND-HEAT TYPE

SUMMER HEAT DAMP TYPE

GENERAL

Constipation

In both Western and Eastern medicine, constipation is attributed to a variety of causes. In the East, constipation can be associated with an excess of Heat leading to Dryness, an excess of Cold, qi stagnation, or qi and Blood deficiency, among others. Many of the following recipes help cool the body with ingredients such as cucumbers and moisten the Intestines with ingredients such as sesame seeds, almonds, and pine nuts.

Cough/Asthma

In traditional Chinese medicine, dry coughs are treated with foods and herbs that moisten the Lungs, such as pear and fritillaria. Other patterns associated with coughs include Lung qi deficiency, yin deficiency, phlegm, and so on, which call for different types of remedies.

FROM DRYNESS

FROM OTHER CAUSES

Dehydration/Thirst

Dryness and Heat can challenge the body. The following dishes are among those that help moisten and cool.

Diabetes/High Blood Sugar

Patients with diabetes and prediabetes often exhibit patterns of Stomach Heat or yin deficiency according to traditional Chinese medicine. Such foods as pumpkin, bitter melon, mushrooms, wood ear, lotus, and Chinese yam can help address these patterns. Also, don't forget to watch your portion sizes.

Dizziness

People with chronic or intermittent dizziness can show patterns of internal Wind of the Liver, Liver Fire, obstruction from phlegm or Dampness, Blood deficiency, or yin deficiency, among others in traditional Chinese medicine. These recipes address some of these problems.

Edema/Fluid Retention

Fluid retention and edema can often be linked to patterns of Spleen qi deficiency or Kidney yang deficiency, leading to an accumulation of Dampness. Dishes that drain Dampness include ingredients such as seaweed, winter melon, and coix, and beverages such as green tea.

Emotional Distress (depression, irritability, stress)

In traditional Chinese medicine, the Heart is seen as governing the consciousness and spirit, the Liver as ensuring the smooth flow of qi throughout the body, and the Kidneys as providing the foundation of qi, so all three can be involved in emotional distress. The following dishes help counteract disturbances of the spirit (Heart), Liver qi stagnation, and Kidney deficiency, and to build resilience and calm the spirit.

Fatigue

No matter what country you're from, a healthy diet is important in maintaining your energy level and combating fatigue. Here are some recipes that counteract patterns of qi or yang deficiency, qi stagnation, or Damp accumulation, associated in traditional Chinese medicine with fatigue.

General Health, Strength, Vitality

*In China, good health and vitality is associated with balance, harmony, and the "three treasures"—*jing *(essence),* qi *(life force or energy), and* shen *(spirit). Most recipes in this book promote these qualities, but here are a few that highlight them.*

Hangover

Hangovers have no doubt been a problem since the invention of alcoholic beverages. Here are some recipes that harmonize the Middle Burner according to traditional Chinese medicine to help bring you back to normal if you have indulged too heavily. Of course, prevention is the best cure.

High Cholesterol/Atherosclerosis/Coronary Artery Disease

While there is no concept of "cholesterol" in traditional Chinese medicine, there is a related concept of Damp and Blood stasis, exacerbated by Spleen deficiency (among other patterns that could relate to this diagnosis). Dishes with such ingredients as seaweed, mushrooms, wood ear, and sesame seeds aim to counteract these problems by invigorating the Blood, draining Dampness, and supplementing the Spleen.

High Blood Pressure

The ancients did not measure blood pressure, but they did note such patterns as Liver yang rising, deficiency of Kidney yin and yang, and obstruction of phlegm Damp. These recipes help these and related conditions by balancing yin and yang, draining Dampness, and clearing Heat.

Hot Weather/Tendency to Feel Hot

*Many people in East Asia tailor their diet according
to the seasons, to try to optimize their health. In the
summer, cooling foods and herbs, such as cucumber,
greens, lotus root, and honeysuckle, counteract the
warm weather in the environment. Individuals also
eat according to their constitution, so people who tend
to run hot include cooling foods in their diet.*

Indigestion/Stomach Upset/ Nausea/Diarrhea

*Much emphasis is put on good digestion in traditional
Chinese medicine, as properly absorbing food is key
to supporting the body's other functions. Poor digestion
can be caused by an excess or deficiency of Cold, Heat,
or Dampness, as well as by qi stagnation. Here are
some recipes to promote digestion and soothe your
stomach, which should be chosen according to your
condition.*

GENERAL

FROM EXCESS HEAT

FROM EXCESS COLD

Insomnia

Insomnia is not considered one condition in traditional Chinese medicine; rather, many, depending on each individual's pattern, which might include Heart Fire, Heart Blood deficiency, Liver qi stagnation, Kidney yin deficiency, food stagnation, and many others. Here are some recipes that clear Heat, nourish yin, regulate the qi, or calm the spirit.

Longevity and Good Health in Old Age

In traditional Chinese medicine, strengthening the Kidneys is considered vital to achieving longevity. Kidney-strengthening dishes such as those listed here often include such ingredients as walnuts, sesame seeds, chestnuts, and beans.

Masses/Lumps (goiter, ovarian cysts, breast lumps, lymph node swelling, fibroids, etc.)

People with soft masses often exhibit patterns of phlegm accumulation, qi stagnation, and/or Blood stasis, according to traditional Chinese medicine. Recipes with seaweed are particularly good at addressing these patterns. Of course, check in with your physician, too.

Menopause

Women going through menopause are often struggling with Kidney yin deficiency or Kidney yang deficiency, often complicated by stagnation of Liver qi, according to traditional Chinese medicine. These dishes help counteract these problems.

Menstrual Disorders (such as irregular bleeding, premenstrual syndrome)

East Asian medicine tends to excel in treating female problems, which are linked to a plethora of traditional diagnoses, including Blood stasis, Cold stagnation, Heat, phlegm obstruction, Liver and Kidney deficiency, and Blood deficiency, among others. In addition to seeing a traditional Chinese medical practitioner and your physician, consider some of these recipes. For premenstrual syndrome, see also Edema/Fluid Retention.

Prevention of and Recovery from Illness

The Western concept of "immunity" is close to the Chinese concept of "wei qi" or defensive energy. These recipes are among those that build the body's wei qi, as well as other types of qi and Blood.

Postpartum Recovery/Lactation

Childbirth, postpartum recovery, and lactation have been topics of concern throughout the ages. In traditional East Asian medicine, women are advised of the need to rebuild qi and Blood, such as with these recipes, after giving birth.

Reproductive Health/Urinary Problems

Here are some recipes that address reproductive and urinary problems, which may be associated with Kidney qi deficiency, Kidney yang deficiency, or phlegm

Damp obstruction, among other patterns in traditional Chinese medicine.

Vision

Such ingredients as goji berries, chrysanthemum, cassia seeds, and mulberry fruit are considered particularly good at helping to address or prevent vision problems, which are associated with patterns including Liver yin deficiency, Blood deficiency, and Liver yang rising in traditional Chinese medicine.

Weight Loss/Weight Control

Although throughout much of history getting enough to eat was a major challenge, today obesity and excess weight gain is a common problem, especially in the West. In traditional Chinese medicine, excess weight is often associated with a pattern of Spleen qi deficiency with an accumulation of Dampness, sometimes complicated by Heat or Liver qi stagnation. This condition can be addressed with such foods as mung beans and seaweed. Also, remember the East Asian saying, "Stop eating when the food tastes best."

Youthful Appearance

To maintain a youthful appearance, including natural hair color and a smooth complexion, traditional Chinese medicine advises strengthening the Kidneys and building Blood. Dishes with such ingredients as black sesame seeds, mushrooms, wood ear, and many types of beans help reach these goals.

CONVERSION CHART

THE RECIPES IN THIS BOOK have not been tested with metric measurements, so some variations might occur.

Remember that the weight of dry ingredients varies according to the volume or density factor: 1 cup of flour weighs far less than 1 cup of sugar, and 1 tablespoon doesn't necessarily hold 3 teaspoons.

GENERAL FORMULA FOR METRIC CONVERSION

OUNCES TO GRAMS	MULTIPLY OUNCES BY 28.35
GRAMS TO OUNCES	MULTIPLY GRAMS BY 0.035
POUNDS TO GRAMS	MULTIPLY POUNDS BY 453.5
POUNDS TO KILOGRAMS	MULTIPLY POUNDS BY 0.45
CUPS TO LITERS	MULTIPLY CUPS BY 0.24
FAHRENHEIT TO CELSIUS	SUBTRACT 32 FROM FAHRENHEIT TEMPERATURE, MULTIPLY BY 5, DIVIDE BY 9
CELSIUS TO FAHRENHEIT	MULTIPLY CELSIUS TEMPERATURE BY 9, DIVIDE BY 5, ADD 32

VOLUME (LIQUID) MEASUREMENTS

1 TEASPOON = ⅙ FLUID OUNCE = 5 MILLILITERS

1 TABLESPOON = ½ FLUID OUNCE = 15 MILLILITERS

2 TABLESPOONS = 1 FLUID OUNCE = 30 MILLILITERS

¼ CUP = 2 FLUID OUNCES = 60 MILLILITERS

⅓ CUP = 2⅔ FLUID OUNCES = 79 MILLILITERS

½ CUP = 4 FLUID OUNCES = 118 MILLILITERS

1 CUP OR ½ PINT = 8 FLUID OUNCES = 250 MILLILITERS

2 CUPS OR 1 PINT = 16 FLUID OUNCES = 500 MILLILITERS

4 CUPS OR 1 QUART = 32 FLUID OUNCES = 1,000 MILLILITERS

1 GALLON = 4 LITERS

VOLUME (DRY) MEASUREMENTS

¼ TEASPOON = 1 MILLILITER

½ TEASPOON = 2 MILLILITERS

¾ TEASPOON = 4 MILLILITERS

1 TEASPOON = 5 MILLILITERS

1 TABLESPOON = 15 MILLILITERS

¼ CUP = 59 MILLILITERS

⅓ CUP = 79 MILLILITERS

½ CUP = 118 MILLILITERS

VOLUME (DRY) MEASUREMENTS (CONTINUED)

⅔ CUP = 158 MILLILITERS
¾ CUP = 177 MILLILITERS
1 CUP = 225 MILLILITERS
4 CUPS OR 1 QUART = 1 LITER
½ GALLON = 2 LITERS
1 GALLON = 4 LITERS

WEIGHT (MASS) MEASUREMENTS

1 OUNCE = 30 GRAMS
2 OUNCES = 55 GRAMS
3 OUNCES = 85 GRAMS
4 OUNCES = ¼ POUND = 125 GRAMS
8 OUNCES = ½ POUND = 240 GRAMS
12 OUNCES = ¾ POUND = 375 GRAMS
16 OUNCES = 1 POUND = 454 GRAMS

LINEAR MEASUREMENTS

½ IN = 1⅓ CM
1 INCH = 2½ CM
6 INCHES = 15 CM
8 INCHES = 20 CM
10 INCHES = 25 CM
12 INCHES = 30 CM
20 INCHES = 50 CM

OVEN TEMPERATURE EQUIVALENTS, FAHRENHEIT (F) AND CELSIUS (C)

100°F = 38°C
200°F = 95°C
250°F = 120°C
300°F = 150°C
350°F = 180°C
400°F = 205°C
450°F = 230° C

SUGGESTED SUBSTITUTIONS

Substitute an equivalent amount, unless otherwise noted.

INGREDIENT	SUBSTITUTION
CHICKEN	Other poultry (such as Rock Cornish hen); red meat (lamb, pork, or beef); shrimp; tofu, tempeh, mushrooms, or black beans (for vegetarians)
CINNAMON STICK, 1	Ground cinnamon, ¾ teaspoon
BEEF	Other meat, such as lamb, pork, or chicken; tofu, tempeh, mushrooms or black beans (for vegetarians)
GALANGAL, FRESH, 1 TABLESPOON	Galangal, dried, ½ tablespoon
GARLIC, 1 CLOVE	Chopped garlic, 1 teaspoon; minced garlic, ½ teaspoon; or garlic powder, ⅛ teaspoon
GINGER ROOT, FRESH, 1 TABLESPOON	Ground ginger, ½ tablespoon, plus ½ teaspoon lemon juice
GREEN ONION	Leek
HERBS, FRESH, 1 TABLESPOON	Same variety of herb, dried, 1 teaspoon; ground, ½ teaspoon
HONEY	Maple syrup, rock sugar, agave syrup, other natural sweetener, white sugar (if necessary). The strength of different sweeteners varies slightly, so taste as you go along.
KABOCHA PUMPKIN	Other pumpkin or winter squash, such as butternut or acorn squash

KUDZU ROOT, POWDERED	Arrowroot, tapioca (thickens quickly), rice starch, potato starch, chestnut starch, cornstarch (not good for freezing or dairy dishes), flour (double the amount)
LEEK	Green onion
LEMON JUICE, 1 TEASPOON	Rice vinegar or white vinegar, ½ teaspoon
MIRIN	Sherry
MUSHROOMS, DRIED, 3 OUNCES	Mushrooms, fresh, 1 pound (no need to soak these ahead of cooking)
MUSHROOMS, FRESH, 1 POUND	Mushrooms, dried, 3 ounces (soak for 20 to 30 minutes before using)
PORK	Other meat, such as lamb, beef, or chicken; tofu, tempeh, mushrooms, or black beans (for vegetarians)
PUMPKIN	Winter squash, such as butternut or other variety
RICE VINEGAR	Cider vinegar; white wine vinegar (dilute slightly with water)
ROCK SUGAR	Honey, maple syrup, granulated white sugar (if necessary). The strength of different sweeteners varies slightly, so taste as you go along.
SAKE	Rice wine (especially Shaoxing wine or *jeongju*), white wine, vermouth
SCALLOPS	Shrimp or other seafood
SHIITAKE MUSHROOMS, DRIED AND WHOLE, 3	Shiitake mushrooms, dried and sliced, ½ cup or 0.3 ounces
SOY SAUCE	Light or reduced-sodium soy sauce (for those concerned about salt consumption); tamari (for those with a wheat allergy or intolerance; be sure to read the label)
TANGERINE PEEL, DRIED	Fresh grated tangerine or orange peel (about double the volume)
WOOD EAR	Cloud ear

RESOURCES

Brick-and-Mortar Asian Food and Herb Shops

Because individual stores come and go, we are pointing you to Asian food chains and sources that can help identify individual Asian supermarkets and herb stores in your area. In addition to the Yellow Pages for your locale and, of course, an Internet search for your area, try the sources listed below.

- 99 Ranch, a chain of pan-Asian grocery stores in California, Arizona, Nevada, Washington, and Georgia. See http://www.99ranch.com/ for store locations.
- H-Mart (also known as Han Ah Reum and Super H), a Korean food store with locations in California, Colorado, New York, New Jersey, Pennsylvania, Maryland, Virginia, Washington, Illinois, Texas, Georgia, and Oregon, as well as British Columbia and Ontario, Canada. For more information, see http://www.hmart.com/.
- Hong Kong Supermarket, a Chinese American supermarket in California, New Jersey, New York, Pennsylvania, and Texas. See http://www.hongkongsupermarketinc.com/ for more information.
- Kam Man Food, a chain of Chinese American supermarkets in New York, New Jersey, and Massachusetts. For more information on the Quincy, Massachusetts, store, see http://www.kammanshops.com/.
- Mitsuwa Marketplace, a chain of Japanese food stores in California, New Jersey, and Illinois. See http://www.mitsuwa.com/english/index.html.
- Nijiya Market, a chain of Japanese food stores in California, Hawaii, and New York. See http://www.nijiya.com/.
- T&T Supermarket, a chain of pan-Asian supermarkets throughout Canada. See http://www.tnt-supermarket.com/big5/index.php? for store locations and information.

- Wikipedia entry on Asian supermarkets, which includes a list of major Asian supermarkets in North America and their locations, at http://en.wikipedia.org/wiki/Asian_supermarkets.

Online Herb and Asian Food Suppliers

You may want to consider purchasing Asian food and herbs online. In addition to using Google to conduct your own up-to-the-minute search for online Asian food and herb suppliers (online or otherwise), here are some resources:

- Asianwok.com, http://www.asianwok.com (Asian ingredients)
- Asiamex, http://www.asiamex.com/ (Asian and Mexican ingredients)
- Ancient Way Acupuncture and Herbs, http://www.ancientway.com/catalog/ (herbs)
- Asian Food Grocer, asianfoodgrocer.com
- Eastern Chinese Medicine Export Company, http://www.tcmtreatment.com/herbs.htm (herbs)
- EthnicFoodsCo.com, http://store.ethnic foodsco.com/ (Asian groceries)
- Global Herbal Supplies, http://www. globalherbalsupplies.com (herbs)
- Gold Mine Natural Foods, http://www. goldminenaturalfood.com/default.aspx (macrobiotic and Japanese)
- Koa Mart, http://www.koamart.com/ (Asian groceries)
- Kushi Institute Store, http://www.kushi store.com/acatalog/Food.html (macrobiotic)
- Natural Import Company, http://www .naturalimport.com (Japanese ingredients)

- MyEthnicWorld.com, http://www.my ethnicworld.com/ (Asian groceries)
- Oriental Food Master, http://store .asianfoodstuff.com/index.html
- Pacific Rim Gourmet, http://www .pacificrimgourmet.com/gourmet_ ingredients.aspx (Asian groceries)

Plant and Seed Suppliers

If you have a green thumb, you may want to consider growing your own herbs and vegetables. Here are a few sources you may find useful to explore this option.

- Botanical.com, http://www.botanical.com/
- Bountiful Gardens, http://www.bountiful gardens.org
- Companion Plants, http://www.companion plants.com/
- Evergreen Seeds, http://www.evergreen seeds.com/vegetableseeds.html
- Ozark Botanical Garden, http://www .one-garden.org
- Penny's Herb Company, http://www .pennysherbco.com/
- Plant It Herbs, specializing in Chinese medicinal plants, http://www.plantitherbs.com
- Seeds of Change, http://www.seedsofchange .com

Recommended Reading

Beinfield, Harriet, and Efrem Korngold. *Between Heaven and Earth: A Guide to Chinese Medicine*. New York: Ballantine Books, 1992.

Bittman, Mark. *Food Matters: A Guide to Conscious Eating*. New York: Simon & Schuster, 2009.

Gao, Duo with Barbara Bernie. *Chinese Medicine*. New York: Thunder's Mouth Press, 1997.

Holland, Alex. *Voices of Qi: An Introductory Guide to Traditional Chinese Medicine*. Berkeley, CA: North Atlantic Books, 2000.

Kaptchuk, Ted J. *The Web That Has No Weaver: Understanding Chinese Medicine*. Chicago: Contemporary Books, 2000.

Pollan, Michael. *The Omnivore's Dilemma: A Natural History of Four Meals*. New York: Penguin, 2007.

———. *In Defense of Food: An Eater's Manifesto*. New York: Penguin, 2008.

Zhu, Hong Zhen. *Better Health with Chinese Medicine*. Toronto: Penguin Group, 2001.

Bibliography

Andoh, Elizabeth. *Washoku: Recipes from the Japanese Home Kitchen*. Berkeley, CA: Ten Speed Press, 2005.

Batmanglij, Najmieh. *Silk Road Cooking: A Vegetarian Journey*. Washington, DC: Mage Publishers, 2008.

Bellame, John, and Jan Bellame. *Japanese Foods That Heal: Using Traditional Japanese Ingredients to Promote Health, Longevity & Well-Being*. Tokyo: Tuttle Publishing, 2007.

Bensky, Dan, and Andrew Gamble, eds., with Ted Kaptchuk. *Materia Medica*, Revised Edition. Seattle, WA: Eastland Press, 1993.

Bensky, Dan, and Randall Barolet. *Chinese Herbal Medicine Formulas & Strategies*. Seattle, WA: Eastland Press, 1990.

Campbell, T. Colin, and Thomas M. Campbell II. *The China Study: The Most Comprehensive Study of Nutrition Ever Conducted and the Startling Implications for Diet, Weight Loss, and Long-Term Health*. Dallas, TX: Benbella Books, 2004.

Chen, John K., and Tina T. Chen. *Chinese Medical Herbology and Pharmacology*. City of Industry, CA: Art of Medicine Press, 2004.

Cost, Bruce. *Asian Ingredients: A Guide to the Foodstuffs of China, Japan, Korea, Thailand, and Vietnam*. New York: HarperCollins, 2000.

Downer, Lesley. *At the Japanese Table: New and Traditional Recipes*. San Francisco, CA: Chronicle Books, 1993.

Flaws, Bob. *The Tao of Healthy Eating: Dietary Wisdom According to Chinese Medicine*. Boulder, Colorado: Blue Poppy Press, 1998.

Fujii, Mari. *The Enlightened Kitchen: Fresh Vegetable Dishes from the Temples of Japan*. Tokyo: Kodansha International, 2005.

Hepinstall, Hi Soo Shin. *Growing Up in a Korean Kitchen: A Cookbook*. Berkeley, CA: Ten Speed Press, 2001.

Hong, I-nang. *Stories About Chinese Herbal Medicine*. Hong Kong: Chinese University Press, 1999.

Hu, Shiu-ying. *Food Plants of China*. Hong Kong: Chinese University Press, 2005.

Kastner, Joerg. *Chinese Nutrition Therapy: Dietetics in Traditional Chinese Medicine (TCM)*. Stuttgart, Germany, and New York: Thieme, 2004.

Kohnstadt, Ingrid, ed. *Food and Nutrients in Disease Management*. Boca Raton, FL: CRC Press, 2009.

Li, Xu, and Wang Wei. *Chinese Materia Medica: Combinations & Applications*. Hertfortshire, UK: Donica Publishing, 2002.

Ling, Kong Foong, ed. *The Food of Asia: Authentic Recipes from China, India, Indonesia, Japan, Singapore, Malaysia, Thailand and Vietnam*. Singapore: Periplus Editions, 1998.

Liu, Jilin, and Gordon Peck, eds. *Chinese Dietary Therapy*. Edinburgh: Churchill Livingstone, 1995.

Lu, Henry. *Chinese System of Food Cures: Prevention & Remedies*. New York: Sterling, 1986.

Maciocia, Giovanni. *The Foundations of Chinese Medicine: A Comprehensive Text for Acupuncturists and Herbalists*. London: Churchill Livingstone, 2005.

Ni, Maoshing, and Cathy McNease. *The Tao of Nutrition*. Los Angeles: Seven Star Communications, 1987.

Peiwen, Li. *Management of Cancer with TCM*. St. Albans, Hertfordshire (UK): Donica Publishing, 2003.

Roberts, Jeremy. *Chinese Mythology A to Z*. New York: Facts on File, 2004.

Schneider, Elizabeth. *Uncommon Fruits & Vegetables: A Commonsense Guide*. New York: Harper & Row, 1986.

Shimbo, Hiroko. *The Japanese Kitchen: 250 Recipes in a Traditional Spirit*. Boston, Harvard Common Press, 2000.

Simonds, Nina. *A Spoonful of Ginger: Irresistible, Health-Giving Recipes from Asian Kitchens*. New York: Alfred A Knopf, 2002.

Tan, Terry. *Cooking with Chinese Herbs*. Singapore: Times Books International, 1983.

Tsu, Lao. *Tao Te Ching*. Translated by Gia-Fu Feng and Jane English. New York: Random House, 1989.

Unschuld, Paul. *Medicine in China: A History of Ideas*. Berkeley, CA: University of California Press, 1985.

Wen-wei, Miao. *Herbal Pearls: Traditional Chinese Folk Wisdom*. Translated by Yue Chong-xi and edited and annotated by Steven Foster. Eureka Springs, AR: Boian Books, 2008.

Wu, Yan, and Warren Fischer. *Practical Therapeutics of Traditional Chinese Medicine*. Edited by Jake Fratkin. Brookline, MA: Paradigm Publications, 1997.

Useful Web Sites

- Acupuncture Today,
    http://www.acupuncturetoday.com/mpacms/at/home.php
- Acupuncture.com (information on Chinese medicine),
    http://acupuncture.com/education/tcmbasics/index.htm
- Education Community Online, "Directory of Acupuncture Schools in the United States,"
    http://www.acupunctureschools.com/
- The Herb Research Foundation,
    http://herbs.org/
- Memorial Sloan-Kettering Cancer Center: Information about Herbs, Botanicals and Other Products,
    http://www.mskcc.org/mskcc/html/11790.cfm
- Shen-Nong.com (information on Chinese medicine),
    http://www.shen-nong.com/eng/front/index.html
- TCMpage.com,
    http://www.tcmpage.com
- Tufts University Evidence-based Complementary and Alternative Medicine (EBCAM) site,
    http://www.tufts.edu/med/ebcam/eastAsianMed/
- UCLA History and Special Collections, "Spices: Exotic Flavors and Medicines,"
    http://unitproj.library.ucla.edu/biomed/spice/index.cfm?displayID=15
- University of Maryland Medical Center, "Complementary and Alternative Medicine Index (CAM),"
    http://www.umm.edu/altmed/index.htm

ACKNOWLEDGMENTS

WRITING A BOOK IS A GROUP EFFORT and we would like to extend our deep appreciation to everyone who made this book possible.

Thank you to our smart, savvy, and hard-working agent Ted Weinstein of Ted Weinstein Literary Management.

Thank you to our talented and thoughtful editor at Da Capo Press, Renée Sedlier. We feel extremely fortunate to have her on our team. Thanks, too, to everyone at Da Capo who believed in this book.

Thank you so much to our dedicated group of recipe testers, manuscript readers, and advisors for their efforts and terrific suggestions: Sallie Reynolds Allen, Micah Arsham, David Bandiouski, Jason Socrates Bardi, Patrik Bass, Leila Benedyk, Risa Benedyk, Mark Bielsky, Jean Cheng, Kevin Clark, Jen Cohen, Jann Coury, Bob Damone, Maureen Farley, Esther Gonzalez, Lori Gritz, Maile Helgeson, Diana Held, Claudia Huang, Jennifer Lau, Jessica Law, Peggy Leong, Hiroshi Ono, Ken Ono, Ria Ono, Jin Hee Park, Murray Polson, Erin Silver, Jenny Ono Suttaby, Jack Suttaby, Eva Stuart, Jeff Tien, and Kimberly Woo. A special thanks to linguist Dr. Insup Taylor for help with some of the Korean vocabulary.

Thank you to the faculty, staff, and students of the Pacific College of Oriental Medicine for their enthusiasm and encouragement.

And, of course, thank you to our families and friends for all of their invaluable support.

We welcome your comments on this book. To contact the authors, send an e-mail to ancient-twisdommodernkitchen@gmail.com or visit http://www.ancientwisdommodernkitchen.com.

INDEX

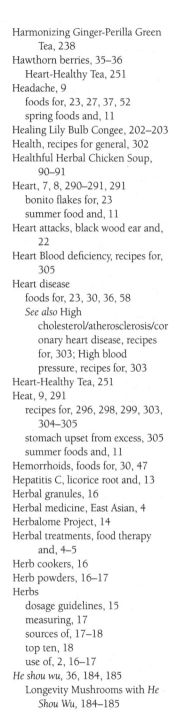